AIDS, DRUGS OF ABUSE, AND THE NEUROIMMUNE AXIS

ADVANCES IN EXPERIMENTAL MEDICINE AND BIOLOGY

Recent Volumes in this Series

Volume 395
OXYTOCIN: Cellular and Molecular Approaches in Medicine and Research
Edited by Richard Ivell and John A. Russell

Volume 396
RECENT ADVANCES IN CELLULAR AND MOLECULAR ASPECTS OF ANGIOTENSIN RECEPTORS
Edited by Mohan K. Raizada, M. Ian Phillips, and Colin Sumners

Volume 397
NOVEL STRATEGIES IN THE DESIGN AND PRODUCTION OF VACCINES
Edited by Sara Cohen and Avigdor Shafferman

Volume 398
RECENT ADVANCES IN TRYPTOPHAN RESEARCH: Tryptophan and Serotonin Pathways
Edited by Graziella Allegri Filippini, Carlo V. L. Costa, and Antonella Bertazzo

Volume 399
DIETARY FATS, LIPIDS, HORMONES, AND TUMORIGENESIS: New Horizons in Basic Research
Edited by David Heber and David Kritchevsky

Volume 400A
EICOSANOIDS AND OTHER BIOACTIVE LIPIDS IN CANCER, INFLAMMATION, AND RADIATION INJURY, Part A
Edited by Kenneth V. Honn, Santosh Nigam, and Lawrence J. Marnett

Volume 400B
EICOSANOIDS AND OTHER BIOACTIVE LIPIDS IN CANCER, INFLAMMATION, AND RADIATION INJURY, Part B
Edited by Kenneth V. Honn, Santosh Nigam, and Lawrence J. Marnett

Volume 401
DIETARY PHYTOCHEMICALS IN CANCER PREVENTION AND TREATMENT
Edited under the auspices of the American Institute for Cancer Research

Volume 402
AIDS, DRUGS OF ABUSE, AND THE NEUROIMMUNE AXIS
Edited by Herman Friedman, Toby K. Eisenstein, John Madden, and Burt M. Sharp

AIDS, DRUGS OF ABUSE, AND THE NEUROIMMUNE AXIS

Edited by

Herman Friedman
University of South Florida College of Medicine
Tampa, Florida

Toby K. Eisenstein
Temple University School of Medicine
Philadelphia, Pennsylvania

John Madden
Emory University
Atlanta, Georgia

and

Burt M. Sharp
Minneapolis Medical Research Foundation
Minneapolis, Minnesota

PLENUM PRESS • NEW YORK AND LONDON

Library of Congress Cataloging-in-Publication Data

AIDS, drugs of abuse, and the neuroimmune axis / edited by Herman Friedman ... [et al.].
p. cm. -- (Advances in experimental medicine and biology ; v. 402)
"Proceedings of the Third Annual Symposium on AIDS, Drugs of Abuse, and the Neuroimmune Axis, held November 9-11, 1995, in San Diego, California"--T.p. verso.
Includes bibliographical references and index.
ISBN-13:978-1-4613-8038-2 e-ISBN-13:978-1-4613-0407-4
DOI:10.1007/978-1-4613-0407-4

1. AIDS (Disease)--Etiology--Congresses. 2. AIDS (Disease)--Risk factors--Congresses. 3. Neuroimmunology--Congresses. 4. Drug abuse--Immunological aspects--Congresses. 5. Drugs of abuse--Immunology--Congresses. 6. Immunosuppression--Congresses. I. Friedman, Herman, 1931- . II. Symposium on AIDS, Drugs of Abuse, and the Neuroimmune Axis (3rd : 1995 : San Diego, Calif.) III. Series.
[DNLM: 1. Immune System--drug effects--congresses. 2. Immunosuppression--congresses. 3. Neuroimmunomodulation--drug effects--congresses. 4. Acquired Immunodeficiency Syndrome--immunology--congresses. 5. Substance Abuse--complications--congresses. 6. Street Drugs--congresses. W1 AD559 v.402 1996 / QW 504 A288 1996]
RC607.A26A3457337 1996
616.97'92071--dc20
DNLM/DLC
for Library of Congress 96-25725
CIP

Proceedings of the Third Annual Symposium on AIDS, Drugs of Abuse and the Neuroimmune Axis, held November 9 – 11, 1995, in San Diego, California

ISBN-13:978-1-4613-8038-2

A Division of Plenum Publishing Corporation
233 Spring Street, New York, N. Y. 10013

10 9 8 7 6 5 4 3 2 1

PREFACE

This volume represents the Proceedings of the Symposium on AIDS, Drugs of Abuse and the Neuroimmune Axis. This meeting was held in San Diego, California, November 11-13, 1995. As in the previous symposia in this series, productive studies were reviewed concerning the relationship between the nervous and the immune systems in regards to the relationship between drugs of abuse and infections, especially infections by the immunodeficiency virus that causes AIDS. In recent years, various investigators have begun to describe the role of illicit drugs and their endogenous counterparts on the brain-immune axis. It is widely recognized that the neuroendocrine system is intimately involved in the effects and manifestations of the interactions of drugs of abuse and the immune system. The meeting on which the chapters in this book are based brought together many biological scientists from an array of various scientific disciplines whose work is focused on the effects of drugs of abuse on the neuroendocrine-immune axis and its relationships to immunodeficiency caused by the AIDS virus. As in the past, the symposium was unique in focusing on the brain-immune axis from the viewpoint of drugs of abuse rather than from the viewpoint of immunity or the brain itself. One of the aims of this series of conferences was to clarify the consequences of immunomodulation induced by drugs of abuse on susceptibility and pathogenesis of infectious diseases in various model systems, including those associated with the AIDS virus. The recreational use of drugs of abuse, such as morphine, cocaine and marijuana, as well as alcohol, by large numbers of individuals in this country and around the world has aroused serious concern about the consequences of use of such drugs. For example, it is widely known that marijuana is used by tens of millions of individuals in this country and abroad. Furthermore, use of cocaine, especially crack cocaine, is now considered to be epidemic, as well as the use of other illicit recreational drugs. Alcoholism is also considered a major problem in this country, as well as elsewhere, and it is estimated there are at least 10 million alcoholics in the U.S.A. alone. A significant proportion of those individuals hospitalized for infectious diseases are known to be alcoholics. Recently there have been reports of association between use of drugs such as marijuana and cancer. Such observations encourage laboratory studies aimed at determining the nature and mechanism of how these drugs affect the immune system, as well as the neuroendocrine system which, in turn, has effects on immunity.

There are now very strong concerns that if drugs of abuse are indeed immunosuppressive, individuals who use such drugs may be prone to infectious diseases and develop increased mortality to such infections. Although many investigators believe that acute infections are not directly associated with use of drugs of abuse, there are suggestive clinical observations indicating that chronic diseases, including infections, may be more frequent in drugs abusers. It is also now widely accepted that many illicit drugs, including marijuana, morphine, and cocaine, as well as alcohol, detrimentally influence the immune response.

With the onset of the AIDS epidemic in the United States and worldwide, attempts have been made to search for possible "co-factors" which interact with the human immunodeficiency virus. It is known that approximately one fifth of all AIDS patients in this country are i.v. drug abusers and it has been shown that the AIDS virus is readily spread by contaminated needles or equipment used by such drug abusers. In addition, in many instances, these drugs are now known to be immunosuppressive . However, it is also well known that many AIDS patients are not i.v. drug abusers but are known to utilize other drugs such as marijuana and cocaine. Thus there is a probability that such drugs may indeed act as cofactors in AIDS progression, and therefore, there has been a concerted effort to examine in detail the mechanisms whereby such drugs may compromise the immune system in general.

It is widely acknowledged that the immune system of humans is continually exposed to a variety of environmental agents and toxic substances. Drugs of abuse are known to consitute one of many such groups of toxic agents. As reported in this symposium by various investigators, drugs of abuse may impact and modulate the function of the immune system either directly or by effects on the neuroendocrine system. Although many of the drug-induced alterations in immune and neuroendocrine functions have been defined, there is still much to be learned concerning the molecular and cellular basis for these changes. Furthermore, the acute and chronic public health implications of the effects of such drugs on immunity and increased risks for infections are not fully appreciated. The first section of this book contains summaries of presentations at the meeting concerning the effect of opiates, including morphine, on the brain-immune axis and the immune response, as well as effects on altering susceptibility to HIV infection, including AIDS in monkey models. On the other hand, there has been an explosion of interest concerning receptors for opiates on brain cells as well as on lymphoid cells. Pharmacological characterization of such opiate receptors has been well studied and some of the papers presented discuss such receptors and the antagonists for these receptors.

The second section of the symposium summarized newer information concerning cannabinoids and immunity. The first receptor for cannabinoids found on immune cells was recently described, as well as the ligand for such receptors. The effect of cannabionoids on immunity to infectious organisms as well as the effect of such cannabinoids on the biochemistry and cytokine formation by immune cells was also discussed. The third section of the book summarizes some of the presentations concerning the effects of cocaine on immunity, including effects of cocaine on the function of immune cells, including macrophages, as well as production of cytokines by lymphocytes and macrophages treated with cocaine. The effect of alcohol on HIV infection, as well as summaries of effects of other drugs, including isobutyl nitrate, on immune cells is also presented. Studies concerning cytokines in immunity and AIDS as affected by drugs of abuse are also presented. There were several workshops presented at the symposium as well as a panel discussion concerning drugs of abuse and progression of AIDS.

It is the hope of the organizers of this series of conferences, including the conference in San Diego on which this proceedings is based, as well as the editors of the proceedings that these publications will further inspire interest in this rapidly developing field of biomedical science and result in a better understanding of the impact of drugs of abuse on the brain-immune axis and their relationship to immunodeficiency, especially that caused by the AIDS virus. It is anticipated that future meetings on the subject will be held periodically and publication of the proceedings of these conferences will continue to stimulate interest in the field of the brain-immune axis and substance abuse. The authors thank the organizing committee and its administrator, Ms. Suzanne Ingalls, for invaluable assistance that contributed to the success of the symposium. The editors also thank Ms. Ilona Friedman for invaluable assistance as editorial coordinator and managing editor for preparation of this volume of the symposium proceedings. We also thank the National Institute for Drug Abuse for financial support and Dr. Charles Sharp, Project Director of NIDA for Immunology, for continuing interest and valuable advice.

H. Friedman
T. K. Eisenstein
J. Madden
B. M. Sharp

CONTENTS

1

AIDS, DRUGS OF ABUSE AND THE NEUROIMMUNE AXIS

Introduction and Perspectives

Herman Friedman

University of South Florida College of Medicine
Tampa, Florida

The use of recreational drugs of abuse by large numbers of individuals in this country and worldwide has aroused serious concerns about the consequences of this activity. For example, it is now well known that illicit drugs such as marijuana is a widely used recreational drug, not only in adults but also in younger individuals. Furthermore, it is widely accepted that cocaine, especially crack cocaine, is used in epidemic amounts. The "war on drugs" by the U.S. Government was directly aimed at use of cocaine, marijuana and opiates, as well as other illicit drugs. In addition, alcohol abuse is also considered a major problem in this country as it is in many other countries. Over the last few decades various studies have shown that drugs of abuse, including marijuana, cocaine, and opiates, as well as alcohol, can alter both neurophysiological as well as pathological responses of individuals. Recently illicit drugs have also been shown to alter immune functions, both *in vivo* and *in vitro*. The influence of such altered immune function has physiological and physical consequences on drug abusers.

Much data has now accumulated showing that drugs of abuse can markedly affect immune responses in human populations as well as in experimental animals, both *in vivo* and *in vitro*. Furthermore, studies on microbial infections has supported imperical observations reported earlier that use of many drugs of abuse is often associated with enhanced susceptibility to infectious diseases. In addition, the mechanism whereby illicit drugs increase the likelihood of infection in humans as well as in experimental animals have begun to be delineated. In particular, it has now been shown that drugs such as morphine, marijuana or cocaine, as well as alcohol, enhances the susceptibility of animals as well as humans to infections by bacteria, viruses, protozoa, or fungi when given to experimental animals or to lymphoid cells *in vitro* challenged with the infectious agents. Thus, it is now appropriate to focus attention on the accumulating new information concerning the effects of recreational drugs in modulating the immune response as it pertains to resistance mechanisms important in infectious diseases as well as resistance to malignancy and autoimmune phenomena. Studies concerning how illicit drugs can affect immunity are now even more urgent because of the world-wide epidemic of AIDS, which is caused by the human immunodeficiency virus.

AIDS, Drugs of Abuse, and the Neuroimmune Axis, Edited by Friedman *et al.*
Plenum Press, New York, 1996

This virus results in collapse of the immune system making an individual highly susceptible to opportunistic organisms which would otherwise not cause disease in healthy individuals.

The onset of the AIDS epidemic in the USA and other countries stimulated attempts to search for possible co-factors which result in a more rapid progression of the disease in individuals infected with the AIDS virus. A significant number of all AIDS patients in the U.S.A. as well as in many other countries are i.v. drug abusers and it has been shown that the AIDS virus is often spread by contaminated needles or equipment used by such drug users. In addition, it is now widely accepted that many illicit drugs taken either by the i.v. route or by other routes are immunosuppressive. Although many AIDS patients are known to be non-i.v. drug abusers, they often utilize other drugs, such as marijuana, cocaine or even alcohol. Thus there is concern that such drugs may serve as possible co-factors for AIDS progression. Therefore there have been various studies in the past few years to examine in detail the mechanisms whereby drugs of abuse may compromise the immune system in general and specifically result in enhanced susceptibility to infection. There is now much interest concerning the possible relationship among the drugs of abuse such as morphine, marijuana, cocaine or alcohol on immune respone function and altered resistance to microorganisms, especially opportunistic ones including the AIDS virus. Among the possible mechanisms involved are the effects of these drugs of abuse on the brain-immune axis important in immunity and homostation. The brain-immune axis is now known to be highly complex and to evince a highly dynamic homostatic mechanism. The effects of various drugs of abuse, especially morphine and cocaine, on this interactive system has multiple consequences, depending upon the specific sites of action of the drug, duration of exposure, and underlying neuroendocrine, neuro and behavioral status of the individual exposed to the drug. Further understanding the effects of drugs of abuse on the immune system and especially the neuro-immune axis, as well as on the neuroendocrine system in general, emphasizes the critical role of interdisciplinary studies incorporating behavioral, pharmacological, neurologic, anatomical and cellular and molecular approaches necessary for elucidating interactions of illicit drugs with the brain-immune axis.

To characterize the mechanisms of action such drugs on the complex interactions of the neurologic and immune systems require rigorous experimental methodology applied by many different disciplinary groups of investigators. For example, the effects of drugs of abuse on environmental and behavioral factors must be understood in more detail. There are also new findings concerning the importance of cytokines not only in the immune system but also on the neurologic system and this has direct bearing on undestanding the mechanism whereby drugs of abuse affect the immune response and in particular affect on susceptibility to infectious agents, including the AIDS virus. The discovery of specific receptors on both neurologic as well as immune cells, including receptors for opiates as well as cannabinoids, indicate that newer knowledge can now be exploited to investigate how illicit drugs affect the brain-immune system. The effect of drugs such as morphine as well as cannabinoids on production of cytokines, both *in vitro* and *in vivo*, by the immune system is also now widely recognized. However, the consequences of these drug/cytokine interactions on immune and neurologic physiology has not yet been completely elucidated. Neither has the effect of illicit drug exposure on endogenous cytokine production by neurological cells been yet thoroughly investigated. In particular, there is little known about the interactions between illicit drugs and cytokines, both circulating and endogenous, with respect to modulation of the endocrine system and the brain-immune axis. Furthermore, the effects of interferon and the cytokines promoting enhanced immunity and neurologic functions in terms of resisting infectious and autoimmune diseases still must be elucidated. These subjects are now being investigated in some detail, as well as the effects of various inflammatory cytokines such as IL-6, IL-10, and TNF on both immunity and the brain.

The effects of endocrine hormones such as corticosteroids and ACTH on both the immune and nervous sytems is another area of investigation which has direct bearing upon study of alteration and susceptibility to infectious agents, especially the AIDS virus. The potential effects of illicit drugs such as morphine and cannabinoids, as well as cocaine, on different responses of either immune or neurologic cells is now being investigated in detail in many laboratories. It can be predicted that in the not too distant future a better understanding of the interactions in the brain-immune axis in regards to altered susceptibility to infectious agents, including the AIDS virus, will be forthcoming, especially in regards to the effects of drugs of abuse on their responses.

2

THE EFFECT OF NOVEL OPIOIDS ON NATURAL KILLER ACTIVITY AND TUMOR SURVEILLANCE *IN VIVO*

Daniel J. J. Carr,[1,2] Mace Scott,[1] Linda L. Brockunier,[3] Jerome R. Bagely,[3] and Charles P. France[2]

[1] Department of Microbiology, Immunology, and Parasitology
[2] Department of Pharmacology
LSU Medical Center, New Orleans, Louisiana
[3] Ohmeda Pharmaceutical Products Division Inc.
The BOC Group
Murray Hill, New Jersey

INTRODUCTION

Morphine and fentanyl (oral or transdermal administration) are used widely to treat pain in a diverse population of patients including those with cancer.[1-3] However, both of these compounds are potently immunosuppressive particularly with regard to cell-mediated immunity. Relative to cytolytic effector cells, the acute administration of morphine (25.0 mg/kg, s.c.) has been shown to suppress natural killer (NK) activity.[4] The suppression is reportedly mediated by central (brain) pathways[5] located in the periaqueductal gray matter of the mesencephalon[6] that involve both μ-opioid receptors and adrenergic-associated processes.[7,8] Central activation of the adrenergic system as well as actions at opioid receptors may ultimately stimulate the hypothalamic pituitary adrenal axis to release adrenocorticotropin hormone (ACTH) which can then act on the adrenals to secrete corticosterone which has recently been implicated in acute morphine-induced suppression of NK activity.[9]

At the cellular level, morphine has been shown to suppress conjugate formation between NK effectors ($NK1.1^+$) and target cells as well as reduce the number of active killer cells within the conjugates.[8] Acute admininstration of morphine (50.0 mg/kg) also has been shown to modestly reduce the expression of 2B4 antigen on $NK1.1^+$ cells.[8] The 2B4 antigen has been suggested to be a component of a signal-transducing complex that may be important for initiating cytolysis of target cells.[10] Taken together, these studies strongly suggest that the acute admininstration of morphine reduces the cytolytic machinery of the NK cell without modifying the absolute number of NK effector cells.[8]

Studies on the effects of opioids on NK activity in humans have been restricted to parenteral heroin abusers which have a dramatically reduced NK activity as compared to normal controls.[11] Unfortunately, these results are difficult to interpret in that many opioid

AIDS, Drugs of Abuse, and the Neuroimmune Axis, Edited by Friedman *et al.*
Plenum Press, New York, 1996

abusers administer a variety of other drugs, including non-opioids, which could also influence NK activity. However, a more controlled study in rhesus monkeys receiving morphine (3.2 mg/kg) daily over a three year period also showed a significant decrease (35-40%) in peripheral blood mononuclear cell NK activity that also correlated with a substantial decrease (50%) in the percentage of effector cells (defined as $CD8^+CD16^+$) in the circulation.[12]

In addition to its potent antinociceptive effects, fentanyl, also has been used widely for inducing anethesia largely because of its high potency (100 times greater than morphine), fast onset, and relatively short duration of action.[13,14] Recently, transdermal administration of fentanyl has proven to be effective in controlling chronic pain in cancer patients,[2] indicating an alternative treatment regimen for the current opioid of choice (i.e., morphine) to control chronic pain in cancer patients.[1] However, similar to morphine, fentanyl suppresses NK activity[15] and this suppression is naltrexone (opioid antagonist)-sensitive and does not appear to be due to acidosis or changes in O_2 levels in the blood[16] which are known to occur following fentanyl administration.[17] Taken together, considerable literature suggests that most opioids are immunosuppressive as indicated by decreases in NK activity.

NK cells are a population of large granular lymphocytes which have been associated with the surveillance of tumor growth and metastasis.[18,19] In response to cytokines such as IL-2, NK cells become "transformed" into lymphokine-activated-killer (LAK) cells which subsequently can kill NK-resistant targets. Moreover, LAK cells have provided a valuable therapeutic mechanism for attenuating the development of some metastatic tumors including malignant melanoma or renal cell carcinoma,[20,21] thereby substantiating the central role these cells play in tumor surveillance. Changes in the cytolytic activity of NK cells (either to enhance or suppress) are predicted to reflect changes in the resistance to tumor growth and development. Since opioids that typically are used to control pain in cancer patients also suppress NK activity, these compounds would appear to be contraindicated in cancer patients.

Experimentally, it has been shown that daily administration of morphine (10.0 mg/kg, s.c.) in mice promotes the growth of EL-4 (leukemia), sarcoma 180 (carcinoma), P815 (mastocytoma), and Meth-A (fibrosarcoma) cells through a naloxone (opioid receptor antagonist)-sensitive pathway.[22] However, this same study showed morphine not to have any direct effect on the growth of these cell lines *in vitro*, suggesting that the effects are mediated indirectly (i.e., through a secondary mechanism) perhaps involving the sympathetic nervous system or the hypothalamic-pituitary adrenal axis. However, other studies suggest opioids (methadone or bremazocine) may act to reduce the growth of tumor (adenocarcinoma and squamous) cell lines *in vivo*[23] or *in vitro*.[24] Although these studies might appear contradictory, the site of drug administration seems to play a significant role in determining the outcome of these studies. Specifically, intrathecal administration has been found to have deleterious effects on the host immune system or to promote tumor burden while oral or subcutaneous routes have been found to have beneficial effects.[25,26] Moreover, the dose of the drug may also influence the outcome (specifically as it pertains to NK activity and by inference, tumor surveillance) since low (10.0 mg/kg, s.c.) and high (100.0 mg/kg, s.c.) doses of morphine can be without effect on NK activity while intermediate doses (25.0 - 56.0 mg/kg, s.c.) can decrease NK activity.[27]

Collectively, these data suggest a relationship between opioids and tumor development and growth. However, a comprehensive evaluation of the types (δ, κ, and μ) of opioid receptors[28] that are involved in the immune response (specifically cell-mediated) as it relates to tumor biology has not been undertaken. Studies showing that the antinociceptive effects of morphine are critically important in the control of tumor metastasis following surgery[29] seem to reinforce the potential utility of opioids in alleviating tumor burden. Consequently, it would seem that opioids that induce analgesia without immunosuppression may have the most promise for treating pain in cancer patients. This laboratory has begun to investigate the characteristics of a novel series of compounds, the 4-(heteroanilido) piperidines, some of which have antinociceptive effects without suppressive effects on NK activity. Reported below are the first series of studies.

METHODS AND RESULTS

Since the discovery of fentanyl, a potent *mu*-receptor selective opioid that shares many pharmacological actions with morphine, a variety of fentanyl derivatives (phenylpiperidines) have been synthesized and evaluated for their antinociception and other behavioral effects.[30] In addition to a wide variety of morphine-like opioids that have been discovered for use in clinical medicine (e.g., sufentanil), are several fentanyl derivatives that appear to have novel mechanism(s) of action in producing *mu*-opioid antinociceptive effects in non-human primates[31]. Two of these compounds identified for their unique behavioral and antinociceptive effects, mirfentanil and OHM3295, were found to have either no effect on splenic NK activity[32] or enhance splenic NK activity[33] at doses that also have antinociceptive effects. The antinociceptive and/or immune effects were blocked by opioid antagonists indicating the action of these compounds is mediated through opioid receptors.[32,33] Similarly, a third compound in this series, OHM3507, has also been found to have antinociceptive effects (Fig. 1) but not to have any apparent detrimental effect on splenic NK activity (Fig. 2) following acute administration. Based on the preliminary data generated, we initiated a study to investigate the long-term effects of opioid exposure on splenic NK activity as well as address the potential anti-tumor effects of the novel fentanyl-derivatives using a tumor-laden mouse model.

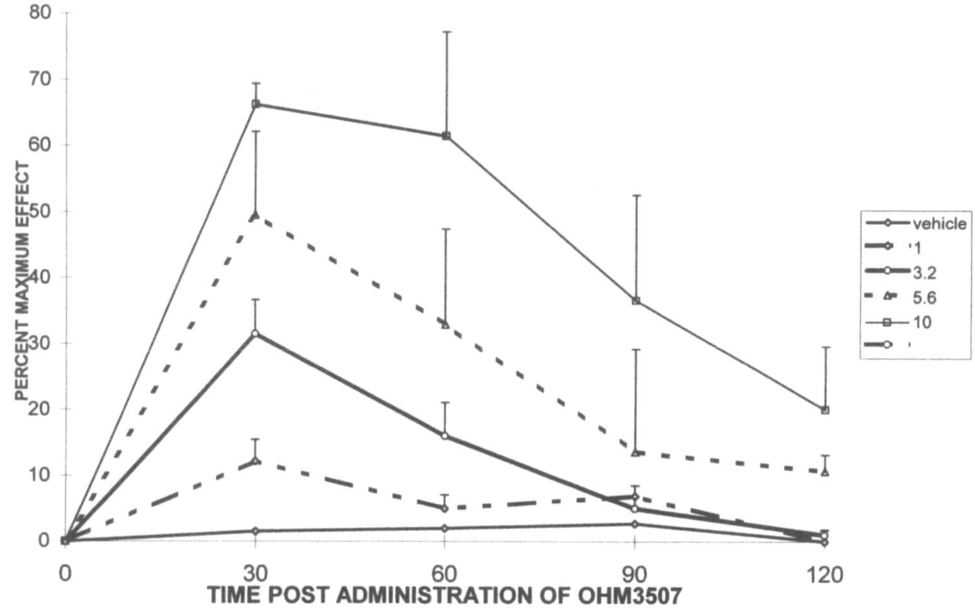

Figure 1. OHM3507 induces antinociception in a dose-dependent fashion. ICR Swiss mice (n=6/group) were administered vehicle or the indicated dose (mg/kg) of OHM3507 (s.c.) and tail flick latencies were determined at 30 min intervals for 120 min. Bars represent SEM.

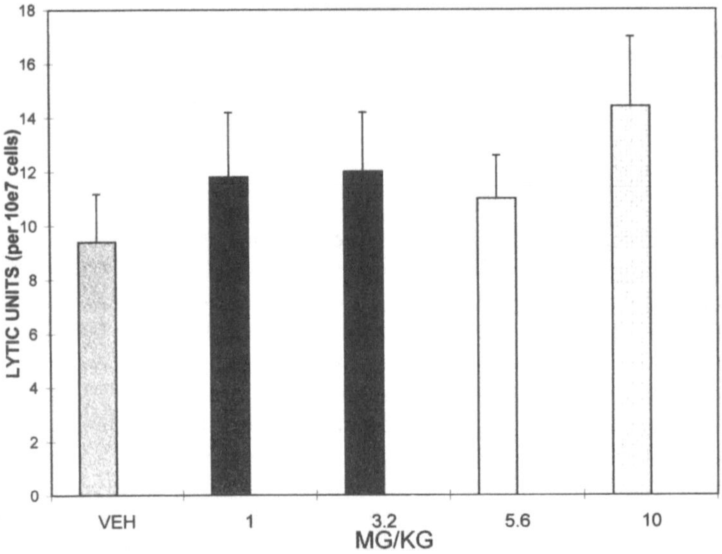

Figure 2. OHM3507 has no effect on splenic NK activity. Mice treated as described in the legend of Fig. 1 were sacrificed 120 min after receiving vehicle or OHM3507. Splenic lymphocytes were prepared and assayed for NK activity using a 4-hr ^{51}Cr-release microcytotoxicity assay with YAC-1 cells as targets. Bars represent SEM.

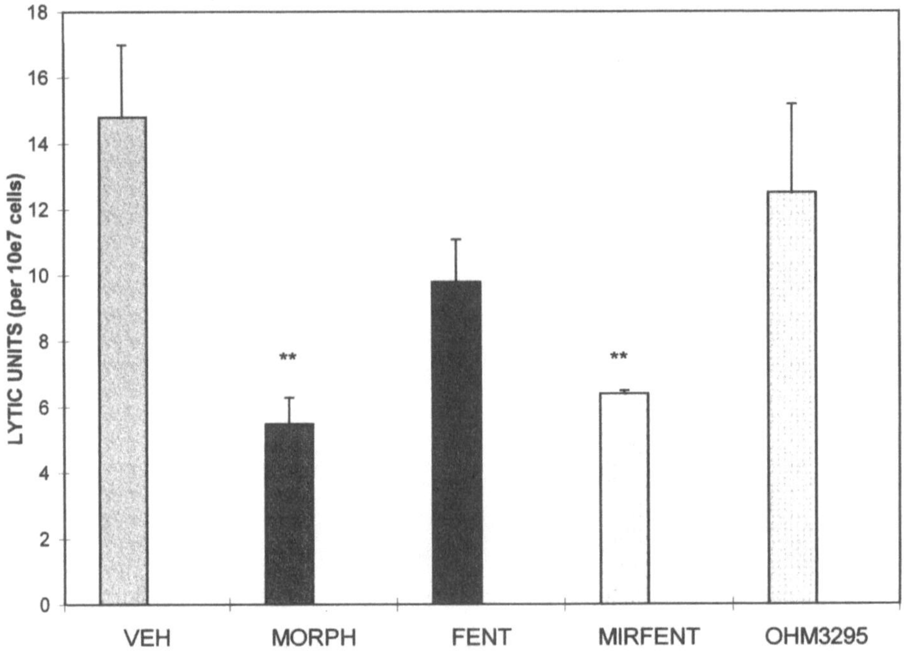

Figure 3. Chronic morphine and mirfentanil exposure suppresses splenic NK activity. C57BL/6 mice (n=5/group) were administered (s.c.) morphine, fentanyl, mirfentanil, OHM3295, or vehicle (Hank's balanced salt solution, HBSS) daily for 21 days. The mice were then sacrificed and splenocytes were isolated and assayed for NK activity in a 4-hr ^{51}Cr-release microcytotoxicity assay using YAC-1 cells as targets. Bars represent the mean ± SEM.

In the first experiment, C57BL/6 mice received equianalgesic doses of morphine (32.0 mg/kg, s.c.), fentanyl (1.0 mg/kg, s.c.), OHM3295 (32.0 mg/kg, s.c.), mirfentanil (10.0 mg/kg, s.c.) or vehicle daily for 21 days. The mice were subsequently sacrificed and splenic lymphocytes assayed for NK activity. The results show that morphine and mirfentanil significantly suppressed splenic NK activity whereas fentanyl modestly suppressed and OHM3295 had no significant effect relative to vehicle-treated controls (Fig. 3).

To assess the potential anti-tumor effect of OHM3295, DBA/2 mice simultaneously received the mastocytoma, P815, along with either morphine (32.0 mg/kg, s.c.), fentanyl (1.0 mg/kg, s.c.), OHM3295 (32.0 mg/kg, s.c.), mirfentanil (10.0 mg/kg, s.c.) or vehicle. Drug or vehicle was administered daily over the next 20 days and mice were monitored for survival. Unexpectedly, the results show that compared to vehicle treatment, only morphine increased the survivability among P815-laden mice while the other compounds either had no effect (fentanyl or mirfentanil) or were detrimental (OHM3295). Moreover, the casual observation showed that the physical appearance of the morphine-treated mice is obviously more favorable relative to the other treated groups including the vehicle controls (data not shown).

These results tend to support previous observations[26,29] showing the beneficial effects of morphine on tumor growth in pulmonary and intestinal tumor models. Future studies will attempt to elucidate the mechanism(s) that are responsible for the beneficial effects of morphine treatment and tumor growth. It is tempting to speculate that the action of morphine (due to the duration of the effect) may be to reduce the stress level (i.e., the activity of the hypothalamic pituitary adrenal axis) in animals undergoing a significant disease process.

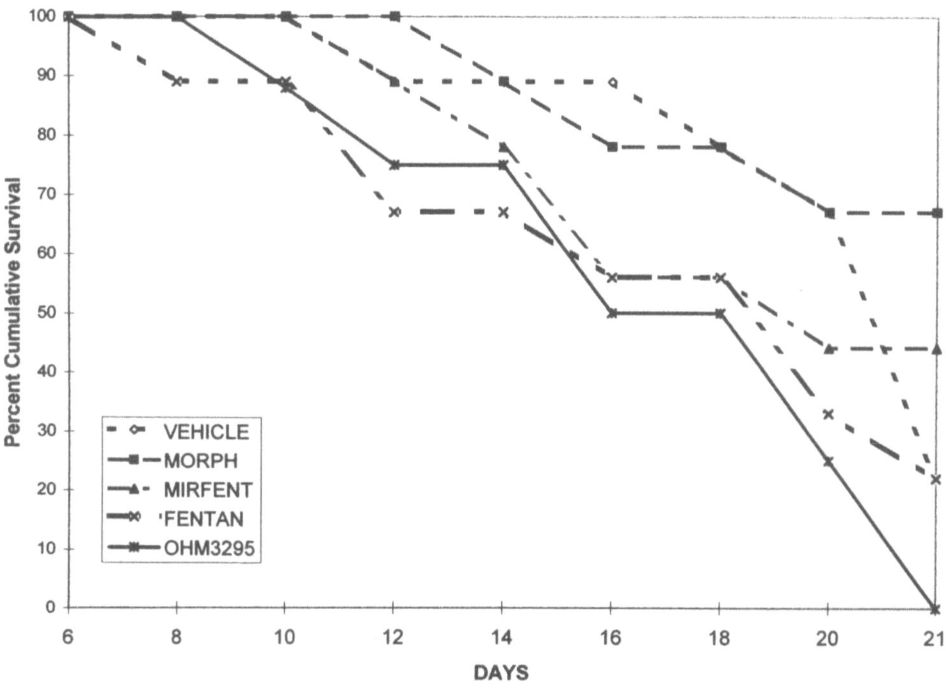

Figure 4. Morphine enhances the survival of tumor (P815) laden-DBA/2 mice *in vivo*. DBA/2 mice (n=9/group) were inoculated with 1×10^6 P815 mastocytoma cells i.p. and subsequently admininstered (s.c.) morphine, fentanyl, OHM3285, mirfentanil, or vehicle (HBSS). The mice were subsequently admininstered drug or vehicle daily and the survival and physical appearance of each mouse was recorded.

ACKNOWLEDGMENTS

This work was supported by a grant from the LSU Medical Center Stanley S. Scott Cancer Center and The Cancer Association of Greater New Orleans. CPF is the recipient of a Research Scientist Development Award from the National Institute on Drug Abuse (DA00211).

REFERENCES

1. Hanks, GW, RG, Twycross, & JM Bliss. 1987. Controlled release of morphine tablets: a double-blind trial in patients with advanced cancer. *Anaesthesia* 42:840-844.
2. Portenoy, RK, MA Southam, SK Gupta, J Lapin, M Layman, CE Inturrisi, & KM Foley. 1993. Transdermal fentanyl for cancer pain. *Anesthesiology* 78:36-43.
3. Twycross, TG. 1982. Morphine and diamorphine in the terminally ill patient. *Acta. Anaesth.* 74S:128-134.
4. Bayer, BM, S Daussin, M Hernandez, & L Irvin. 1990. Morphine inhibition of lymphocyte activity is mediated by an opioid dependent mechanism. *Neuropharmacol.* 29:369-374.
5. Shavit, Y, A Depaulis, FC Martin, GW Terman, RN Pechnick, CJ Zane, RP Gale, & JC Liebeskind. 1986. Involvement of brain opiate receptors in the immune-suppressive effect of morphine. *Proc. Natl. Acad. Sci. USA.* 83:7114-7117.
6. Weber, RJ & A Pert. 1989. The periaqueductal gray matter mediates opiate- induced immunosuppression. *Science* 245:188-190.
7. Carr, DJJ, BM Gebhardt, & D Paul. 1993. Alpha adrenergic and mu-2 opioid receptors are involved in morphine-induced skuppression of splenocyte natural killer activity. *J. Pharmacol. Exp. Ther.* 264:1179-1186.
8. Carr, DJJ, S Mayo, BM Gebhardt, & J Porter. 1994. Central α-adrenergic involvement in morphine-mediated suppression of splenic natural killer activity. *J. Neuroimmunol.* 53:53-63.
9. Freier, DO & BA Fuchs. 1994. A mechanism of action for morphine-induced immunosuppression: Corticosterone mediates morphine-induced suppression of natural killer activity. *J. Pharmacol. Exp. Ther.* 270:1127-1133.
10. Garni-Wagner, BA, A Purohit, PA Mathew, M Bennett, & V Kumar. 1993. A novel function-associated molecule related to non-MHC-restricted cytotoxicity mediated by activated natural killer cells and T cells. *J. Immunol.* 151:60-70.
11. Novick, DM, M Ochshorn, V Ghali, TS Croxson, WD Mercern, N Chiorazzi, & MJ Kreek. 1989. Natural killer cell activity and lymphocyte subsets in parenteral heroin abusers and long-term methadone maintenance patients. *J. Pharmacol. Exp. Ther.* 250:606-610.
12. Carr, DJJ & CP France. 1993. Immune alterations in morphine-treated rhesus monkeys. *J. Pharmacol. Exp. Ther.* 267:9-15.
13. Cookson, RF & GDW Towse. 1981. The search for new analgesics. *Clin. Res. Rev.* 1:219-225.
14. Marshall, BE & DE Longnecker. 1990. General anesthetics. In *The Pharmacolgical Basis of Therapeutics* (eds. LS Goodman & A Gilman), MacMillan, New York, pp. 285-297.
15. Beilin, B, FC Martin, Y Shavit, RP Gale, & JC Liebeskind. 1989. Suppression of natural killer cell activity by high-dose narcotic anesthesia in rats. *Brain Behavior Immun.* 3:129-137.
16. Beilin, B, Y Shavit, S Cohn, & E Kedar. 1992. Narcotic-induced suppression of natural killer cell activity in ventilated and nonventilated rats. *Clin. Immun. Immunopath.* 64:173-176.
17. Bailey, PL, GB Streisand, KA East, TD East, S Isern, TW Hansen, EFM Posthuma, FW Rosendaal, NL Pace, & TH Stanley. 1990. Differences in magnitude and duration of opioid-induced respiratory depression and analgesia with fentanyl and sufentanil. *Anesth. Analg.* 70:8-15.
18. Poste, G & IJ Fidler. 1980. The pathogenesis of cancer metastasis. *Nature (London)* 283:139-146.
19. Herberman, RB & JR Ortaldo. 1981. Natural killer cells: their role in defenses against disease. *Science* 214:24-30.
20. Lafreniere R, SA Rosenberg. 1985. Adoptive immunotherapy of murine hepatic with lymphokine activated killer (LAK) cells and recombinant interleukin 2 (RIL2) can mediate the regression of both immunogenic and nonimmunogenic sarcomas and an adenocarcinoma. *J. Immunol.* 135:4273- 4280.
21. Schwarz, RE, NL Vujanovic, JC Hiserodt. 1986. Enhanced antimetastatic activity of lymphokine-activated killer cells purified and expanded by their adherence to plastic. *Cancer Res.* 49:1441-1446.

22. Ishikawa, M, K Tanno, A Kamo, Y Takayanagi, & K-I Sasaki. 1993. Enhancement of tumor growth by morphine and its possible mechanism in mice. *Biol. Pharm. Bull.* 16:762-766.
23. Reubi, JC. 1985. Central nervous system-mediated growth inhibition of a rat prostate carcinoma by an opioid. *J. Endocrinol.* 107:247-250.
24. Maneckjee, R, JD Minna. 1992. Nonconventional opioid binding sites mediate growth inhibitory effects of methadone on human lung cancer cells. *Proc. Natl. Acad. Sci. USA.* 89:1169-1173.
25. Provinciali, M, G Di Stefano, W Raffaeli, G Pari, F Desiderio, N Fabri. 1991. Evaluation of NK and LAK cell activities in neoplastic patients during treatment with morphine. *Intern. J. Neurosci.* 59:127-133.
26. Yeager, MP, TA Colacchio. 1991. Effect of morphine on growth of metastatic colon cancer in vivo. *Arch. Surg.* 126:454-456.
27. Carr, DJJ, LR Gerak, CP France. 1994. Naltrexone antagonizes the analgesic and immunosuppressive effects of morphine in mice. *J. Pharmacol. Exp. Ther.* 269:693-698.
28. Pasternak, GW. 1993. Pharmacological mechanisms of opioid analgesics. *Clin. Neuropharmacol.* 16:1-18.
29. Page, GG, S Ben-Eliyahu, JC Liebeskind. 1994. The role of LGL/NK cells in surgery-induced promotion of metastasis and its attenuation by morphine. *Brain Behavior Immun.* 8:241-250.
30. Bagley, JR, LV Kudzma, NL Lalinde, JA Colapret, B-S Huang, B-S Lin, TP Jerussi, MJ Benvenga, BM Doorley, MH Ossipov, TC Spaulding, HK Spencer. 1991. Evolution of the 4-anilidopiperidine class of opioid analgesics. *Med. Res. Rev.* 11:402-436.
31. France, CP, G Winger, R Medzihradsky, MR Seggel, KC Rice, JH Woods. 1992. Mirfentanil: pharmacological profile of a novel fentanyl derivative with opioid and nonopioid effects. *J. Pharmacol. Exp. Ther.* 258:502-510.
32. Carr, DJJ, LL Brockunier, M Scott, JR Bagley, CP France. 1996. Mirfentanil antagonizes morphine-induced suppression of splenic NK activity in mice. *Immunopharmacol.* in press.
33. Baker, ML, LL Brockunier, JR Bagley, CP France, DJJ Carr. 1995. Fentanyl- related 4-heteroanilido piperidine OHM3295 augments splenic natural killer activity and induces analgesia through opioid receptor pathways. *J. Pharmacol. Exp. Ther.* 274:1285-1292.

3

KAPPA OPIOID RECEPTORS ON IMMUNE CELLS AS STUDIED BY FLUORESCENT LIGANDS

Jean M. Bidlack, Diane M. P. Lawrence, and Tracey A. Ignatowski

Department of Pharmacology and Physiology
University of Rochester, School of Medicine and Dentistry
Rochester, New York 14642-8711

1. INTRODUCTION

Despite both functional (1-4) and molecular biological (5-8) evidence for the presence of opioid receptors on lymphocytes, the search for opioid binding sites on leukocytes has been difficult. Opioid binding sites possessing all the characteristics of the classical brain opioid receptors had not been detected until the identification of the κ opioid receptor on the mouse R1.1 thymoma cell line (9,10). Possible reasons why opioid receptors have been difficult to detect on mixed cell populations from the immune system include: 1) opioid receptors may be expressed on only a small population of lymphocytes; 2) the expression of opioid receptors on lymphocyte changes during lymphocyte maturation; and 3) radioreceptor binding methodology is not sufficiently sensitive to detect opioid receptors present at a low density. While the R1.1 cell line was useful in establishing that a lymphocyte could express an opioid receptor, interest still lies in determining if lymphocytes from a mixed cell population, such as thymus and spleen, express opioid receptors. To address this question, we developed an indirect immunofluorescent method that is more sensitive than radioreceptor binding assays (11,12).

Studies over fifteen years have demonstrated the ability to couple fluorescent moieties to opiates while retaining affinity. However, some opioids autofluoresce, and coupled with tissue and cell autofluorescence, this has limited the use of fluorescently labeled opioids. Another major difficulty is the low density of opioid receptors on cells from the immune system. The use of phycoerythrin (PE) in an amplification protocol may overcome these problems. Generally, compounds and tissue autofluoresce at a lower wavelength than is used to detect PE. The fluorescent intensity of PE approaches the theoretical detection of a single molecule (13).

An indirect immunofluorescence method to visualize the κ opioid receptor was developed, using a high affinity, κ-selective fluorescein-conjugated arylacetamide opioid FITC-AA, shown in Fig. 1, with the amplified signal being measured with the PE fluorophore (11). The mouse thymoma cell line, R1E/TL8x.1.G1.OUA^r.1 (R1EGO), which expresses the

AIDS, Drugs of Abuse, and the Neuroimmune Axis, Edited by Friedman *et al.*
Plenum Press, New York, 1996

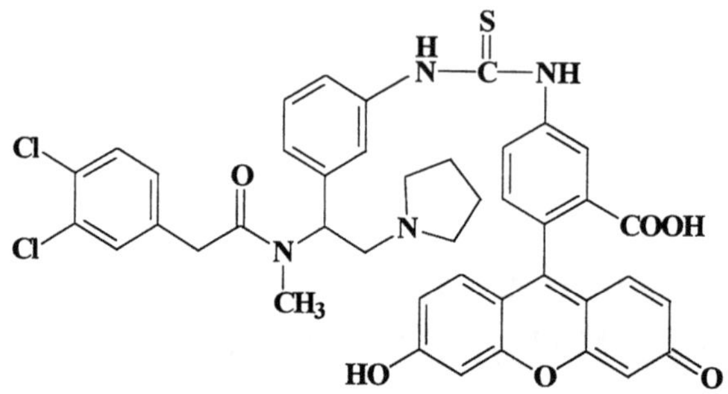

FITC-AA

Figure 1. Structure of the fluorescein-conjugated κ opioid FITC-AA.

κ but not μ or δ opioid receptors (14), was used as a positive control for fluorescence labeling. The R1EGO cell line is a derivative of the R1.1 thymoma, but R1EGO cells express six times more κ receptors than the parent R1.1 cell line (14). FITC-AA displayed high affinity for the κ opioid receptor, having a K_i value less than 10 nM for the inhibition of the binding of the κ-selective ligand [^{3}H]U69,593 to either guinea pig brain membranes or R1EGO cell membranes (11). When R1EGO cells were incubated with FITC-AA, followed by a biotinylated antibody directed against fluorescein and then extravidin conjugated to PE, specific opioid binding to the cells was 73 ± 6%, as defined as PE fluorescence that was blocked by the κ-selective antagonist nor-binaltorphimine (nor-BNI) (11,15). Similarly, mouse thymocytes from C57Bl/6ByJ mice showed 58 ± 1% specific binding (11). Without the amplification procedure, no specific opioid binding was detected to either the R1EGO thymoma cells or the mouse thymocytes. These experiments demonstrated that the κ ligand FITC-AA, followed by the amplification procedure could be used to detect κ opioid receptors on mouse thymocytes.

The study described here is directed at determining if FITC-AA, followed by the amplification procedure could be used to detect κ opioid receptors on mouse splenocytes, and to determine if the entire amplification protocol was required to achieve optimal labeling of the κ receptor.

2. MATERIALS AND METHODS

2.1. Preparation of Mouse Splenocytes

Male C57Bl/6ByJ mice, aged 6-8 weeks, were sacrificed by CO_2 inhalation, and spleens were removed aseptically. Splenocytes were dissociated in cold HEPES-balanced salt solution (HEPES-BSS), consisting of 15 mM HEPES, 3.4 mM K_2HPO_4, 0.6 mM KH_2PO_4, 150 mM NaCl, 5 mM KCl, 2.5 mM $CaCl_2$, 1.2 mM $MgSO_4$, and 1% (w/v) bovine serum albumin, pH 7.4. The cell suspension was passed over a sterile glass wool column to remove dead cells and debris. After centrifugation at 200 x g for 10 min at 4°C, the cell suspension was treated with a cold isotonic ammonium chloride solution, to lyse erythrocytes. In some experiments, the cell suspension was passed over a nylon wool column immediately after passage through the glass wool column. The nylon wool column was eluted with 37°C HEPES-BSS. After centrifugation at 200 x g for 10 min at 4°C, fluorescent opioid binding to the cells was measured as described below. Viable cells as determined by trypan blue exclusion, were counted in a hemacytometer.

2.2. Cell Culture

The R1EGO cells, obtained from the American Type Culture Collection (Rockville, MD), were cultured in a humidified atmosphere of 5% CO_2/95% air at 37°C. The media used was RPMI 1640 buffered with 12.5 mM HEPES, pH 7.2, and containing 10% (vol/vol) iron-supplemented bovine calf serum, 300 μg/ml L-glutamine, 100 units/ml penicillin, 100 μg/ml streptomycin, 50 μM 2-mercaptoethanol and 60 μM 2-aminoethanol.

2.3. Indirect Immunofluorescence of Kappa Opioid Receptors on Splenocytes

The structure of the κ-selective arylacetamide compound, FITC-AA, is shown in Fig. 1. FITC-AA was synthesized as previously described (11) and was obtained from Dr. S. Archer (Rensselaer Polytechnic Institute, Troy, NY). The labeling of the κ receptor on splenocytes passed through both glass wool and nylon wool columns was compared with the labeling obtained from splenocytes that had been passed through only the glass wool column. For all fluorescence studies, the buffer used was HEPES-BSS. Unfixed cells were washed twice by centrifugation at 200 x g for 10 min at 4°C, followed by resuspension in HEPES-BSS. In a final volume of 200 μl HEPES-BSS, 2 x 10^6 cells per sample were incubated with 30 μM FITC-AA for 30 min at 25°C for optimal staining. The κ-selective antagonist nor-BNI at a final concentration of 500 μM was included to measure nonspecific fluorescence. Samples were then chilled on ice, diluted with 1 ml of HEPES-BSS, and centrifuged at 400 x g for 3 min at 4°C. After aspirating the supernatants, cells were washed two additional times, followed by resuspension in a final volume of 100 μl of HEPES-BSS. This volume included 10 μl of biotinylated rabbit anti-fluorescein IgG (Molecular Probes, Eugene, OR), except in FITC-AA only and PE only controls. After incubation for 30 min on ice, samples were diluted with 1 ml of HEPES-BSS followed by centrifugation at 400 x g for 3 min at 4°C. The supernatants were aspirated, and the cells were washed again. Cells were then resuspended in 40 μl of HEPES-BSS and 10 μl of extravidin-R-phycoerythrin (Sigma Chemical Co. St. Louis, MO) for 15 min on ice. The cells were washed twice as described above and were resuspended in a final volume of 500 μl HEPES-BSS.

2.4. Labeling Kappa Receptors with Naltrexamine Derivatives

In order to determine if the entire PE amplification was necessary for the labeling of κ receptors, a FITC-labeled derivative of naltrexamine (FITC-NTXamine) and biotin-labeled naltrexamine, shown in Fig. 2, were synthesized as previously described (12). Naltrexamine, containing an amino group in the C-6β position, is a derivative of the opioid antagonist naltrexone (Fig. 2). One-step direct fluorescence with FITC-NTXamine was compared with a two-step method that used biotin conjugated to naltrexamine followed by extravidin-conjugated PE. The three-step method used FITC-NTXamine, followed by a biotinylated antibody directed against fluorescein and then extravidin-conjugated PE. The R1EGO cell line which expresses κ receptors was used to compare the three methods for labeling of the receptor.

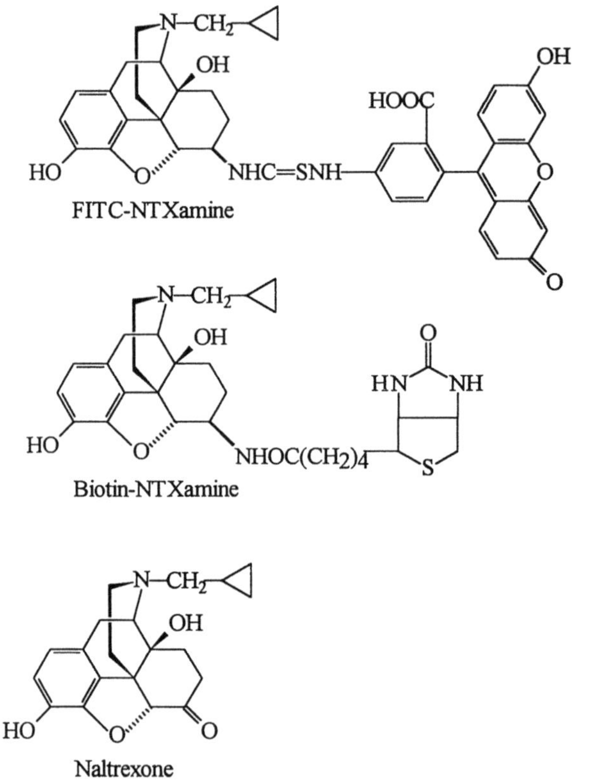

Figure 2. Structures of FITC-NTXamine, biotin-NTXamine and naltrexone.

2.4.1. Direct Labeling of the Kappa Receptor with FITC-Labeled Naltrexamine. R1EGO cells were washed twice by centrifugation at 200 x g for 10 min at 4°C, followed by resuspension in HEPES-BSS. In a final volume of 200 µl HEPES-BSS, 2 x 10^6 cells per sample were incubated with 30 µM FITC-NTXamine for 30 min at 25°C for optimal staining. Nonspecific fluorescence was measured by including 500 µM nor-BNI. Autofluorescence was measured by incubating the cells with buffer alone during each incubation step. Samples were then chilled at 4°C, diluted with 1 ml of HEPES-BSS, and centrifuged at 400 x g for 3 min at 4°C. After aspirating the supernatants, cells were washed twice more, then resuspended in a final volume of 1 ml of HEPES-BSS.

2.4.2. Two-Step Indirect Immunofluorescence with PE. Cells were prepared as described above and incubated with 30 µM biotin-NTXamine for 30 min at 25°C, in a final volume of 200 µl of HEPES-BSS. Controls included the addition of 500 µM nor-BNI to measure nonspecific fluorescence, and the omission of biotin-NTXamine to measure the extravidin-PE background. Samples were then chilled at 4°C, washed twice in 1 ml of HEPES-BSS as described above, and resuspended in a final volume of 50 µl of HEPES-BSS, including 10 µl of extravidin-PE. This incubation took place for 15 min at 4°C in the dark; the cells were then washed twice as described above. The samples were resuspended in a final volume of 1 ml of HEPES-BSS.

2.4.3. Three-Step Indirect Immunofluorescence with PE. R1EGO cells were prepared as described above and incubated with 30 µM FITC-NTXamine for 30 min at 25°C, in a final volume of 200 μl of HEPES-BSS. To measure nonspecific fluorescence, 500 μM nor-BNI was included, and FITC-NTXamine was omitted for the biotin-anti-fluorescein IgG/extravidin-PE background control. Samples were then chilled at 4°C, washed twice in 1 ml of HEPES-BSS as described above, and resuspended in a final volume of 100 μl, including 10 μl of biotin-conjugated anti-fluorescein IgG. After incubation for 30 min at 4°C, samples were washed twice with 1 ml of HEPES-BSS as described above and resuspended in a volume of 50 μl of HEPES-BSS, including 10 μl of extravidin-PE. The cells were incubated for 15 min at 4°C in the dark, then washed twice as described above. The cells were resuspended in a final volume of 1 ml of HEPES-BSS.

2.5. Visualization of Fluorescence

Samples were analyzed by flow cytometry with a Becton-Dickinson FACScan (San Jose, CA) equipped with a 15-mW argon-ion laser for excitation at 488 nm. In each sample, 25,000 splenocytes or 10,000 R1EGO cells were analyzed. The fluorescence was measured on a logarithmic scale, with band pass filters of 530 ± 15 nm for fluorescein and 585 ± 21 nm for PE. Data were collected with a computer, using Becton-Dickinson Lysis II or Cell Quest software. Median values of fluorescence intensity distributions were used to compare the fluorescence among samples, which assumed that only a single population was labeled. Unlabeled cells ("autofluorescence") and cells labeled only with FITC-labeled opioid were used as negative controls to insure that fluorescein did not contribute to the PE signal as measured by flow cytometry. For the naltrexamine samples, the compensation was set so that when PE fluorescence was measured, the intensity of cells labeled with only FITC-NTXamine was identical to that of the autofluorescence controls. In the three-step staining procedure, background PE controls were also included, where FITC-NTXamine was omitted; cells were incubated only with biotin-conjugated anti-fluorescein IgG and extravidin-PE. This control provided baseline PE emission including the nonspecific staining of both the anti-fluorescein IgG and the extravidin-PE.

3. RESULTS

3.1 Labeling the Kappa Opioid Receptor on Splenocytes with FITC-AA

Previously, FITC-AA (Fig. 1) as part of the three-step amplification procedure, using PE as the fluorophore, resulted in 58 ± 1% specific labeling of the κ opioid receptor on mouse C57Bl/6ByJ thymocytes (11). In the current study, this labeling procedure was used with splenocytes from C57Bl/6ByJ mice to determine if κ receptors were present on a mature population of lymphocytes. As shown in the flow cytometric tracing in Fig. 3A, when splenocytes were dissociated and passed only through a glass wool column, two PE peaks were obtained. The antagonist nor-BNI reduced the labeling of the first and second peaks by only 18 ± 7% and 8 ± 1%, respectively. In order to obtain a higher level of specific labeling of the κ receptor and a single PE peak, splenocytes were first passed through a glass wool column, followed by a nylon wool column. After passage through the nylon wool column, only one PE peak was obtained for splenocytes (Fig. 3B) and nor-BNI displaced 55 ± 9% of the labeling. This result is similar to the amount of specific labeling obtained with the thymocytes. While B cells and some monocytes are eluted along with T cells from the nylon wool column, this procedure enhanced the specific labeling of the κ receptor. This study demonstrates that both thymocytes and splenocytes obtained from C57Bl/6ByJ mice express κ opioid receptors.

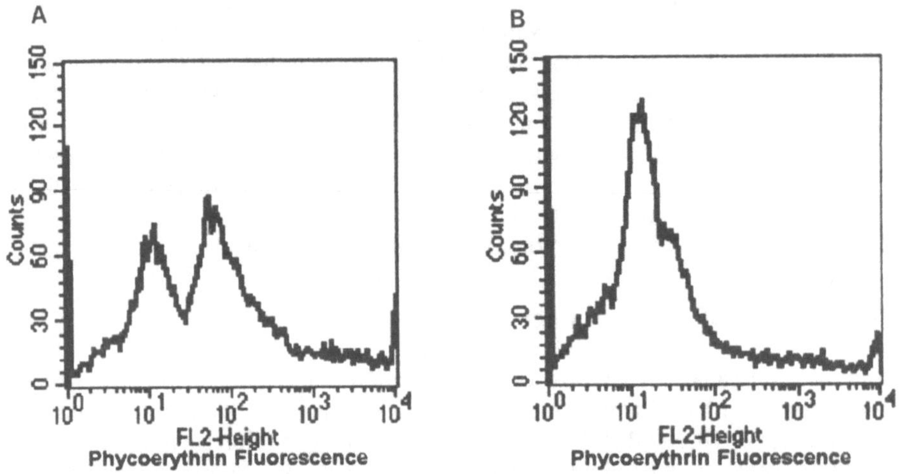

Figure 3. Phycoerythrin fluorescent labeling the κ opioid receptor on splenocytes. Mouse splenocytes were separated by either a glass wool column (A) or by a glass wool column followed by a nylon wool column (B). The splenocytes prepared by the two methods were labeled with FITC-AA in the absence and presence of nor-BNI as described under Materials and Methods. Only total fluorescence is shown. The first peak in panel A was reduced by 18 ± 7% with nor-BNI. The second peak in panel A was reduced by 8 ± 1% in the presence of nor-BNI. In panel B, the PE peak was reduced by 55 ± 8% in the presence of nor-BNI.

3.2. Comparing One-Step, Two-Step and Three-Step Amplification Methods for Labeling the Kappa Opioid Receptor

The PE amplification procedure, used with FITC-AA to label κ receptors, involved three steps with fluorescein used as a hapten not as a fluorophore in the procedure. Using FITC-NTXamine and biotin-NTXamine, shown in Fig. 2, three procedures to label the κ receptor were compared. Both compounds had high affinity for the κ receptor with K_i values less than 10 nM for the inhibition of [^{3}H]U69,593 binding to the κ receptor on guinea pig brain membranes (12). Figure 4 shows schematic representations of the three different methods used to fluorescently label the κ opioid receptor on the R1EGO thymoma cell line. When R1EGO cells were incubated with 30 μM FITC-NTXamine (Fig. 4A), the resulting fluorescein staining was only slightly reduced in the presence of nor-BNI, indicating that primarily nonspecific staining was observed. Flow cytometric analysis showed that although the average of median fluorescence intensity values for the total and nonspecific staining were different, as shown in Table 1, the fluorescence intensity distributions overlapped almost completely (12). To determine whether a switch from fluorescein to PE would enhance the fluorescence sufficiently to visualize the receptor, R1EGO cells were incubated with biotin-NTXamine in the absence or presence of nor-BNI, followed by extravidin-PE, as shown in Fig. 4B. When PE fluorescence intensity was measured, both total and nonspecific staining were minimal, and not significantly different from the background staining of extravidin-PE alone. No specific binding was observed in the two-step amplification (Table 1). Finally, the three-step method was tested, using FITC-NTXamine, biotin-anti-fluorescein IgG, and extravidin-PE (Fig. 4C). Compared to the two-step method, the relative PE staining intensity was much greater. When nor-BNI was included, PE staining was reduced by almost 40% (Table 1). These results demonstrate that the three-step method is the most sensitive method to visualize fluorescence staining of the κ opioid receptor. Like

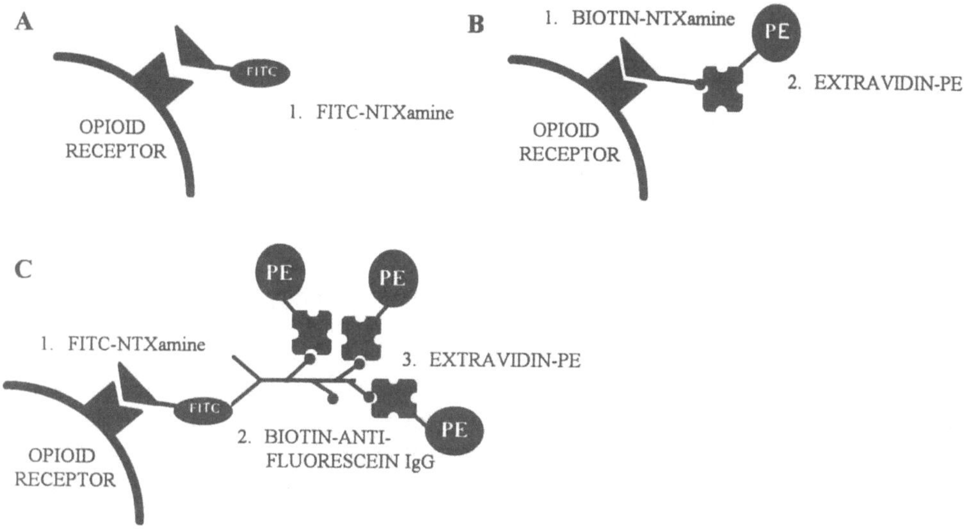

Figure 4. Schematic representation of the fluorescent labeling methods. One-step direct labeling of opioid receptors involve the direct measurement of FITC-NTXamine binding to the cell surface (A). With two-step indirect labeling, cells were incubated with biotin-NTXamine, followed by extravidin-conjugated PE; the intensity of PE fluorescence was measured (B). In the three-step indirect staining protocol, cells were first incubated with FITC-NTXamine, followed by biotin-conjugated anti-fluorescein IgG, and finally extravidin-PE. The intensity of the PE fluorescence was measured independently of FITC fluorescence (C).

Table 1. Comparison of fluorescence staining of κ opioid receptor on R1EGO thymoma cells using three methods

One-Step	FITC fluorescence above autofluorescence (n=2)	Percent Specific Binding
FITC-NTXamine	116 ± 1*	15 ± 1
FITC-NTXamine + nor-BNI	98 ± 2*†	
Two-Step	**PE fluorescence intensity above background (n=3)**	**Percent Specific Binding**
Biotin-NTXamine	1.2 ± 0.4	not detectable
Biotin-NTXamine + nor-BNI	3.8 ± 1.0*	
Three-Step	**PE fluorescence intensity above background (n=7)**	**Percent Specific Binding**
FITC-NTXamine	311 ± 30*	36 ± 7
FITC-NTXamine + nor-BNI	200 ± 33*†	

R1EGO cells were fluorescently stained as described under "Materials and Methods" for each of the three protocols. The data are expressed as the mean ± S.E. of the median fluorescence intensity values, in arbitrary units, above background from *n* experiments. Background staining levels were as follows: One-step, autofluorescence = 5.7; two-step, extravidin-PE background = 6.9 ± 0.6; three-step, biotin-anti-fluorescein IgG plus extravidin-PE background = 88 ± 6. Percent specific staining was calculated as the mean ± S.E. of (total-nonspecific)/total fluorescence intensity. *significantly different from background (P<.05); †significantly less than total staining (P<.05).

FITC-AA, FITC-NTXamine also labeled the κ receptor when the three-step amplification procedure was used.

4. DISCUSSION

Previous studies have shown that FITC-AA labeled the κ opioid receptor on the R1EGO cells (11), mouse thymocytes (11), and human microglia (16). The R1EGO cell line is a homogenous cell line. Thymocytes contain multiple cell types, but still represent a more homogenous population of cells than splenocytes. Splenocytes passed over a glass wool column to remove dead cells and debris, followed by red blood lysis, demonstrated two PE peaks, suggesting a complexity in labeling the κ receptor (Fig. 3). In addition, the PE fluorescence in the two peaks was only slightly reduced with nor-BNI, indicating that the labeling was primarily the result of nonspecific labeling. In contrast, after passage of splenocytes through a nylon wool column, one single PE peak was observed. Also, this PE fluorescence was reduced by 55% in the presence of nor-BNI. Specific binding to splenocytes eluted from the nylon wool column was similar to the 58% specific labeling previously obtained with thymocytes (11). These results indicate that the κ opioid receptor is expressed on mouse thymocytes and splenocytes. Double labeling experiments, using antibodies directed against specific cell surface markers, will lead to a mapping of which cells from the immune system express the κ opioid receptor. Preliminary data suggest that CD4+ and CD8+ thymocytes express the κ receptor (data not shown).

The three-step amplification procedure described here with FITC-AA and splenocytes, and used previously with FITC-AA and thymocytes (11), uses the fluorescein conjugated to the opioid as a hapten in order to amplify the signal. In this method, multiple PE molecules are associated with a single receptor because the biotinylated antibody directed against fluorescein contains multiple biotin molecules. Extravidin-conjugated PE can then bind to these multiple biotin sites, thereby amplifying the signal. In order to determine if the full amplification was required to label the receptor, the naltrexamine derivatives FITC-NTXamine and biotin-NTXamine were tested to determine if the receptor labeling procedure could be reduced to fewer steps. Naltrexamine derivatives were used because both fluorescein and biotin could be conjugated to this opioid antagonist in the C-6β position (12). When FITC-NTXamine staining of R1EGO cells was measured, a slight reduction in staining was observed when nor-BNI was included. This result is consistent with a study that demonstrated 2.5-6% specific labeling of opioid receptors on rat peripheral leukocyte subpopulations when fluorescein conjugated to naltrexone hydrozone was used as the probe (17). The reason for the low specific labeling of leukocyte opioid receptors using fluorescein-labeled opioids may be that fluorescein emits too weak a signal to detect the number of receptors per cell. Alternatively, autofluorescence of the cells may be sufficiently high and occurring in the same emitting wavelength as fluorescein to mask the signal, or the signal may be quenched when bound to the opioid receptors. Because PE is a molecule with a higher quantum yield and higher molar absorptivity than fluorescein (18,19), it seemed more likely that the opioid receptors could be detected by PE. However, PE is a large phycobiliprotein (18), so it is expected that a PE-conjugated opioid ligand would have poor affinity due to steric hindrance. Biotin-NTXamine was used in combination with extravidin-PE to determine whether changing the fluorophore was sufficient to detect fluorescent staining. This method resulted in one biotin and one PE molecule being associated with one receptor. This approach, however, did not result in the detection of the κ opioid receptor. Only the three-step amplification procedure, which resulted in multiple biotin and PE molecules being associated with one receptor, was successful in specifically labeling the κ receptor. FITC-AA resulted in approximately 70% specific labeling of the κ receptor expressed on R1EGO cells

(11) in comparison to 40% labeling obtained with FITC-NTXamine in the identical amplification procedure. The greater specific labeling with FITC-AA may be due to lower nonspecific binding of this compound to cells. Despite the differences in the percentage of fluorescence labeling that was blocked by nor-BNI, both compounds can be used to detect the κ receptor. In addition, FITC-NTXamine, which is a relatively nonselective opioid, may be useful in labeling μ and δ receptors. If the compounds used to measure nonspecific binding are selective for one type of opioid receptor, then it may be possible to use a nonselective fluorescein-conjugated opioid to label μ, δ and κ opioid receptors.

Molecular biological studies have demonstrated the presence of mRNA encoding the δ (6) and κ (20) opioid receptor in human and rhesus monkey peripheral blood lymphocytes and human lymphoma cell lines (6,7,20). The μ opioid receptor gene has been detected in rat peritoneal macrophages (8) and in human and monkey lymphocytes (21). However, the molecular approach alone does not address whether functional receptors are expressed on the cell surface. Fluorescent opioid labeling allows for the detection of receptors on the cell surface, and the identification of the cell type expressing those receptors. Using antibodies directed against cell surface markers in combination with FITC-conjugated opioids and the PE amplification procedure, it will be possible to determine which types of immune cells express which types of opioid receptors.

5. ACKNOWLEDGEMENTS

This work was supported by U.S. Public Health Service Grants DA04355, DA07232 and DA09676 from the National Institute on Drug Abuse.

6. REFERENCES

1. Wybran, J., Appelboom, T., Famaey, J.-P. and Govaerts, A. Suggestive evidence for receptors for morphine and methionine-enkephalin on normal human blood T lymphocytes. *J. Immunol.* 123:1068-1070 (1979).
2. Sharp, B. M., Keane, W. F., Suh, H. J., Gekker, G., Tsukayama, D. and Peterson, P.K. Opioid peptides rapidly stimulate superoxide production by human polymorphonuclear leukocytes and macrophages. *Endocrinology* 117: 793-795 (1985).
3. Taub, D. D., Eisenstein, T. K., Geller, E. B., Adler, M. W. and Rogers, T.J. Immunomodulatory activity of μ- and κ-selective opioid agonists. *Proc. Natl. Acad. Sci. U.S.A.* 88: 360-364 (1991).
4. Linner, K.M., Quist, H.E. and Sharp, B.M. Met-enkephalin-containing peptides encoded by proenkephalin A mRNA expressed in activated murine thymocytes inhibit thymocyte proliferation. *J. Immunol.* 154: 5049-5060 (1995).
5. Belkowski, S.M., Zhu, J.M., Liu-Chen, L.-Y., Eisenstein, T.K., Adler, M.W. and Rogers, T.J. Sequence of kappa-opioid receptor cDNA in the R1.1 thymoma cell line. *J. Neuroimmunol.* 62: 113-117 (1995).
6. Chuang, L.F., Chuang, T.K., Killam, K.F., Jr., Chuang, A.J., Kung, H., Yu, L. and Chuang, R.Y. Delta opioid receptor gene expression in lymphocytes. *Biochem. Biophys. Res. Commun.* 202: 1291-1299 (1994).
7. Gaveriaux, C., Peluso, J., Simonin, F., LaForet, J. and Kieffer, B. Identification of kappa- and delta-opioid receptor transcripts in immune cells. *FEBS Lett.* 369: 272-276 (1995).
8. Sedqi, M., Roy, S., Ramakrishnan, S., Elde, R. and Loh, H.H. (1995) Complementary DNA cloning of a μ-opioid receptor from rat peritoneal macrophages. *Biochem. Biophys. Res. Comm.* 209: 563-574, 1995.
9. Bidlack, J.M., Saripalli, L.D. and Lawrence, D.M.P. κ-Opioid binding sites on a murine lymphoma cell line. *Eur. J. Pharmacol.* 227: 257-265 (1992).
10. Lawrence, D.M.P. and Bidlack, J.M. The kappa opioid receptor expressed on the mouse R1.1 thymoma cell line is coupled to adenylyl cyclase through a pertussis toxin-sensitive guanine nucleotide-binding protein. *J. Pharmacol. Exp. Ther.* 266: 1678-1683 (1993).

11. Lawrence, D.M.P., El-Hamouly, W., Archer, S., Leary, J.F. and Bidlack, J.M. Identification of κ opioid receptors in the immune system by indirect immunofluorescence. Proc. Natl. Acad. Sci. U.S.A. 92: 1062-1066 (1995).
12. Lawrence, D.M.P., Hutchison, I., Seyed-Mozaffari, A., Archer, S. and Bidlack, J.M. Improved fluorescent staining of kappa opioid receptors in the immune system using naltrexamine derivatives and phycoerythrin. Submitted.
13. Mathies, R.A. and Stryer, L. Single-Molecule Fluorescence Detection: A Feasibility Study Using Phycoerythrin. in *Applications of Fluorescence in the Biomedical Sciences* (D.L. Taylor, A.S. Waggoner, R.F. Murphy, F. Lanni and R.R. Birge, ed.), Alan R. Liss, NY, pp. 129-140 (1986).
14. Lawrence, D.M.P., Joseph, D.B. and Bidlack, J.M. Kappa opioid receptors expressed on three related thymoma cell lines: differences in receptor-effector coupling. *Biochem. Pharmacol.* 49:81-90 (1995).
15. Portoghese, P.S., Lipkowski, A.W. and Takemori, A.E. Binaltorphimine and nor-binaltorphimine, potent and selective κ-opioid receptor antagonists. *Life Sci.* 40:1287-1292 (1987).
16. Chao, C.C., Gekker, G., Hu, S., Sheng, W.S., Bu, D.-F., Archer, S., Bidlack, J.M. and Peterson, P.K. Kappa opioid receptors in human microglia downregulate human immunodeficiency virus-1 expression. Submitted.
17. Lang, M.E., Jourd'Heuil, D., Meddings, J.B. and Swain, M.G. Increased opioid binding to peripheral white blood cells in a rat model of acute cholestasis. *Gastroenterology* 108:1479-1486 (1995).
18. Aubin, J.E. Autofluorescence of viable cultured mammalian cells. *J. Histochem. Cytochem.* 27:36-43 (1979).
19. Oi, V.T., Glazer, A.N. and Stryer, L. Fluorescent phycobiliprotein conjugates for analyses of cells and molecules. *J. Cell Biol.* 93:981-986 (1982).
20. Chuang, L.F., Chuang, T.K., Killam, K.F., Jr., Qiu, Q., Wang, X.R., Lin, J.-J., Kung, H.-F., Sheng, W., Chao, C., Yu, L. and Chuang, R.Y. Expression of kappa opioid receptors in human and monkey lymphocytes. *Biochem. Biophys. Res. Commun.* 209:1003-1010 (1995).
21. Chuang, T.K., Killam, K.F., Jr., Chuang, L.F., Kung, H.-F., Sheng, W.S., Chao, C.C., Yu, L. and Chuang, R.Y. Mu opioid receptor gene expression in immune cells. *Biochem. Biophys. Res. Commun.* 216:922-930 (1995).

4

PRESENCE OF OPIATE ALKALOID-SELECTIVE μ_3 RECEPTORS IN CULTURED ASTROCYTES AND IN BRAIN AND RETINA

M. H. Makman,[1] K. Dobrenis,[2] S. Downie,[3] W. D. Lyman,[3] and B. Dvorkin[1]

[1] Departments of Biochemistry and Molecular Pharmacology
[2] Department of Neuroscience
[3] Department of Pathology
Albert Einstein College of Medicine
New York, New York 10461

ABSTRACT

Opiate alkaloid-selective receptors, insensitive to opioid peptides and differing from classical opioid receptors in other respects, mediate inhibition by morphine of activation of human peripheral blood monocytes and are present on other macrophage cell types as well, including microglia. This receptor has been tentatively designated as a μ_3 subtype. The present studies provide evidence for the presence of this receptor in cultures of astrocytes derived from human fetal brain, in cultures of feline astrocytes and in an immortalized feline astrocyte cell line. Also, neonatal and adult rat striatum and other brain regions, assayed in the presence of agents that blocked classical μ, δ and κ binding sites, were found to contain additional saturable ^{3}H-morphine binding sites that exhibited the pharmacology of μ_3 receptors. Additionally, μ_3 receptor sites were present in rat retina and in the avascular guinea pig retina, retinas that lack endogenous opioid peptides and that do not contain classical opioid peptide-sensitive μ, δ or κ binding sites. For each of these preparations, with ^{3}H-morphine as ligand, binding sites were saturable and displaced by morphine, etorphine, naloxone, diprenorphine and morphine 6-glucuronide, but not by morphine 3-glucuronide, fentanyl, benzomorphans, or by enkephalins, dynorphin, β-endorphin or other opioid peptides. These sites also could be distinguished from other (μ, δ and κ) sites on the basis of sensitivity to sulfhydryl compounds. It is proposed that μ_3 receptors occur on astrocytes as well as on microglia in brain and retina, where they function to modulate responses to injury and infection, as has been proposed previously for these receptors in the immune system.

INTRODUCTION

Opiate alkaloid-selective μ_3 receptors mediate inhibition by morphine of activation of human peripheral blood monocytes and granulocytes (1, 2). In addition, these receptors are present in the J774.2, BAC1.2F-5 and RAW 264 murine macrophage cell lines (3, 4) and also in several other macrophage cell types, including rat Kupffer cells and cat microglia (4). Effects of opiate alkaloids on microglial morphology appear to be mediated by this receptor (5). Essentially identical receptors were also found to be present in mouse N18 neuroblastoma cells, and a detailed pharmacological characterization of the N18 receptors has been carried out (6). Recently, evidence was obtained for the presence of this receptor on primary feline astrocytes and rat C6 glioma cells in culture (5). The present report provides further characterization of astrocyte μ_3 receptors, and evidence for the presence of this receptor in primary cultures of astrocytes derived from human fetal brain, and in a clonal immortalized feline astrocyte cell line. In addition, evidence is presented for the presence of this receptor in adult and newborn rat brain, as well as in rat retina and in the avascular guinea pig retina.

METHODS

Highly purified astrocyte cultures derived from neocortex of 1, 8 and 19 day-old cats were prepared and maintained in culture as previously described (5). Immunocytochemistry indicated that nearly all cells were positive for glial fibrillary acidic protein (GFAP), and in addition microglial contamination was far less than 1%, based on the rare presence of cells positive for binding of peroxidase-conjugated *Griffonia simplificolia* I-B_4 isolectin and uptake of dioctadecyl-tetramethyl-indocarbocyanate-labeled low density lipoproteins (di-iacLDL). Human fetal astrocyte cultures were derived from brain of 16-22 week-old fetuses and tissues were available within ten minutes of fetal demise. The cultures, prepared according to the protocol of McCarthy and deVellis (7), contained predominantly GFAP-positive cells. The GCC1-3C clonal astrocyte cell line, developed from a single cell, was derived from immortalized cells produced by transfection with an adenovirus type 5/origin-defective simian 40 viral construct of primary astrocyte cultures from feline cerebral cortex. GCC1-3C cells maintained under differentiating conditions exhibit astrocytic morphology and are GFAP-positive, but lack neuronal (neuron-specific enolase; neurofilament 68kD, 160 kD & 200kD) or oligodendroglial (galactocerebroside) markers. Receptor binding assays of membrane preparations with ^{3}H-morphine, ^{3}H-D-ala^2,N-Me-Phe^4,Gly^5(ol)enkephalin (DAGO) or other opioid as radioligand were carried out for the above cell cultures as well as for preparations of adult and 1-2 neonatal day rat striatum and retina and for guinea pig retina as previously described (5,6). Radioligand concentration was 3 nM for competition studies.

RESULTS

Membranes from fetal human astrocytes, with ^{3}H-morphine as ligand, exhibited distinct saturable binding sites, comparable in affinities and receptor density to the sites previously reported to be present on feline astrocyte membranes (5). Human astrocyte ^{3}H-morphine binding was displaced by morphine, etorphine, naloxone, diprenorphine and morphine 6-glucuronide, but not by morphine 3-glucuronide, fentanyl, benzomorphans, or by enkephalins, dynorphin, β-endorphin or other opioid peptides (e.g., Fig. 1). Similar results

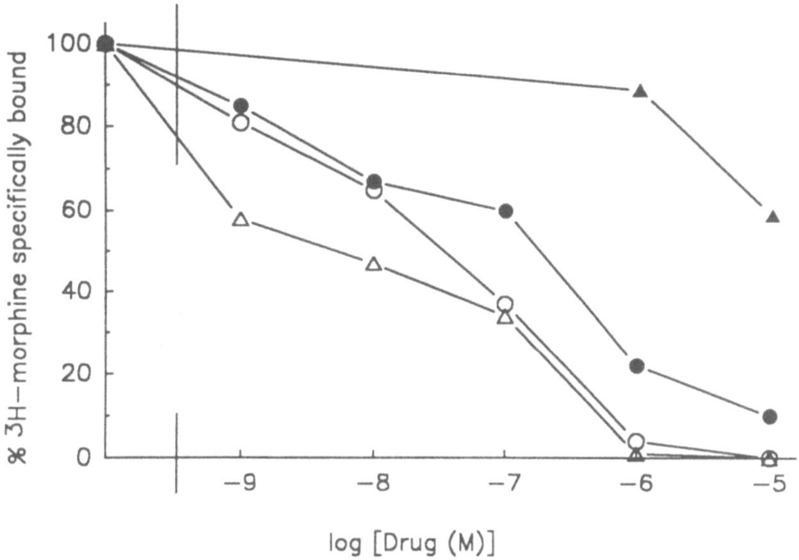

Figure 1. Concentration dependence for drug displacement of ^{3}H-morphine (3 nM) from human fetal astrocyte membranes. Each value is the mean of 2 -4 experiments. Morphine, open circles; morphine 6-glucuronide, closed circles; etorphine, open triangles; morphine 3-glucuronide, closed triangles. Specific binding was 310 fmoles/mg protein.

were obtained for the immortalized GCC1-3C astrocyte cell line (data not shown). In contrast to the C6 astrocytoma cell line, for which binding was dependent on preteatment of cells with desipramine (5), with the primary astrocyte culture preparations or the GCC1-3C cells binding was not dependent on or influenced by desipramine treatment.

Membranes from adult rat striatum and other brain regions (frontal cortex, hippocampus, cerebellum, hypothalamus) as well as from 1 -3 day old rat brain regions, assayed in the presence of agents that blocked classical μ, δ and κ binding sites, were found to contain additional saturable ^{3}H-morphine binding sites (K_d 20 -35 nM) that exhibited the pharmacology of μ_3 receptors, i.e., pharmacology previously found for peripheral blood monocytes, microglia and astrocytes. Thus, for rat striatum, in the presence of D-ala^2,D-Leu^5-enkephalin (DADLE) plus DAGO plus ethylketocyclazocine (EKC), each at 1 μM, a considerable component of the remaining ^{3}H-morphine binding was displaced by unlabeled morphine (K_i 30 nM) (Fig. 2), morphine 6-glucuronide, etorphine or naloxone, but not by opioid peptides, fentanyl or morphine 3-glucuonide. Similar results were obtained when fentanyl alone was present in place of DADLE plus DAGO plus EKC (not shown). In contrast, with ^{3}H-DAGO as ligand, morphine competed only for those sites also displaced by DAGO or fentanyl, and affinity for morphine was in the 1 - 3 nM range (not shown).

Retinas of mammalian species examined thus far generally have not been found to contain endogenous opioid peptides or opioid peptide-sensitive μ, δ or κ receptor sites. Thus, it was of interest to assess the possible presence of μ_3 receptors in rat retina. In addition, the avascular guinea pig retina (8) was examined as part of an attempt to determine the cell types containing μ_3 receptors in the CNS (see Discussion). In agreement with previous studies, no specific binding of ^{3}H-DAGO to rat retinal membranes could be detected, with DAGO, morphine or fentanyl as competitor. In contrast, with ^{3}H-morphine as ligand, saturable binding was readily detected, with a B_{max} of 2900 fmole/mg and K_d of 27 nM. In competition

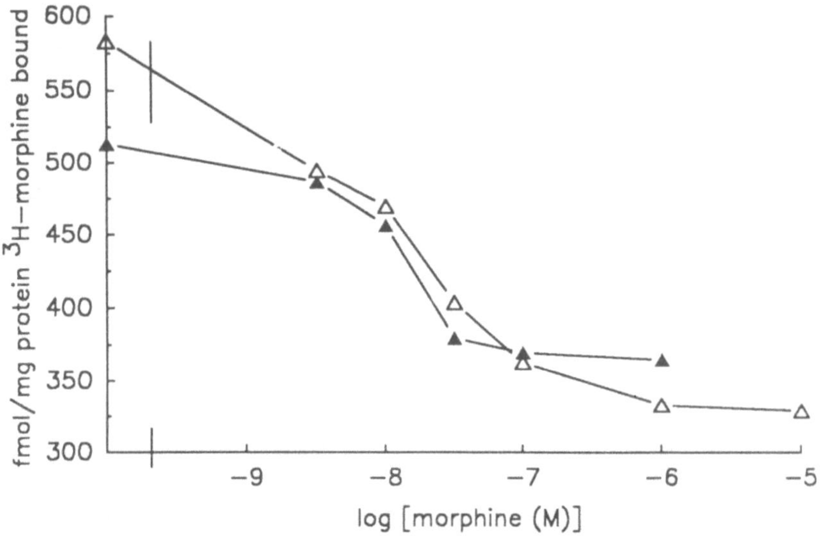

Figure 2. Concentration dependence for displacement of ^{3}H-morphine (3 nM) from rat striatal membranes by unlabeled morphine. Each value is the mean of 3 -4 experiments. Assays were carried out both in the absence (open triangles; standard assay conditions) and in the presence (closed triangles) of 1 μM DADLE + 1 μM DAGO + 1 μM EKC.

studies, these sites were not influenced by opioid peptides, and in other respects also exhibited the properties of μ_3 receptors (e.g., Fig. 3). Similar results were obtained with the guinea pig retina: with ^{3}H-morphine as ligand, B_{max} was 1600 fmole/mg and K_d was 37 nM.

For each of the preparations examined, binding sites characterized as μ_3 receptors were found to be highly sensitive to certain sulfhydryl reagents such as reduced glutathione

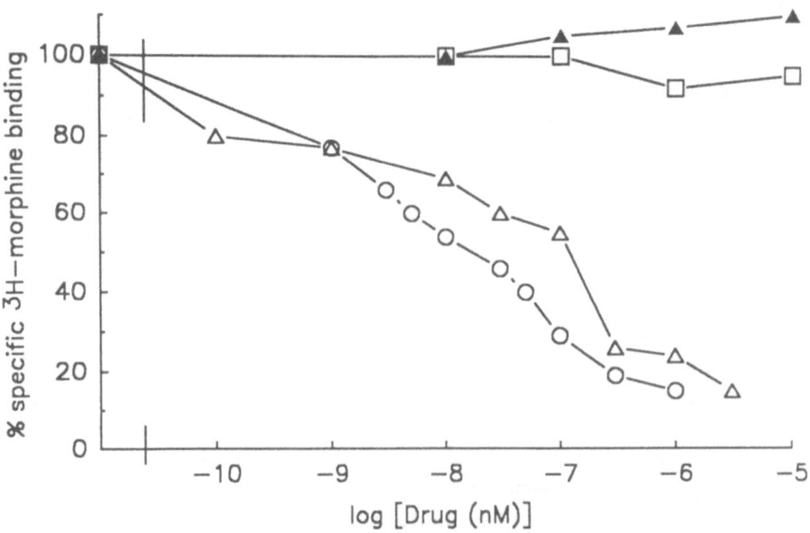

Figure 3. Concentration dependence for drug displacement of ^{3}H-morphine (3 nM) from rat retinal membranes. Each value is the mean of 3 -4 experiments. Morphine, open circles; morphine 6-glucuronide, open triangles; morphine 3-glucuronide, closed triangles; fentanyl, open squares. Specific binding was 370 fmoles/mg protein.

(GSH). Thus, μ_3 receptor binding to astrocyte, striatal and retinal membrane preparations was reduced to less than 5% of control values upon incubation of these membrane preparations with 10 μM GSH; nonspecific binding was unaffected, and also oxidized gluthathione had no effect on specific binding. In contrast, 10 μM GSH had no effect on specific binding of ^{3}H-DAGO to striatal peptide-sensitive μ receptors, binding of ^{3}H-EKC to striatal κ receptors or binding of ^{3}H-DADLE to δ receptors assayed under the same conditions.

DISCUSSION

The present studies provide additional evidence for the presence of the opiate alkaloid-selective μ_3 receptor in astrocytes. The presence of this receptor in astrocytes represents a significant addition to the cell types found to contain this receptor, previously detected and characterized predominantly in macrophages (including microglia) and other immunocyte cell types. Another exception was the earlier finding of this receptor in the murine N18 neuroblastoma cell line (Cruciani et al., 1994). Based on the present as well as our previous studies, the μ_3 receptor occurs in both feline and human astrocytes in primary culture as well as in rat C6 glioma cells and in the GCC1-5C immortalized astrocyte cell line. The evidence reported here for this receptor in rat and human brain, as well as in rat and gunea pig retina raises the question of which cell types contain the μ_3 receptor in the CNS. While the presence of the μ_3 receptor in the neuroblastoma cells suggests that it might be present in CNS neurons as well, its presence in nontransformed neurons remains to be demonstrated, and in preliminary studies other neuroblastoma cell lines and primary neurons in culture did not contain the μ_3 receptor. Nevertheless, the presence of this receptor on CNS neurons has not yet been ruled out. The presence of μ_3 receptors in rat and guinea pig retina is of particular interest, since in this CNS tissue classical opioid peptide-sensitive μ, δ or κ sites were not detected. Also, since the guinea pig retina is avascular, it therefore contains Müller cells but not other astrocytic cell types (8). Furthermore, guinea pig retina would not contribute to the binding assay membrane from peripheral blood cells or vascular tissue. It may be noted that μ_3 receptor density was lower in guinea pig that in rat retina, possibly due to a species diference but alternatively, possibly due to the absence of astrocytes other than Müller cells.

In previous studies, the 6-glucuronide but not the 3-glucuronide metabolite of morphine was shown to bind to the μ_3 receptor; also, the potent opiate fentanyl did not bind (3, 5). Similar results were obtained for the astrocyte, brain and retinal preparations examined in the present study. The inactivity of drugs such as fentanyl and the opioid peptides had been utilized previously as well as in the present study to distinguish the μ_3 receptor from other receptor subtypes. This was of particular importance for studies of brain where classical opioid receptor subtypes are routinely also present. In addition, the present studies indicate that the μ_3 receptor differs from previously described opioid receptors not only in cell type of occurrence and pharmacological properties, but also in its biochemical properties including sensitivity to GSH. Thus, it is possible to interfere with μ_3 receptor binding or to inactivate μ_3 receptors without causing alteration in binding to other receptor subtypes.

In conclusion, the μ_3 receptor appears to be present in the mammalian CNS. In the CNS it is likely that μ_3 receptors are present on astrocytes as well as on microglia, while a possible presence on neurons remains to be demonstrated. Although the functions of the μ_3 receptor in the CNS remain to be elucidated, it is proposed that this receptor participates in the interrelated roles of astrocytes and microglia in the response of the CNS to infection and injury (9 - 11). Thus, it will be of interest to compare the presence and role of these receptors in the normal CNS (i.e., in the absence of infection, lesion or trauma) and in the presence of CNS pathology.

REFERENCES

1. Stefano, G. B., Digenis, A., Spector, S., Leung, M. K., Bilfinger, T., Makman, M. H., Scharrer, B. and Abumrad, N. N. (1993). Opiate-like substances in an invertebrate, an opiate receptor on invertebrate and human immunocytes, and a role in immunosuppression. Proc. Natl. Acad. Sc.i U.S.A. 90:11099-11103.
2. Makman, M. H., Bilfinger, T. V. and Stefano, G. B. (1995) Human granulocytes contain an opiate alkaloid-selective receptor mediating inhibition of cytokine-induced activation and chemotaxis. J. Immunol. In Press 154:1323-1330.
3. Makman, M. H., Dvorkin, B. and Stefano, G. B. (1995) Murine macrophage cell lines contain μ_3 opiate receptors. Eur. J. Pharmacol. 273:R5-R6.
4. Makman, M. H. (1994) Morphine receptors in immunocytes and neurons. Adv. Neuroimmunol. 4:69-82.
5. Dobrenis, K., Makman, M. H. and Stefano, G. B. (1995) Occurrence of the opiate alkaloid-selective μ_3 receptor in mammalian microglia and astrocytes in culture and in Kupffer cells. Brain Res. 686:239-248.
6. Cruciani, R. A., Dvorkin, B., Klinger, H. P. and Makman, M. H. (1994) Presence in neuroblastoma cells of a μ_3 receptor with selectivity for opiate alkaloids but without affinity for opioid peptides. Brain Res. 667:229-237.
7. McCarthy, K. D. and deVellis, J. (1980) Preparation of separate astroglial and oligodendroglial cell cultures from rat cerebral tissue. J. Cell Biol. 85: 890-902.
8. Small, R. E., Watkins, B. A., Munro, P.M. and Liu, D. (1993) Functional properties of retinal Müller cells following transplantation to the anterior eye chamber. Glia 7:158-169.
9. Benveniste, E.N. (1993) Astrocyte - microglia interactions. Chapter in S. Murphy, ed.:*Astrocytes - Pharmacology and Function*, Academic Press, NY, pp. 355-382.
10. Eddleston, M. And Mucke, L. (1993) Molecular profile of reactive astrocytes - implications for their role in neurologic disease. Neuroscience 54:15-36.
11. Landis, D. M. D. (1994) The early reactions of non-neuronal cells to brain injury. Annu. Rev. Neurosci. 17:133-151.

5

OPIATES, GLIA, AND NEUROTOXICITY

Chun C. Chao,* Shuxian Hu, and Phillip K. Peterson

Minneapolis Medical Research Foundation and the University of Minnesota Medical School
Minneapolis, Minnesota 55404

Activated glial cells (microglia and astrocytes) are a histopathologic feature of numerous neurodegenerative diseases. Microglial cells have been demonstrated to migrate to and to proliferate and differentiate at sites of inflammation (1). In the cerebral cortex, glia comprise greater than 85% of the total population of brain cells. Of these, astrocytes account for about 85% of the glial cell population, while microglia constitute up to 10 to 15% of brain glial cells. Functional evidence has suggested that glial cells express receptors for opiates, such as morphine (2, 3) and endogenous opioids, such as dynorphin (4). A rapidly growing body of studies suggests that activated glial cells cause neuronal injury via releasing immune mediators, such as cytokines, reactive oxygen or nitrogen intermediates, and toxins (5). Results of these studies have raised an interesting question regarding the potential role of opiates in modulating neuronal injury.

INVOLVEMENT OF TUMOR NECROSIS FACTOR (TNF)-α AND NITRIC OXIDE (NO)

It has been shown that murine microglia stimulated with lipopolysaccharide (LPS) will induce neuronal injury through a mechanism involving generation of NO (6, 7). Furthermore, we have demonstrated that TNF-α is involved in LPS-induced microglial cell activation and neuronal injury (8). Since human microglia are incapable of generating substantial amounts of NO in response to LPS and cytokines, it appears that human microglia are not neurotoxic via the NO-related mechanism reported in murine species (9). Using human brain cell cultures, we have found that TNF-α is neurotoxic (10). By inhibiting astrocyte glutamine synthetase and glutamate uptake activity, TNF-α potentiates glutamate-induced neurotoxicity via NMDA receptors. Since morphine potentiates LPS-induced TNF-α release (2, 11), this opiate may affect microglia-mediated neuronal injury. Pretreatment of murine microglial/neuronal cell cocultures with morphine, however, failed to alter signifi-

* Correspondence: Chun C. Chao, Ph.D., Minneapolis Medical Research Foundation, 914 S. 8th Street, D3, Minneapolis, Minnesota 55404.

AIDS, Drugs of Abuse, and the Neuroimmune Axis, Edited by Friedman *et al.*
Plenum Press, New York, 1996

cantly microglia-mediated neuronal loss (unpublished data). This finding suggests that other mechanisms may also be involved in microglia-mediated neuronal injury associated with morphine treatment. In parallel studies, we have found that morphine reduced murine microglial cell production of NO when cells were stimulated with interferon (IFN)-γ plus LPS (12). The mechanisms underlying morphine-induced suppression of NO production in enriched murine microglial cell cultures is unknown. It is possible that morphine antagonizes the activating effect of interferon (IFN)-γ.

INVOLVEMENT OF IL-4 AND TRANSFORMING GROWTH FACTOR (TGF)-β

Deactivation of microglia has been proposed to have a beneficial effect against neuronal injury. Anti-inflammatory cytokines such as interleukin (IL)-4 have been shown to suppress murine microglial cell NO production (8). IL-4 also has been demonstrated to be protective against murine microglia-mediated neuronal injury (8).

Several *in vitro* studies using murine cell cultures have shown that TGF-β, another anti-inflammatory cytokine, is neuroprotective (13, 14). Interestingly, we have found that morphine potentiates LPS-stimulated microglial cell release of TGF-β (Fig. 1). A potential mechanism underlying morphine-induced enhanced release of TGF-β may involve morphine's ability to upregulate LPS-induced TNF-α, as reported previously (2). Our most recent studies have demonstrated that TNF-α plays a key role in inducing microglial cell release of TGF-β (15). If TGF-β exerts a neuroprotective effect as reported (13, 14), then it is not surprising to find that morphine fails to potentiate neuronal injury due to the increased release of neuroprotective cytokines, such as TGF-β. Potentiation of both a pro-inflamma-

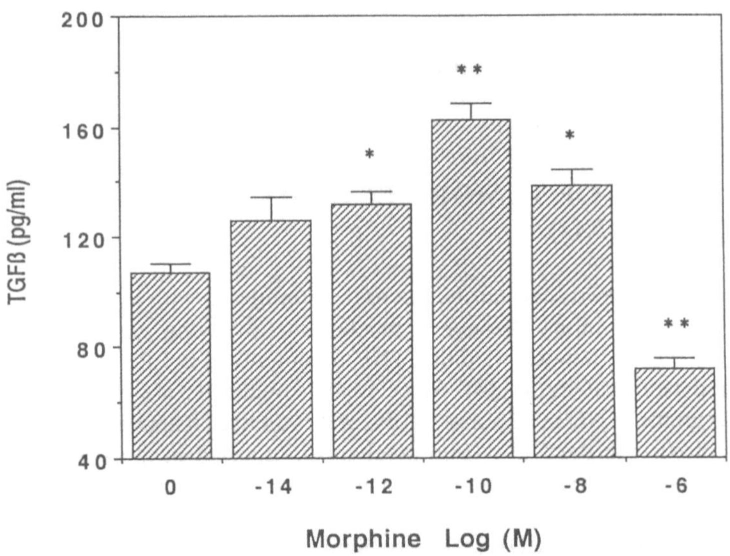

Figure 1. Dose-response effects of morphine on TGF-β release. Murine microglial cell cultures were treated with indicated concentrations of morphine for 24 h prior to stimulation with LPS (1 μg/ml) for an additional 24 h. Supernatants were then collected for TGF-β bioassay using an IL-4-dependent HT-2 cell line (15). Data (mean±SEM of triplicate values) are representative of three separate experiments. $^{*}P<0.05$, $^{**}P<0.01$ vs control value.

tory cytokine (TNF-α) and an anti-inflammatory cytokine (TGF-β) by morphine underscore the complex biological role of this opiate in the brain.

In addition to a neuroprotective role of TGF-β, we have shown using murine neuronal cell cultures that this cytokine potentiates N-methyl-D-aspartate (NMDA) receptor-mediated neurotoxicity (16). Since TGF-β alone does not appear to induce a direct injury to neurons, an indirect metabolism underlying TGF-β-mediated neurotoxicity has been proposed. Mechanisms underlying neuronal injury associated with TGF-β involve suppression of astrocyte glutamine synthetase activity and glutamate uptake transporter function (16).

ROLE OF ASTROCYTES IN NEURONAL INJURY

Astrocytes, the major cell type in the brain, play an important role in neurotransmitter metabolism and in maintaining homeostasis of the central nervous system. Under certain pathologic conditions, murine glial cells have been found to be activated with cytokines for production of substantial amounts of NO, which is neurotoxic (6, 7). Astrocyte NO may potentiate NMDA receptor-mediated neurotoxicity. Studies in our laboratory have shown that human astrocytes activated with the cytokines IFN-γ plus interleukin (IL)-1β (17, 18) generate substantial amounts of NO which in turn kills neurons via a NMDA receptor-related mechanism. Our studies suggest that the mechanisms associated with glial cell NO-mediated neuronal injury are different in human and murine species.

Treatment of cytokine-stimulated human astrocytes with anti-inflammatory cytokines (i.e., IL-4, IL-10 or TGF-β) downregulates NO production, suggesting a potential therapeutic value (19). In figure 2, a schematic representation is given of the potential involvement of cytokines and human glia in cytokine-mediated neuronal injury. Since opiates are generally immunosuppressive and glial cells possess opiate receptors, whether

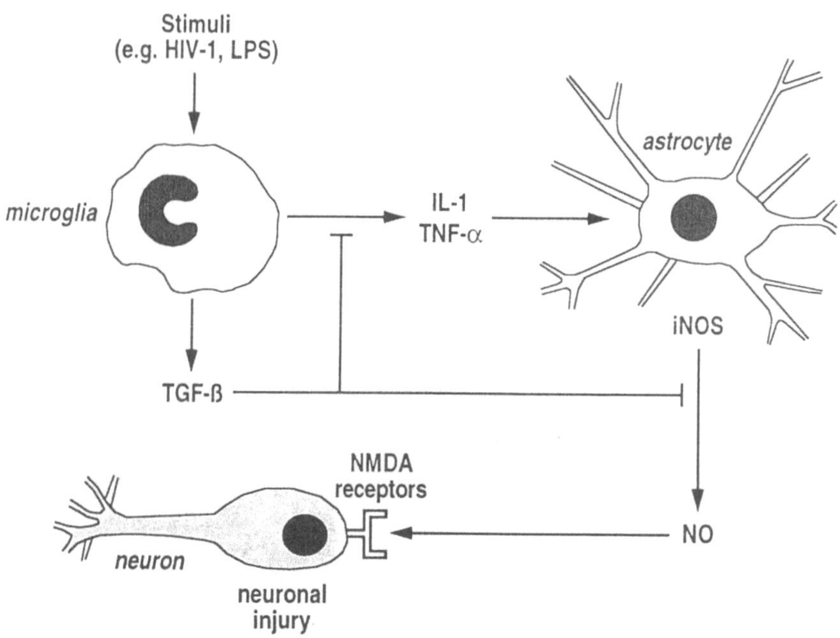

Figure 2. Proposed mechanisms underlying glia-mediated neuronal injury.

opiates would affect glia-mediated neuronal injury merits investigation. In this regard, both morphine and naloxone at mM concentrations have been reported to be protective in murine cortical neuronal cell cultures against NMDA receptor-mediated neurotoxicity (20). Further studies are warranted to elucidate the role of opiates or opioid antagonists in the pathogenesis of and protection against glia-induced neuronal injury in relevant *in vitro* and animal models of human neurodegenerative diseases.

ACKNOWLEDGMENTS

This work was supported in part by U.S. Public Health Service Grants DA09924, DA04381, and T32-DA07239 from the National Institute on Drug Abuse.

REFERENCES

1. del Rio-Hortega, P. (1932) Microglia. In: Penfield, W., Ed. *Cytology and Cellular Pathology of the Nervous System*. vol. 2. New York: Paul P. Hocker, pp 481-584.
2. Peterson, P. K., Gekker, G., Hu, S., Anderson, W. R., Kravitz, F., Portoghese, P. S., Balfour, H. H., Jr., and Chao, C. C. (1994) Morphine amplifies HIV-1 expression in chronically infected promonocytes cocultured with human brain cells. *J. Neuroimmunol.* 50: 167-175.
3. Peterson, P. K., Gekker, G., Hu, S., Sheng, W. S., Molitor, T. W., and Chao, C. C. (1995) Morphine stimulates phagocytosis of *Mycobacterium tuberculosis* by human microglial cells: involvement of a G protein-coupled opiate receptor. *Adv. Neuroimmunol.* in press.
4. Chao, C. C., Gekker, G., Hu, S., Sheng, W. S., Portoghese, P. S., and Peterson, P. K. (1995) Upregulation of HIV-1 expression in cocultures of chronically infected promonocytes and human brain cells by dynorphin. *Biochem. Pharmacol.* 50: 715-722.
5. Chao, C. C., Hu, S., and Peterson, P. K. (1995) Glia, cytokines, and neurotoxicity. *Crit. Rev. Neurobiol.* in press.
6. Boje, K. M., and Arora, P. K. (1992) Microglia-produced nitric oxide and reactive nitrogen oxides mediate neuronal cell death. *Brain Res.* 587: 250-256.
7. Chao, C. C., Hu, S., Molitor, T. W., Shaskan, E. G., and Peterson, P. K. (1992) Activated microglia mediate neuronal cell injury via a nitric oxide mechanism. *J. Immunol.* 149: 2736-2741.
8. Chao, C. C., Molitor, T. W., and Hu, S. (1993) Neuroprotective role of IL-4 against activated microglia. *J. Immunol.* 151: 1473-1481.
9. Peterson, P. K., Hu, S., Anderson, W. R., and Chao, C. C. (1994) Nitric oxide production and neurotoxicity mediated by activated microglia from human versus mouse brain. *J. Infect. Dis.* 170: 457-460.
10. Chao, C. C., and Hu, S. (1994) Tumor necrosis factor-α potentiates glutamate neurotoxicity in human fetal brain cell cultures. *Dev. Neurosci.* 16: 172-179.
11. Chao, C. C., Gekker, G., Sheng, W. S., Hu, S., Tsang, M., and Peterson, P. K. (1994) Priming effect of morphine on the production of tumor necrosis factor-α by microglia: implications in respiratory burst activity and human immunodeficiency virus-1 expression. *J. Pharmacol. Exp. Ther.* 269: 198-203.
12. Chao, C. C., Hu, S., Sheng, W. S., Gekker, G., and Peterson, P. K. (1995) Morphine and toxoplasmosis. In Drugs of Abuse and the Immune Response, eds. H. Friedman, T. Klein, and S. Specter, CRC Press, Boca Raton, in press.
13. Chao, C. C., Hu, S., Kravitz, F. H., Tsang, M., Anderson, W. R., and Peterson, P. K. (1994) Transforming growth factor-β protects human neurons against β-amyloid-induced injury. *Molec. Chem. Neuropathol.* 23: 159-178.
14. Prehn, J. H., Peruche, B., Unsicker, K., and Kreiglstein, J. (1993) Isoform-specific effects of transforming growth factor-beta on degeneration of primary neuronal cultures induced by cytotoxic hypoxia or glutamate. *J. Neurochem.* 60: 1665-1672.
15. Chao, C. C., Hu, S., Sheng, W. S., Tsang, M., and Peterson, P. K. (1995) Tumor necrosis factor-α mediates the release of bioactive transforming growth factor-β in microglial cell cultures. *Clin. Immunol. Immunopathol.* in press.

16. Chao, C. C., Hu, S., Tsang, M., Weatherbee, J., Molitor, T. W., Anderson, W. R., and Peterson, P. K. (1992) Effects of transforming growth factor-β on murine astrocyte glutamine synthetase activity: Implications in neuronal injury. *J. Clin. Invest.* 90: 1786-93.
17. Chao, C. C., Hu S., Erlich, L., and Peterson, P.K. (1995) Interleukin-1 and tumor necrosis factor-α synergistically mediate neurotoxicity: involvement of nitric oxide and of N-methyl-D-aspartate receptors. *Brain Behav. Immun.* in press.
18. Chao, C. C., Hu, S., Sheng, W. S., Bu, D., Bukrinsky., M. I., Peterson, P.\K. Cytokine-stimulated astrocytes damage human neurons via a nitric oxide mechanism. *Glia* in press.
19. Hu, S., Sheng, W. S., Peterson, P. K., and Chao, C. C. (1995) Differential regulation by cytokines of production of nitric oxide by human astrocytes. *Glia* in press.
20. Choi, D. W., and Visekul, V. (1988) Opioids and non-opioid enantiomers selectively attenuate N-methyl-D-aspartate neurotoxicity on cortical neurons. *Eur. J. Pharmacol.* 155: 27-35.

6

MORPHINE AFFECTS THE BRAIN-IMMUNE AXIS BY MODULATING AN INTERLEUKIN-1 BETA DEPENDENT PATHWAY

Sulie L. Chang,[1] Roberta L. Moldow,[1] Steve D. House,[1] and James E. Zadina[2]

[1] Department of Biology
Seton Hall University
400 South Orange Avenue
South Orange, New Jersey 07079
[2] VA Medical Center and Department of Medicine
Tulane University Medical School
New Orleans, Louisiana

1. INTRODUCTION

In response to a pathological condition, cytokines, such as interleukin 1-beta (IL-1β), are released and induce an immune response, i.e. inflammation. In association with the inflammatory response, however, the host often enters a catabolic state because these cytokines can also cause fever and loss of appetite.[1,2] Through its central nervous system (CNS) effects, IL-1β can also stimulate the hypothalamic-pituitary-adrenal (HPA) axis to produce ACTH and glucocorticoids, which are anti-inflammatory.[3] In such a way, both the induction and progression of immune responses are highly regulated through the modulatory actions of cytokines on the CNS[4] as well as on the immune system.[5] It has, therefore, been suggested that the HPA axis may function as a feedback loop between the CNS and the immune system.[6] This intricate interrelationship between the neuroendocrine and immune systems is schematically illustrated in Figure 1.

Modulation of this loop by exogeneous factors, such as morphine, could represent a mechanism underlying the effects of opiate addiction on the neuro-immune axis. Recently, our lab has obtained some evidence showing that chronic exposure to morphine, in addition to attenuating the immune response directly, may impair the HPA axis by attenuating an IL-1β-dependent pathway. The impairment of this axis may, in turn, cause an imbalance in the regulatory interaction between the brain and the immune system.

AIDS, Drugs of Abuse, and the Neuroimmune Axis, Edited by Friedman *et al.*
Plenum Press, New York, 1996

2. IMMUNOCYTOCHEMICAL STAINING OF FOS PROTO-ONCOGENE PROTEIN PROVIDES INFORMATION ABOUT THE SITES OF ACTION OF MORPHINE AND OF IL-1β

Immunocytochemical staining of FOS, the protein product of the immediate early proto-oncogene c-fos, has been used in our lab and others to provide information about the sites of action of various stimuli in the brain.[7,8,9] At the basal level, the expression of FOS, an inducible nuclear phosphoprotein, is low or absent. Induction of FOS expression allows the mapping of sites which contain neurons activated in response to a particular stimulus at the level of single cell resolution. Following acute treatment with morphine (10 μg/rat icv or 20 mg/kg sc), various FOS immunoreactive brain nuclei have been identified and include: the caudate putamen (CPU); the hypothalamic paraventricular (PVN), supraoptic (SON) and ventromedial (VMN) nuclei; the thalamic paraventricular nucleus (PVA); and the central lateral (CL) nuclei in the frontal brain.[10,11] Following an icv injection of IL-1β (100-200 ng),

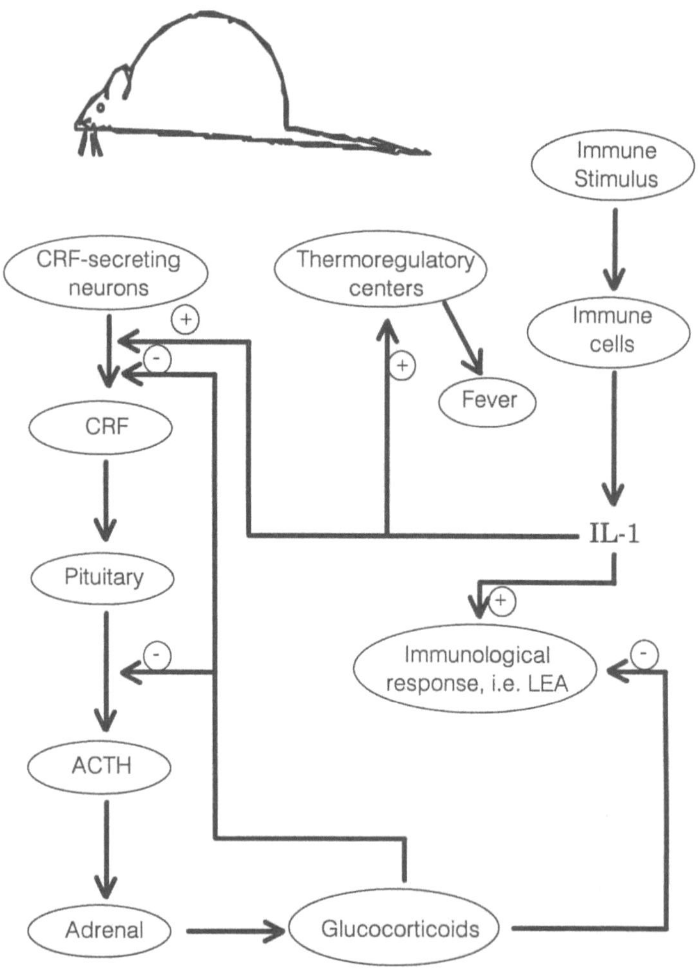

Figure 1. The the hypothalamic-pituitary-adrenal (HPA) axis functions as a feedback loop between the central nervous system (CNS) and immune system.

we and others have demonstrated induction of FOS immunoreactivity (FOSir) in several hypothalamic nuclei, including the PVN and SON.[7] Comparison of the patterns of FOSir induced by morphine and by IL-1β indicates that the PVN and SON may serve as anatomical sites of convergence of the neuronal signal pathways mediated by morphine and by IL-1β. These sites, therefore, can be considered as neuro-anatomical sites in which various biological actions of morphine and IL-1β converge.

3. CHRONIC EXPOSURE TO MORPHINE DESENSITIZES THE RAT BRAIN TO MORPHINE- AND IL-1β-INDUCED FOS IMMUNOREACTIVITY

Numerous studies have shown that chronic use of opiates induces tolerance and dependence at the biochemical, pharmacological, and behavioral levels.[12] After chronic exposure to opioid receptor agonists, desensitization, or a loss of signalling responsiveness to that agonist, is observed. For example, the inhibitory effects of opiates on cAMP[13,14,15] and neuronal firing[16,17] are diminished after chronic exposure to the opiate. We have shown that, after chronic exposure to morphine pellets, subsequent acute icv treatment with morphine failed to induce FOSir in brain nuclei, including the PVN.[18] In addition, we showed that chronic treatment with morphine prevents FOSir induced by IL-1β in the PVN.[18] These data indicate that chronic exposure to morphine results in a loss of FOS responsiveness (desensitization) in specific brain areas that are normally responsive to acute treatment with morphine and to IL-1β. The loss of FOS responsiveness following chronic exposure to morphine demonstrates both homologous and heterologous desensitization. Homologous desensitization refers to the loss of responsiveness to the agonist used for the chronic exposure, or to agonists acting at the same receptor. Thus, chronic exposure to morphine results in homologous desensitization of the FOS response to a challenge dose of morphine. By contrast, heterologous desensitization refers to diminished responsiveness to agonists that act at different receptors but whose signal transduction pathways converge. Pre-treatment with naloxone, an opioid antagonist, does not block IL-1β-induced FOSir in the PVN (unpublished results). Thus, IL-1β-induced FOSir in the PVN may not be due to activation of the opiate receptor, even though some studies suggest that IL-1β can interact with opioid receptors.[19,20] Chronic exposure to morphine dramatically reduces the capacity of both morphine and IL-1β to induce FOSir, possibly by altering a common signaling pathway from morphine to FOS and from IL-1β to FOS. This type of desensitization supports the concept that the PVN and SON are convergent sites of action for morphine and IL-1β in the CNS. It also indicates that the interaction between morphine and IL-1β may be mediated through the regulation of the transcriptional factor, FOS. Our studies have provided the first evidence of both homologous and heterologous desensitization to the FOS response following chronic opiate treatment, and suggests that chronic use of morphine may result in a decrease in IL-1β activity at the level of gene regulation in the central nervous system.

4. ANTISENSE OLIGODEOXYNUCLEOTIDE ATTENUATES IL-1β INDUCED FOS IMMUNOREACTIVITY IN THE PVN AND CRF mRNA EXPRESSION IN THE HYPOTHALAMUS

As indicated in the above section, chronic pre-treatment with morphine appears to prevent the activity of IL-1β in the PVN. One of the functions of IL-1β is to modulate the expression of corticotropin releasing factor (CRF) in the PVN.[21,22] CRF stimulates the release of ACTH from the anterior pituitary, and increases the subsequent release of glucocorticoids from the adrenal gland.

FOS functions as a transcriptional factor by forming a complex with the JUN protein which then binds to AP-1 sites on target genes.[23] The gene for the precursor of CRF contains many AP-1 sites. It is possible, therefore, that the desensitization of IL-1-β-induced FOS responsiveness may extend to the gene regulation of CRF and, in turn, to the regulation of the HPA axis. We infused a c-fos antisense oligonucleotide (5'-GAA-CAT-CAT-GGT-CGT-3')[24] into the PVN bilaterally, followed by injection of IL-1β into the right lateral ventricle (LV) in order to examine the causal relationship between the expression of FOS and IL-1β-mediated CRF mRNA expression in the hypothalamus.

The animals receiving antisense control vehicle (6 μl 75 mM TRIS buffer containing 1% BSA three times during a 24 hour period) followed by an IL-1β injection clearly show FOS immunoreactivity in the PVN. However, the rats receiving antisense oligonucleotide (6 nmoles three times during a 24 hour period) into both sides of the PVN, followed by an icv injection of IL-1β (100 ng) into the lateral ventricle do not show FOS immunoreactivity in the PVN after 3 hours.

In a preliminary study, using reverse transcriptase-polymerase chain reaction (RT-PCR), we examined the CRF mRNA levels in the hypothalamus of rats with and without pre-treatment with a c-fos antisense, as indicated above. An icv injection of IL-1β increased the RT-PCR CRF products in the hypothalamus of the rats infused with the antisense control vehicle, but not in the hypothalamus of the rats infused with the antisense oligonucleotide. There was no difference in RT-PCR β-actin products between the animals treated with antisense and those treated with only the antisense control vehicle. Taken together, these data indicate that IL-1β does not induce either FOS immunoreactivity in the PVN nor CRF mRNA expression in the hypothalamus of the rats pre-treated with a c-fos antisense in both sides of the PVN. These data suggest that there may be a causal relationship between FOS activation in the PVN and CRF mRNA expression in the hypothalamus. Morphine-tolerant rats fail to release ACTH or corticosterone in response to further treatment with the opiate, or to stress.[25] It has also been shown that the hypothalamus in the tolerant rats fails to release CRF in response to various stimuli.[26] Since chronic exposure to morphine attenuates the IL-1β-induced FOS immunoreactivity in the PVN, which may regulate CRF expression in the hypothalamus, one can argue that chronic exposure to morphine could suppress the CRF-mediated activation of the HPA axis by attenuating the IL-1β-induced FOS-mediated pathways in the PVN.

5. BOTH FMLP AND IL-1β INCREASE LEUKOCYTE-ENDOTHELIAL ADHESION (LEA) IN THE RAT MESENTERY

To study the actions of morphine directly on the immune system, we examined the modulatory effects of chronic exposure to morphine on leukocyte-endothelium adhesion (LEA) in the rat mesentery. During normal physiological conditions, some white blood cells (leukocytes) travel along the vessel wall, particularly in a venule, at a constant velocity, intermittently coming in contact with the endothelium.[27,28] During inflammatory conditions, the leukocytes may adhere to the endothelium in the venules.[27,29] This leukocyte-endothelium adhesion (LEA) is the prelude to all of the following cellular immune events, including migration toward a chemotactic stimulus, phagocytosis, intracellular degradation and cytokine release. This complex physiological process is regulated by various adhesion receptors found on both leukocytes and vascular endothelium,[30] and can be enhanced by several factors, including chemotactic factors such as the bacterial peptide, FMLP, and immunocytokines, such as IL-1β.

Many studies have shown that the action of FMLP is transient (minutes)[31], and that it causes LEA by increasing adhesion receptors on the surface of the leukocytes. By contrast, the action of IL-1β is long-lasting (hours or days), and causes LEA by inducing the expression of cell adhesion molecules[30] including intercellular adhesion molecule-1 (ICAM-1), on the vascular endothelium.

In the current study, topical suffusion of 10^{-7} M FMLP increases LEA in the mesenteric venules of rats. This increase is observed within minutes, and is reproducible. Intraperitoneal (ip) injection of IL-1β (1μg human recombinant IL-1β) also increases LEA in the rat mesenteric venules approximately 3-4 hours after the initiation of IL-1β treatment. The degree of LEA induced by combined FMLP and IL-1β administration appears to be additive. This suggests that the mechanisms of action of FMLP and of IL-1β are independent.

6. CHRONIC EXPOSURE TO MORPHINE ATTENUATES THE LEA RESPONSE TO FMLP AND POTENTIATES THE RESPONSE TO IL-1β

The effects of FMLP seem to be confined to the immune system via circulating leukocytes, and to be independent of neuroendocrine regulatory actions. IL-1β causes LEA by inducing the expression of cell adhesion receptors, including ICAM-1, on the vascular endothelium. However, the expression of ICAM-1 has been shown to be negatively regulated by circulating glucocorticoids.[32] Taken together, these data indicate that the actions of IL-1β on LEA could be modulated through the HPA axis. The net effect of IL-1β on LEA would, therefore, reflect the balance between its stimulatory effect on ICAM-1 expression, and its inhibitory effects through glucocorticoids.

Since we have shown that chronic exposure to morphine may attenuate HPA activity, we, therefore, examined the effects of chronic morphine on the LEA response to FMLP and to IL-1β. Under basal conditions, LEA is not significantly different between morphine- and placebo-treated rats.[33] This may be due to "adaptation" in an opiate tolerant state, and is consistent with our findings that there is no significant difference in the glucocorticoid levels between placebo- and morphine-treated rats, as determined by radioimmunoassay (unpublished data). However, during acute inflammation in response to FMLP, the LEA in morphine-treated rats is lower than in animals administered placebo. This suggests that the circulating leukocytes of the rats given chronic morphine may not respond to the challenge of FMLP as do the leukocytes of the placebo rats. Thus, morphine appears to render leukocytes refractory to FMLP, and to inhibit the expression of adhesion receptors or inflammatory mediators.

In a second study, we examined the LEA response to IL-1β in morphine-treated rats versus placebo rats. LEA in the rats given chronic morphine followed by an IL-1β injection was found to be significantly higher than in the rats given placebo followed by an IL-1β injection, in both basal and inflammatory conditions. These data indicate that chronic exposure to morphine potentiates the LEA response to IL-1β with and without topical suffusion of FMLP. Two conclusions can be drawn from these data. First, IL-1β is able to overcome the morphine-induced loss of responsiveness to FMLP, which is consistent with cytokine reversal of morphine-induced suppression of antibody production,[34] and also with direct effects of morphine on the immune system. Second, chronic exposure to morphine potentiates the effects of IL-1β on the LEA response. This potentiation could occur by augmenting its stimulatory effects, for example on ICAM-1, or by attenuating its inhibitory effects, such as on IL-1β-mediated release of ACTH and glucocorticoids, which can suppress the LEA response. Thus, chronic exposure to morphine may potentiate the LEA response to IL-1β by attenuating IL-1β-induced activity of the HPA axis.

7. SUMMARY

In the neuroendocrine system, chronic exposure to morphine causes a desenstitization of FOS responsiveness in the PVN, and may impair the HPA axis by attenuating IL-1β-induced FOS activation and CRF expression in the PVN. In the immune system, chronic exposure to morphine attenuates the LEA response in the FMLP-induced acute inflammatory condition, which may contribute to the suppression of the immunological response. However, in response to systemic challenge with IL-1β, chronic exposure to morphine potentiates the LEA response to IL-1β. This may reflect the impairment of the HPA axis in the rats given chronic morphine. The modulatory loop in the brain-immune axis may be interrupted by chronic exposure to morphine, as shown in Figure 2. In this model, chronic exposure to

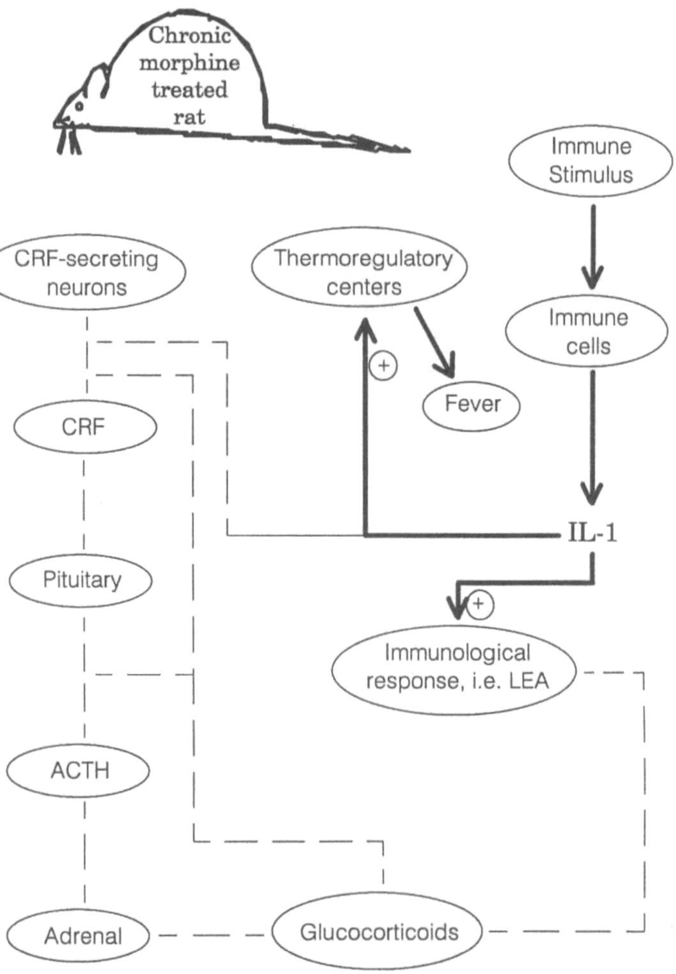

Figure 2. Chronic exposure to morphine may interrupt the modulatory loop in the brain-immune axis.

morphine could attenuate the IL-1β-stimulated release of ACTH and glucocorticoids, which serve in an inhibitory feedback loop on immunological responses, such as LEA. In conclusion, our studies suggest that morphine interrupts the brain-immune axis by modulating an IL-1β-dependent pathway.

8. ACKNOWLEDGEMENTS

This work is supported by RO1DA-07058 (SLC), R29HL-44914(SDH), and VA (JEZ). The authors thank Immunex, Inc. (Seattle, WA) for the generous gift of recombinant human interleukin-1β, and the technical assistance of Suzanne Quercia, Gao-de Wu, James Bersig and Dino Espineli.

9. REFERENCES

1. Dinarello, C.A. 1984 Interleukin-1. *Rev. Infect. Dis.*, 6:51-58.
2. Dinarello, C.A. 1988 Biology of interleukin-1. *FASEB J.*, 2:108-115.
3. van de Stolpe, A., Caldenhoven, E., Raaijmakers, J.A.M., van der Saag, P.T. and Koenderman, L. 1993 Glucocorticoid-mediated repression of intercellular adhesion molecule-1 expression in human monocytic and bronchial epithelial cell lines. *Am. J. Respir. Cell. Mol. Biol.*, 8:340-347.
4. Sundar, S.S., Becker, K.J., Cierpial, M.A., Carpenter, M.D., Rankin, L.A., Fleener, S.L., Ritchie, J.C., Simson, P.E. and Weiss, J.M. 1989 Intracerebroventricular infusion of interleukin-1 rapidly decreases peripheral cellular immune response. *Proc. Natl. Acad. Sci. USA*, 86:6398-6402.
5. Cannon, J.G., Tatro, J.B., Reichlin, S. and Dinarello, C.A. 1986 Alpha melanocyte stimulating hormone inhibits immunostimulatory and inflammatory actions of interleukin-1. *J. Immunol.*, 137(7):2232-2236.
6. Bateman, A., Singh, A., Kral, T. and Solomon, S. 1989 The immune-hypothalamic-pituitary-adrenal axis. *Endrocr. Rev.*, 10:92-98.
7. Chang, S.L., Ren, T. and Zadina, J.E. 1993 Interleukin-1 activation of FOS proto-oncogene protein in the rat hypothalamus. *Brain Res.*, 617:123-130.
8. Chang, S.L., Patel, N.A. and Romero, A.A. 1995 Activation and desensitization of Fos immunoreactivity in the rat brain following ethanol administration. *Brain Res.*, 679:89-98.
9. Morgan, J.I. and Curran, T. 1991 Stimulus-transcription coupling in the nervous system: Involvement of the inducible proto-oncogenes *fos* and *jun*. *Annu. Rev. Neurosci.*, 14:421-451.
10. Chang, S.L., Squinto, S.P. and Harlan, R.E. 1988 Morphine activation of c-*fos* expression in the rat brain. *Biochem. Biophys. Res. Commun.*, 157(2):698-704.
11. Chang, S.L. and Harlan, R.E. 1990 The FOS proto-oncogene protein: regulation by morphine in the rat hypothalamus. *Life Sci.*, 46:1825-1832.
12. Cox, B.M. and Werling, L.L. Opioid tolerance and dependence. In: *The Biological Bases of Drug Tolerance and Dependence*. J.A. Pratt, ed., Academic Press. San Diego, 1991, pp. 199-229.
13. Law, P.Y., Hom, D.S. and Loh, H.H. 1983 Opiate receptor down-regulation and desensitization in neuroblastoma x glioma NG108-15 hybrid cells are two separate cellular adaptation processes. *Mol. Pharmacol.*, 24:413-424.
14. Attali, B., Saya, D. and Vogel, Z. 1989 K-opiate agonists inhibit adenylate cyclase and produce heterologous desensitization in rat spinal cord. *J. Neurochem.*, 52:360-369.
15. Makman, M.H., Dvorkin, B. and Crain, S.M. 1988 Modulation of adenylate cyclase activity of mouse spinal cord-ganglion explants by opioids, serotonin, and pertussin toxin. *Brain Res.*, 445:303-313.
16. Andrade, S., Vandermaelen, C.P. and Aghjanian, G.K. 1983 Morphine tolerance and dependence in the locus coeruleus: single cell studies in brain slices. *Eur. J. Pharmacol.*, 91:161-169.
17. Christie, M.J., Williams, J.T. and North, R.A. 1985 Cellular mechanisms of opioid tolerance: studies in single brain neurons. *Mol. Pharmacol.*, 2:633-638.
18. Chang, S.L., Kenigs, V., Moldow, R.L. and Zadina, J.E. Chronic treatment with morphine and ethanol, but not cocaine, attenuates IL-1β activation of Fos expression in the rat hypothalamic paraventricular nucleus. In: *The Brain Immune Axis and Substance Abuse*, B. Sharp, et. al., eds., Plenum Press, New York, 1995, pp. 201-208.

19. Ahmed, M.S., LLanos-Q., J., Dinarello, C.A. and Blatteis, C.M. 1985 Interleukin-1 reduces opioid binding in guinea pig brain. *Peptides*, 6:1149-1153.
20. Wiedermann, C.J. 1988 Interleukin-1 interaction with neuroregulatory systems: selective enhancement by recombinant human and mouse interleukin-1 of in vitro opioid peptide receptor binding in rat brain. *J. Neurosci. Res.*, 22:172-180.
21. Berkenbosch, F., van-Oers, J., del-Rey, A., Tilders, F. and Besedovsky, H. 1987 Corticotropin-releasing factor-producing neurons in the rat activated by interleukin-1. *Science*, 238:524-526.
22. Sapolsky, R., Rivier, C., Yamamoto, G., Plotsky, P. and Vale, W. 1987 Interleukin-1 stimulates the secretion of hypothalamic corticotropin-releasing factor. *Science*, 238:522-524.
23. Thompson, R. C., Seaholtz, A. F. and Herbert, E. 1987 Rat corticotropin-releasing hormone gene: sequence and tissue-specific expression. Mol. Endocrinology., 1: 363-369.
24. Chiasson, B.J., Hooper, M.L., Murphy, P.R. and Robertson, H.A. 1992 Antisense oligonucleotide eliminates in vivo expression of *c-fos* in mammalian brain. *Eur. J. Pharmacol.*, 227:451-453.
25. George, R. and Way, E.L. 1955 Studies on the mechanism of pituitary-adrenal activation by morphine. *British J. of Pharmacology and Chemotherapy*, 10:260-264.
26. Buckingham, J.C. and Cooper, T.A. 1984 Differences in hypothalamic-pituitary-adrenocortical activity in the rat after acute and prolonged treatment with morphine. *Neuroendocrinology*, 38:411-417.
27. House, S.D. and Lipowsky, H.H. 1987 Leukocyte-endothelial adhesion: Microhemodynamics in mesentery of the cat. *Microvasc. Res.*, 34:363-379.
28. Nazziola, E. and House, S.D. 1992 Effects of hydrodynamics and leukocyte-endothelium specificity on leukocyte-endothelium interactions. *Microvasc. Res.*, 44:127-142.
29. Graham, I.L. and Brown, J.E. 1991 Extracellular calcium results in a conformational change in Mac-1 (CD11b/CD18) on neutrophils: Differentiation of adhesion and phagocytosis functions of Mac-1. *J. Immunol.*, 146:685-691.
30. Smith, C.W. 1993 Endothelial adhesion molecules and their role in inflammation. *Canadian J. of Physiol. and Pharmacol.*, 71:76-87.
31. Tonnesen, M.G., Anderson, D.C., Springer, T.A., Knedler, A., Avdi, N. and Henson, P.M. 1989 Adherence of neutrophils to cultured human microvascular endothelial cells. Stimulation by chemotactic peptides and lipid mediators and dependence upon the Mac-1, LFA-1, p150,95 glycoprotein family. *J. Clin. Invest.*, 83:637-646.
32. Van De Stolpe, A., Caldenhoven, E., Raaigmakers, J.A.M., Van Der Saag, P.T. and Koenderman, L. 1993 Glucocorticoid-mediated repression of intercellular adhesion molecule-1 expression in human monocytic and bronchial epithelial cell lines. *Am. J. Respir. Cell Mol. Biol.*, 8:340-347.
33. Chang, S.L., Bersig, J.M., Wu, G.-D., Patel, N.A., Zadina, J.E. and House, S.D. 1995 Chronic exposure to morphine attenuates leukocyte-endothelial interactions in the rat mesentery. *NIDA Research Monogr.*, In press.
34. Bussiere, J.L., Adler, M.W., Rogers, T.J. and Eisenstein, T.K. 1993 Cytokine reversal of morphine-induced suppression of the antibody response. *J. Pharmacol. Exptl. Thr.*, 264:591-597.

7

OPIOID DEPENDENCY AND THE PROGRESSION OF SIMIAN AIDS

Mortality and Behavioral Observations

Keith F. Killam, Jr., Linda F. Chuang, and Ronald Y. Chuang

Department of Medical Pharmacology and Toxicology
School of Medicine
University of California, Davis, California 95616

Studies of the effects of opioids on T lymphocytes have become increasingly important in light of statistical data which suggest that opioid users/abusers are at high risk for developing AIDS. Also, these studies are significant since T lymphocytes play a crucial role in both cellular and humoral immunity in patients with AIDS. The simian model of immunodeficiency virus infection, which has been followed thoroughly in our laboratory in a controlled fashion, has yielded important insights which may not be obtainable from a clinical setting involving human subjects. Using this system, we have studied the consequences of chronic morphine intake on the progression of AIDS in order to model a segment of the human population shown to be at risk. These studies are concerned with the possible modulation of the immuno-responses of primates toward lentiviral as well as opioid challenges. We have found that administration of morphine sulfate to rhesus monkeys may activate the quiescent lymphocyte for proliferation, induce a transient increase in the T cell proliferative response to mitogens, and cause an enhanced interleukin-2 (IL-2) release from the mitogen-stimulated lymphocytes (1). However, longitudinal studies of the animals dependent upon morphine have revealed an overall immunosuppression of both T helper cell functions (T cell proliferation and IL-2 release) and PMN (polymorphonuclear cells) chemotaxis and phagocytosis activities (1,2). In addition to cellular effects, opioid treatment also affects the humoral response of the treated subjects; relative to saline-treated animals, morphine-dependent animals had a lower titer of anti-SIV neutralizing antibody activity after SIV infection (3). Moreover, we have demonstrated that SIV is capable of mutating antigenically in opioid-treated monkeys so that the host is rendered "seronegative" with regard to the infecting virus (4,5). However, the autologous virus can be isolated from the infected animals, and using a SIV-specific PCR procedure developed in our laboratory (6), SIV RNA can be detected in the PBMC of the seronegative monkeys (4,5). The mutated *gag* gene sequence of the mutant virus has also been determined (4,5). The present report describes our general and behavioral observations of the rhesus macaques treated with opioids and experimentally infected with SIV.

AIDS, Drugs of Abuse, and the Neuroimmune Axis, Edited by Friedman *et al.*
Plenum Press, New York, 1996

Behavioral and general health evaluations were used to provide assessment of state type changes as the viremia developed and as changes occurred in the immune system. Animals not infected with the virus but receiving the interactions with personnel and the environment served as control populations.

MATERIALS AND METHODS

Virus

SIVmac239, a pathogenic molecular clone of SIVmac kindly provided by Dr. R. C. Desrosiers of the New England Regional Primate Research Center, was used for this study. The complete nucleotide sequence of this virus has been reported (7).

Animals

A colony of young adult male rhesus monkeys (*Macaca mulatta*) of age 4-5 years old was maintained at the California Regional Primate Research Center for our initial studies. These animals were separated into two groups. The first group received morphine sulfate administrations of 5 mg/kg body weight intramuscularly three times daily. The second group, the control animals, received corresponding saline injections intramuscularly 3 times daily. All animals were housed in accredited facilities in accordance with the NIH "Guide for the Care and Use of Laboratory Animals." For the present study, three morphine-treated monkeys (MMU 23686, MMU 22803 and MMU 23740) and three saline-treated monkeys (MMU 22988, MMU 23750 and MMU 23679) were infected with SIVmac239. Before virus inoculation, all animals were tested for previous exposure to SRV, STLV-1 and SIV by ELISA, and for active virus infection by co-cultivation procedures. All results were negative.

Infection of Rhesus macaques with SIVmac239

A homogeneous virus stock of SIVmac239 (1.58 x 10^3 rhesus monkey infectious dosage$_{50}$/animal) was inoculated into the opioid- or saline-treated animals *via* the intravenous route. The dosage of virus was chosen to ensure 100% infection (8) and an average life expectancy of 18 to 20 months for the infected monkeys (9); these values are in accordance with those reported in most other SIVmac239 studies. Infection was determined by virus isolation through co-cultivation of monkey peripheral blood mononuclear cells (PBMC) with CEM x 174 cells. Viral RNA detection was performed by the polymerase chain reaction (6).

Behavioral Assessment

Rhesus monkeys were housed singly with visual and auditory contact with others of the species and were exposed to general events in the holding area. The monkeys received water ad libitum, were hand fed biscuits twice a day at reasonably precise time intervals, were injected three times per day at eight hour intervals, seven days a week, and were weighed every three days. Two daily sessions to record cage behavior were done five out of seven days on a random basis. Within a day, the first behavioral assessment was after the second feeding and before the second injection. The second behavioral assessment followed the second injection. The cage behavior of male rhesus monkeys was annotated using bar codes (Fig. 1) to describe as many aspects of the behavior of monkeys as possible. The

Table 1. Behavioral descriptors

Goal Directed
Eating and Drinking
Expressions of Aggression
Displacement Behaviors
Grooming
Manipulating Environment
Random Behavior
Drug Induced Behaviors
Depression
Stimulation
Withdrawal Symptoms

observer was prompted by a program on a notebook computer. The observer selected the appropriate descriptive behavior (Table 1) and stroked the bar code with the input wand. The data were stored in the notebook computer until the end of the observation session. The notebook computer was then attached to a larger computer and the data transferred from the notebook computer to the laboratory computer.

RESULTS AND DISCUSSION

General and Behavioral Observations

The research data were characterized and sorted to describe the behavioral events in sequence and with time frames. Consummatory behavior was encoded by the bar-coded descriptor and by the biscuit count. The effectiveness of the consummatory behavior was noted by following the weight alterations. Throughout the study, most animals consumed a standard number of biscuits per day. However, the avidness of the eating behaviors varied between the two daily sessions and these patterns varied with the drug treatment and the progress of the viremia.

Control subjects, i.e., no drug treatment and non-infected, ate with great gusto during the first observation with little attendant displacement behavior. During the second observation period and following the injection of saline, the animals continued to eat their daily ration but with less avidness and with more display of accessory behaviors. Weight gain in these animals was steady and progressive (Fig. 2A). As time progressed, periods of masturbation were observed in most of the animals.

Control subjects injected with saline and then infected with the virus exhibited a progressive change in the consummatory pattern of behavior. Eating behavior was distributed over the two observation periods. Displacement behaviors became more dominant and weight gain progressively slowed (Fig. 2B). It is to be noted that daily intake of biscuits was not significantly affected. As the viremia progressed, the animals became more inattentive, and consummatory behavior became more random. The animals began to have bouts of diarrhea that are not controllable with conventional anti-diarrheal therapy. Masturbating behavior disappeared from the behavioral repertoire. Of special note is the case of one saline-treated and SIVmac239-infected monkey (macaque MMU 22988). During the acute phase of the viremia behavioral signs and the falling-off in weight progress were similar to those of the other infected monkeys. Subsequently, diarrhea stopped, weight gain accelerated

GENERAL BEHAVIOR

inattentive	005
resting	010
attentive	015
retreating	020
cowering	025
threatening	030
presenting	035
eating	040
taste stool	045
drinking	050
taste urine	055
play toy	060
vocalizing	065
grimacing	070
play food	075
lip smacking	080
play collar	085
grinding teeth	090

MOTOR BEHAVIOR

standing	105
sitting	110
prone	115
supine	120
on side	125
asleep	130
non-rousable	135
twitching	140
wet dog sh	143
seizure	145
bobbing	150
rocking	155
jump/acro	160
pacing	165
climbing	170
stretching	175
hanging	180
reaching	185
rub cage	190
pick cage	192
slap cage	194
pull cage	196
throw food	198
throw feces	199

VEGETATIVE BEHAVIOR

salivate	200
retch	210
vomit	220
urinate	230
defecate	240
piloerect.	250
penile erect.	260
masturbate	262
ejaculate	264
cough	270
sneeze	280
yawn	290
tachypnea	300
bradypnea	310
gasping	320
apnea	330

VISUAL BEHAVIOR

stare	340
scan	350
blink	360

LICKING

floor	370
cage	380

GROOMING

head 400 | arm 410 | hand 420 | leg 430 | foot 440

torso 450 | perineum 460 | tail 470 | mouth 480

SCRATCHING

head 500 | arm 510 | hand 520 | leg 530 | foot 540

torso 550 | perineum 560 | tail 570

BITING

arm 600 | hand 610 | leg 620 | foot 630 | torso 640

perineum 650 | tail 660 | cage 670

CAGED 888 | IN CHAIR 889

MEDICATION 9997 | END SESSION 9998 | DELETE ENTRY 9999

INFECTED

23750 | 23679 | 23686 | 22803

22988

NON-INFECTED

23773 | 22801 | 23039 | 23022

23089 | 23587 | 23820 | 24067

25299 | 25727 | 24893 | 25753

Figure 1. Representative bar codes for behavioral assessment.

(Fig. 3), and behavioral depression lifted. The animal survives today (over fifty months after infection), although virus could still be isolated from its peripheral blood mononuclear cells (PBMC).

Opioid-treated subjects before the injections were switched from saline to opioid exhibited the same cage behaviors as the non-infected, saline-injected animals. When the administration of the opioids began, there was a sharp drop in consummatory behavior. Biscuit intake during the first daily observation period stopped. Biscuit intake sporadically occurred during the second daily observation period. The daily biscuit intake did not drop significantly but there was a significant drop in body weight (Fig. 2C). This pattern continued

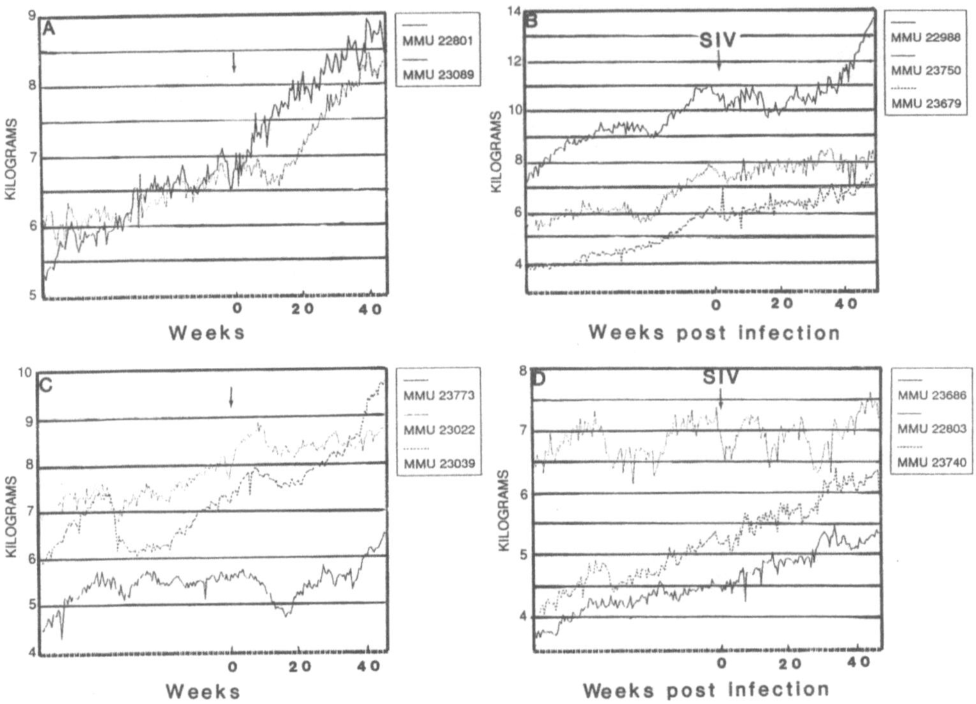

Figure 2. Comparison of weight gains between different groups of experimental animals. A. (NONINFC), noninfected, saline-treated monkeys; B. (INFC), SIVmac239-infected, saline-treated monkeys; C. (NON-INFM), noninfected, morphine-treated monkeys; D. (INFM), SIVmac239-infected, morphine-treated monkeys. Arrows shown in A and C indicate the corresponding time when infected animals (B & D) received the virus SIVmac239.

for a week to ten days. This was followed by a beginning of consummatory behavior during the first daily observation period. The consummatory behavior during this first observation period was accompanied by a variety of displacement behaviors. During the second daily observation period during this phase, consummatory became regularized and was accompanied by a variety of behaviors but with no overt signs of avid eating. Weight gain began to return, but over the next two years, the slope of the weight gains as compared to the control subjects (saline and non-infected) was markedly different (Fig. 2A & 2C). Masturbating behavior decreased in incidence.

Following the infection of the SIV in the opioid-treated animals, there was no significant change in the nature of the consummatory response. The daily intake of biscuits remained within the group response. The slope of the weight curve decreased and then flattened (Fig. 2D). The generalized behavior scores indicated a gradual and overall depression (Fig. 4). Later, the animals exhibited persistent diarrhea that was non-responsive to usual anti-diarrheal treatment even in the face of chronic opioid administration. These data supplement those reported by Murray et al. (10) who described cognitive and motor impairment associated with SIV infection in rhesus monkeys. As with the saline treated and infected animals, masturbating behavior disappeared from the behavioral repertoire.

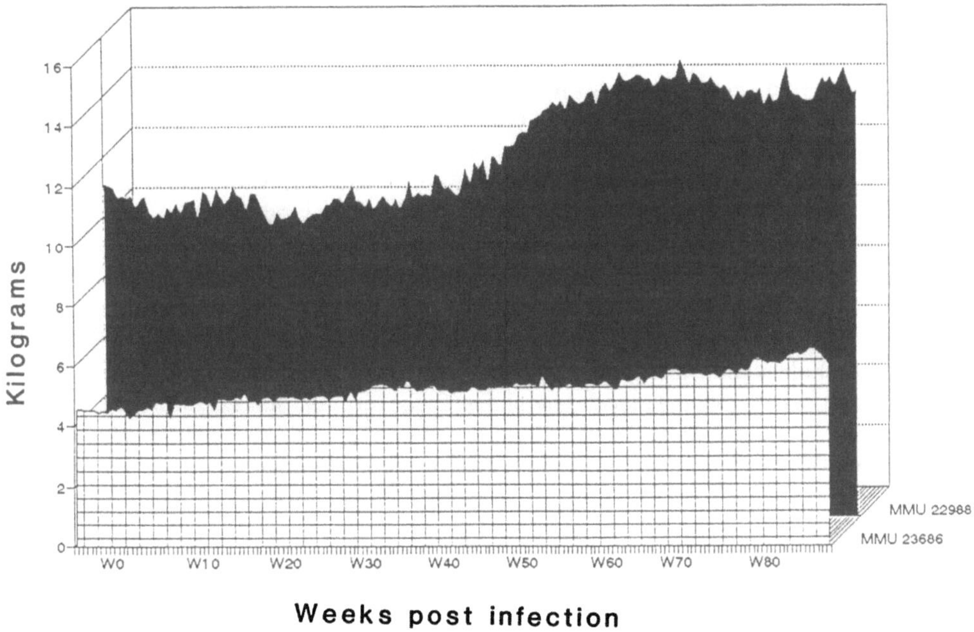

Figure 3. Weight gain of macaque MMU 22988, a long-time survivor of SIVmac239 infection. For comparison, the pattern of weight gains of a morphine-treated animal (MMU 23686) is also shown (open square).

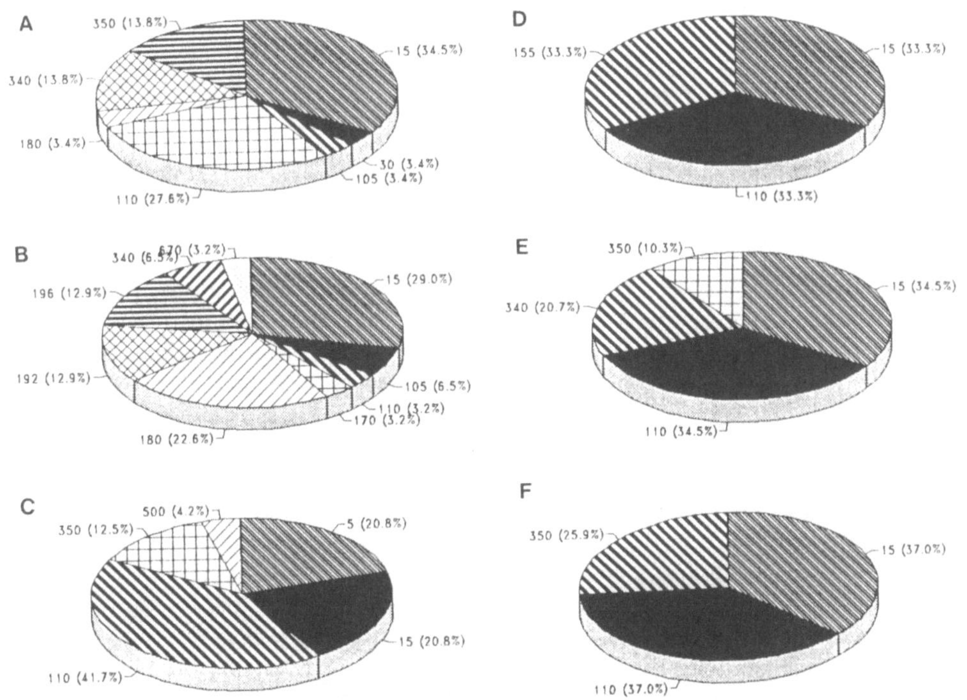

Figure 4. Behavioral patterns of monkeys after SIVmac239 infection. A, B & C, saline-treated monkeys (A, MMU 23679; B, MMU 23750; C, MMU 22988). D, E & F, morphine-treated monkeys (D, MMU 23686; E, MMU 22803, F, MMU 23740). Behavioral assessments were taken eleven days after SIVmac239 infection. The bar code number and its percentage of total behavior (in parenthesis) are shown.

Occurrence of Opportunistic Infections and Mortality Rate

SIV-infected rhesus monkeys have an average life span of 18 to 20 months after infection occurs (9). Opioid-treated animals were found to be more susceptible to opportunistic infections and had a shorter life span than saline treated monkeys. By 17 months post-infection, three of the five opioid-treated animals had died while the other two were undergoing chronic diarrhea, opportunistic infections, and/or viral mutation. In contrast, of the three saline-treated, SIVmac239-infected monkeys, two of the macaques were exhibiting chronic diarrhea (a sign of SIV infection) while the other monkey, macaque MMU 22988, was consistently displaying weight gain (Fig. 3). Within 17 months post-infection, the presence of secondary infections and diseases such as Giardia infection, enterocolitis, amyloidosis, cholecystitis, and lymphoma was much more apparent in opioid-treated monkeys than in similarly infected placebo monkeys. In the terminal stages, animals from all the infected groups, except macaque MMU 22988, a saline-treated animal, were equally affected (Macaque MMU 22988 survived past 50 months post-infection).

CONCLUSION

The above observations, describing behavioral alterations and mortality rate of opioid treated monkeys after SIVmac239 infection, substantiate our biochemical and immunological studies (1-6, 8) which suggest that opioids such as morphine potentiate the pathogenesis of SIV infection. In light of these observations, we have taken the task of searching for opioid receptors on immune cells. Our most recent molecular findings of the presence of all three types of brain-like opioid receptors (*delta, kappa* and *mu)* in cells of the immune system (11-13) may provide a direct mechanism by which opioids modulate host immune functions.

SUMMARY

Behavior and general comportment was measured as an integral part of a study of the possible modulatory effects of opioids on the immune system of rhesus monkeys before and after SIVmac239 infection. Four treatment groups were investigated: 1) saline treatment, 2) saline treatment followed by infection with SIV, 3) opioid treatment and 4) opioid treatment followed by infection with SIV. The results showed that the animals established initial consummatory patterns which were altered on a short lived basis upon opioid treatment but later re-established. The slope of weight gain of the opioid-treated animals, however, was depressed throughout the project period. Post-infection of SIV produced an interruption in the consummatory pattern of all animals. After infection masturbating behavior disappeared from the infected monkeys' behavioral repertoire. As the immune functions exhibited alterations, chronic diarrhea appeared intermittently and then persistently in all animals; the persistent diarrhea was non-responsive to the usual anti-diarrheal treatment even in the face of chronic opioid administration. A gradual and overall progression of behavioral depression was noted with the infected animals, particularly with the opioid-treated monkeys. The opioid dependent animals exhibited symptoms and signs of SIV infection earlier than the infected animals treated only with saline. In the terminal stages, animals from all the infected groups, except one saline-treated animal, were equally affected.

ACKNOWLEDGMENT

This research was supported by a research grant DA 05901 from the National Institute on Drug Abuse, NIH.

REFERENCES

1. L.F. Chuang, K.F. Killam, Jr., and R.Y. Chuang. Opioid dependency and T-helper functions in rhesus monkey. In Vivo 7:159-166, 1993.
2. Y. Liu, D.J. Blackbourn, L.F. Chuang, K.F. Killam, Jr., and R.Y. Chuang. The effects of in vivo and in vitro administration of morphine sulphate upon rhesus macaque polymorphonuclear cell phagocytosis and chemotaxis. J. Pharmacol. Exp. Ther. 263:533-539, 1992.
3. R.Y. Chuang, D.J. Blackbourn, L.F. Chuang, Y. Liu and K.F. Killam, Jr. Modulation of simian AIDS by opioids. Adv. Biosci. 86:573-583, 1993.
4. L.F. Chuang, D.J. Blackbourn, A.J. Chuang, K.F. Killam, Jr., X. Liu, Y. Li, H-f. Kung and R.Y. Chuang. Emergence of antigenic variants of simian immunodeficiency virus (SIVmac) in a seronegative macaque after SIVmac239 infection. Cell. Mol. Biol. Res. 40: 661-669, 1994.
5. R.Y. Chuang, L.F. Chuang, Y. Li, H-f. Kung and K.F. Killam, Jr. SIV mutations detected in morphine-treated *Macaca mulatta* following SIVmac239 infection. p. 175-181. In: B. Sharp et al. (Eds.) The Brain Immune Axis and Substance Abuse, Plenum Press, NY, 1995.
6. D.J. Blackbourn, L.F. Chuang, S. Sutjipto, K.F. Killam, Jr., P.M. McCready, R.H. Doi, Y. Li and R.Y. Chuang. Detection of simian immunodeficiency virus RNA from infected rhesus macaques by the polymerase chain reaction. J. Virol. Meth. 37:109-118, 1992.
7. D.A. Regier, and R.C. Desrosiers. The complete nucleotide sequence of a pathogenic molecular clone of the simian immunodeficiency virus. AIDS Res. Human Retroviruses 6:1221-1231, 1990.
8. L.F. Chuang, K.F. Killam, Jr. and R.Y. Chuang. Increased replication of simian immunodeficiency virus in CEM x174 cells by morphine sulfate. Biochem. Biophys. Res. Commun. 195:1165-1173, 1993.
9. H. Kestler, T. Kodama, D. Ringler, M. Marthas, N. Pedersen, A. Lackner, D. Regier, P. Sehgal, M. Daniel, N. King, and R. Desrosiers. Induction of AIDS in rhesus monkeys by molecularly cloned simian immunodeficiency virus. Science 248:1109-1112, 1990.
10. E.A. Murray, D.M. Rausch, J. Lendvay, L.R. Sharer, and L.E. Eiden. Cognitive and motor impairments associated with SIV infection in rhesus monkeys. Science 255:1246-1249, 1992.
11. L.F. Chuang, T.K. Chuang, K.F. Killam, Jr., A.J. Chuang, H.F. Kung, L. Yu, and R.Y. Chuang. Delta opioid receptor gene expression in lymphocytes. Biochem. Biophys. Res. Commun. 202:1291-1299, 1994.
12. L.F. Chuang, T.K. Chuang, K.F. Killam, Jr., Q. Qiu, X.R. Wang, J.J. Lin, H.F. Kung, W. Sheng, C. Chao, L. Yu, and R.Y. Chuang. Expression of kappa opioid receptors in human and monkey lymphocytes. Biochem. Biophys. Res. Commun. 209:1003-1010, 1995.
13. T.K. Chuang, K.F. Killam, Jr., L.F. Chuang, H.F. Kung, W.S. Sheng, C.C. Chao, L. Yu, and R.Y. Chuang. Mu opioid receptor gene expression in immune cells. Biochem. Biophys. Res. Commun. 216:922-930, 1995.

8

ENDOGENOUS OPIOIDS AND HIV INFECTION

Kamaraju S. Sundar,[1*] Lakshmi S. Kamaraju,[1] James McMahon,[2]
Robert A. Bitonte,[2] Sastry Gollapudi,[3] William H. Wilson,[1]
Ling-yuan Kong,[4] John S. Hong,[4] and James E. Lee[1]

1 Department of Psychiatry
Duke Medical Center, Durham, North Carolina
2 Eve Clinic
National Boulevard, Los Angeles, California
3 Department of Medicine
University of California at Irvine, California
4 Laboratory of Molecular Neuroscience
National Institute of Environmental Health Sciences
Research Triangle Park, North Carolina

ABSTRACT

Beta endorphin enhanced the HIV-p24 production in fetal microglia infected with HIV-$1_{JR\text{-}CSF}$, a strain that replicates poorly in these cells. Enhancement of HIV-p24 production by beta endorphin was associated with increased tumor necrosis factor a, interleukin-1 and IL6 production. In addition, beta endorphin activated parent HIV promoter. However, this transactivation is diminished when NFkB and SP-1 regions were deleted from HIV-LTR. These data demonstrate that beta endorphin enhances HIV-$1_{JR\text{-}CSF}$ replication in microglia by increased cytokine production and activation of HIV promoter possibly by NFkB and SP-1 transcription factors.

INTRODUCTION

HIV is detected in the brains of asymptomatic patients very early in the course of the disease. In addition, increased replication of HIV has been correlated with the development of AIDS dementia complex (ADC). Endogenous opiate, beta endorphin has been shown to

* Address correspondence to: Kamaraju S. Sundar, Ph. D. , Director, Laboratory of Neuroimmunology, Department of Psychiatry, Box 3552, Duke University Medical Center, Durham, North Carolina 27710. Telephone number: 919-684-6205; Fax: 919-684-3071.

synergistically enhance the synthesis of pro inflammatory cytokines in conjunction with GP-120, as well enhance the replication of a neurotropic HIV-1 in fetal microglia. In addition, beta endorphin enhanced the transactivation of HIV-promoter in microglia (Sundar et al., 1995). Similarly, exogenous opiate, morphine was also shown to enhance the replication of HIV (Peterson et al., 1990, 1991; Chuang et al., 1993). In order to determine whether opiates can contribute to the progression of ADC early in the course of the disease by increasing the replication of HIV, we have selected a neurotropic strain that poorly replicates in brain microglia. HIV-$1_{JR\text{-}CSF}$ strain is known to establish a persistent and low level of infection in primary explant cultures of glial cells (Konayagi et al., 1987; 1988). It replicates less efficiently than HIV-$1_{JR\text{-}FL}$ in primary human mononuclear cells. Since the low level of replication closely mimics the *in vivo* condition, this model can be used to evaluate the agents that can contribute to the progression of the disease. In this study, we investigated the effect of beta endorphin on the synthesis of p-24 antigen and cytokines were evaluated in HIV-$1_{JR\text{-}CSF}$ infected microglia. The results presented here demonstrate that beta endorphin enhanced the replication of this virus and induced the synthesis of cytokines. In addition, beta endorphin-induced transactivation is dependent on the presence of NFkB and SP-1 regions in the HIV promoter.

2. MATERIAL AND METHODS

2.1 Effect of Beta Endorphin on the Replication of HIV-$1_{JR\text{-}CSF}$ in Fetal Microglia

The protocol to obtain fetal tissue has been approved by the Institutional Review Board of the Duke University Medical Center. Fetal microglia were isolated from the brains of legally terminated pregnancies. Microglia were isolated as described earlier (Sundar et al., 1995). Two million microglia were infected with HIV-$1_{JR\text{-}CSF}$ (30 ng of p-24 antigen. This strain of virus was obtained from the AIDS Research and Reference Reagent Program of the NIH). Beta endorphin (10^{-8} M) was added to these cultures. Every four days, one-half medium was replaced with fresh medium containing twice the concentration of beta endorphin. Fourteen days later, cells were lysed with three cycles of freezing and thawing and then analyzed for the presence of P-24 by ELISA (Incstar).

2.2 Effect of Beta Endorphin on the Synthesis of Cytokines in HIV-Infected Cells

The microglia were infected with HIV-$1_{JR\text{-}CSF}$ and treated with beta endorphin as described above. Seven days later, the culture were lysed and analyzed for the presence of interleukin-1, IL6 and tumor necrosis factor α (TNFα) using ELISA (Cistron).

2.3 Mediators of Beta Endorphin-Induced Enhancement of Transactivation of HIV-LTR

In order to determine the transcription factors responsible for the transactivation of HIV-LTR, HIV-LTR mutants were used. In this experiment, microglia were transfected with HIV-LTR mutants in which the regions of NFkB, SP-1 and nef were deleted (These reagents were obtained from the AIDS Research and Reference Reagent Program of the NIH). Transactivation of HIV-LTR were determined by the expression of the reporter gene chloramphenicol acetyl transferase as described earlier (Sundar et al., 1995).

2.4. Statistical Analysis

Each experiment was carried out in duplicate with microglia derived from 4 individual brain samples. Results were examined with paired t-tests.

3. RESULTS

3.1 Enhancement of HIV-$1_{JR\text{-}CSF}$ in the Microglia

HIV-$1_{JR\text{-}CSF}$ infected microglia produced low levels of p-24 antigen 14 days post infection. In sharp contrast, treatment of these HIV-infected cells with 10^{-8} M concentration of beta endorphin resulted in a marked increase in the synthesis of p-24 antigen 14 days post infection ($p \leq 0.05$; Figure 1).

3.2. Beta Endorphin Enhances the Synthesis of Cytokines in HIV-Infected Microglia

Control un-infected cells constitutively synthesized low levels of IL-1, IL6 and TNFα In HIV-infected cells, these cytokine concentrations were elevated significantly. In contrast, beta endorphin significantly enhanced the synthesis of these cytokines in HIV-infected microglia ($p \leq 0.05$; Figure 2).

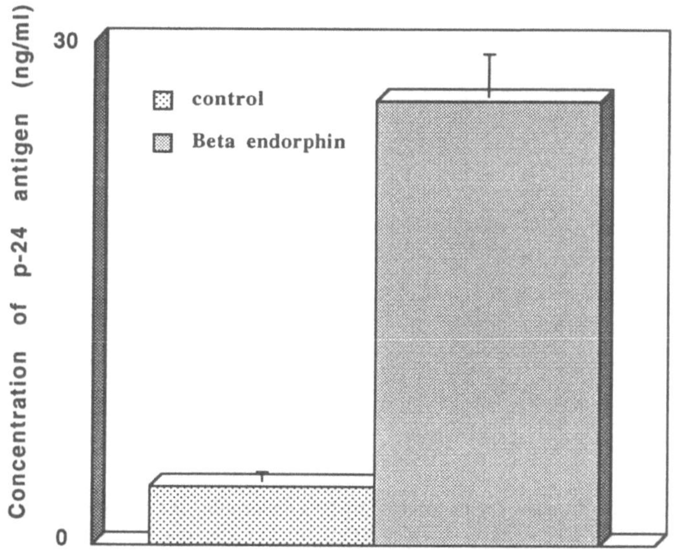

Figure 1. Two million microglia were infected with 30 ng of HIV-$1_{JR\text{-}CSF}$. HIV infected cells were treated with beta endorphin (10^{-8} M). All treatments were tested in duplicate and microglia from 4 brains were examined (N=4). Fourteen days later, the cell lysates were analyzed for the presence of p-24 antigen by ELISA (Incstar). HIV infected controls showed a minimal synthesis of p-24 antigen ($\leq$ 5 ng/ml). In contrast, beta endorphin enhanced the concentration of p-24 antigen significantly (over 20 folds; $p \leq 0.005$).

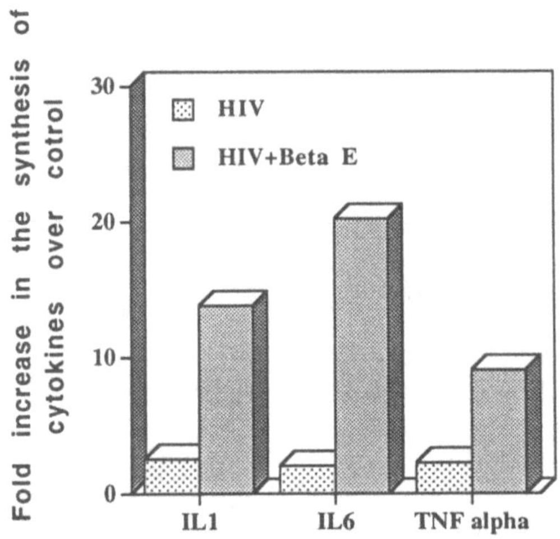

Figure 2. Two million microglia were infected with 30 ng of HIV-$1_{JR\text{-}CSF}$. Infected cells were treated with beta endorphin (Beta E, 10^{-8} M). All treatments were carried out in duplicate, and four brains were tested. Cells were examined for the presence of IL1, IL6 and TNF alpha by ELISA. While control microglia constitutively expressed these cytokines, infection of these cells with HIV resulted in significant increase in the synthesis of these cytokines ($p \leq 0.05$). Beta endorphin significantly enhanced the synthesis of cytokines in HIV infected microglia ($p \leq 0.05$).

3.3 Transactivation of HIV-LTR by Beta Endorphin is Mediated through NFkB Region

Microglia were transfected with parent HIV-LTR and a mutant in which the NFkB,SP-1 and nef region were deleted. Beta endorphin significantly enhanced the transactivation of parent HIV-LTR. When NFkB region and nef region were deleted, transactivation of HIV-LTR by beta endorphin was significantly reduced. However, when NFkB and SP-1 regions were deleted transactivation is completely abrogated ($p \leq 0.05$; Figure 3).

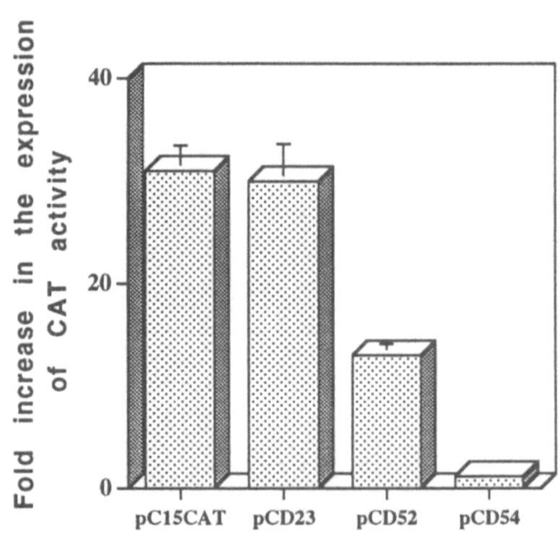

Figure 3. In order to determine the region affected by beta endorphin, one million microglia were transfected with HIV-LTR or with HIV-LTR mutants in which NFkB, SP-1 and nef region were deleted. pC15 CAT=Parent promoter; pCD23= HIV promoter with nef region deleted; pCD52= NfKB and nef regions deleted; pCD54=nef, NFkB and SP-1 regions were deleted. CAT activity was determined by ELISA. As shown before, beta endorphin significantly enhanced the transactivation of HIV-LTR ($p \leq 0.005$). However, when nef and NFkB regions were deleted from parent HIV-LTR, the ability of beta endorphin to transactivate HIV-LTR was significantly diminished ($p \leq 0.05$). Deletion of NFkB and SP-1 resulted in complete loss of transactivation. These data suggest that beta endorphin enhances HIV-LTR primarily by interacting with NFkB and SP-1 regions.

4. DISCUSSION

The results presented here demonstrate that beta endorphin enhanced the replication of this strain of HIV in the fetal microglia. The increased synthesis of p-24 antigen in fetal microglia is accompanied by an increase in the levels of cytokines in beta endorphin-treated HIV infected cells. In addition, transactivation of IV-LTR by beta endorphin appears to require the presence of NFkB and SP-1 regions. Deletion of nef regions has no effect on the transactivation of HIV promoter by beta endorphin. Since cytokines were shown to activate NFkB, it is likely that beta endorphin is enhancing the transactivation of HIV-LTR by activating NFkB region. Whether opiates induce these transcription factors, in the microglia, is yet to be determined. These results indicate that beta endorphin or other opiates can significantly contribute to the progression of AIDS and ADC, particularly in asymptomatic patients.

ACKNOWLEDGMENTS

This research is supported by a grant from the National Institute of Mental Health MH51524.

REFERENCES

Chao, C.C., Gekker, G., Sheng W.S., Hu, S., Tsang, M., Peterson, P.K (1993). Priming effect of morphine on the production of tumor necrosis factor α by microglia: implications in repiratory burst activity and human immunodeficiency virus-1 expression. J. Pharmacol. Exp. Therapeutics. 269:198-203.

Koyanagi, Y., Miles, S., Mitsuyasu, R.T., Merill, J.E., Vinters, H.V., Chen, I.S (1987). Dual infection of the central nervous system by AIDS viruses with distinct cellular tropisms. Science 236: 819-22.

Koyanagi, Y., O'Brien, W.A., Zhao, J.Q., Golde, D.W., Gasson, J.C., Chen, I.S (1988). Cytokines alter production of HIV-1 from primary mononuclear phagocytes. Science 241:1673-5.

Peterson, P.K., Gekker, G., Chao, C.C., Verhoef, J., Balfour, H.H. Jr (1991). Effects of morphine on human immunodeficiency virus-1 expression in the chronically infected cell lines U1 and ACH-2. Immunol Inf. Dis. 1:313- 17

Peterson, P.K., Gekker, G., Schut, R., Hu ,S., Balfour, H,H. Jr., Chao, C.C (1992). Enhancement of HIV-1 replication by opiates and cocaine: The cytokine connection. Adv. Exp. Med. Biol 335:181-8.

Sundar, K.S., Kamaraju, L.S., Dingfelder, J., McMahon, J., Gollpaudi, S., Wilson, W.H., Ling-Yuan Kong., Hoong, J.S., Lee, J. E (1995). Beta-endorphin enhances the replication of neurotropic human immunodeficiency virus in fetal perivascular microglia. J. Neuroimmunol. 61: 97-104.

DISCUSSION

9

METHIONINE ENKEPHALIN USED IN COMBINATION WITH AZIDOTHYMIDINE IN MURINE RETROVIRUS INFECTION

Steven Specter,[1] Nicholas Plotnikoff,[2] Jeong-Im Sin,[1] and Darlene Goodfellow[1]

[1] Department of Medical Microbiology and Immunology
University of South Florida College of Medicine
12901 N. Bruce B. Downs Blvd.
Tampa, Florida 33612
[2] Department of Pharmacodynamics
University of Illinois at Chicago
Box 6998
Chicago, Illinois 60680

1. INTRODUCTION

The neuropeptide, methionine enkephalin (Met-ENK), has been demonstrated to have immunomodulatory activity, most notably increasing CD4+ lymphocyte counts.[1] Based on this information-Met-ENK has been administered to virus infected mice and humans in an attempt to treat retroviral diseases.[2,3] Bihari and coworkers noted that patients infected with the human immunodeficiency virus (HIV), who either have the acquired immunodeficiency syndrome (AIDS) or AIDS related complex, demonstrated increased CD4+ cell counts.[2] However these authors did not report any long term clinical results for these patients. Specter et al. have reported that BALB/c mice infected with Friend leukemia virus (FLV) or C57BL/6 mice infected with BM5 lymphoproliferative virus complex showed reduced disease progression when treated with a combination of azidothymidine (AZT) and Met-ENK.[3] In this study Met-ENK did not provide any benefit when used alone and AZT was about 50% effective compared to the AZT and Met-ENK combination. The data suggest that AZT and Met-ENK used in combination may be effective for reducing morbidity and mortality of retroviral disease in animal and human infections. It was not clear from the studies cited above whether Met-ENK was providing benefit as an antiviral drug or as an immunostimulatory drug working in combination with an antiviral drug (AZT).

Sidwell and coworkers have reported direct antiviral activity for Met-ENK in mice infected with influenza virus.[4] Thus, *in vitro* studies were undertaken to determine if the effects of Met-ENK used in combination were the result of direct antiviral activity or were immune mediated.

AIDS, Drugs of Abuse, and the Neuroimmune Axis, Edited by Friedman *et al.*
Plenum Press, New York, 1996

2. *IN VITRO* INHIBITION OF FLV REPLICATION

In vitro infection with FLV can be accomplished using a susceptible mouse fibroblast cell line designated *Mus dunni* (Dunni) cells. Infection results in the accumulation of cells in foci. These are readily detected 3-5 days after infection by staining cells with a monoclonal antibody directed against the viral envelope glycoprotein gp70. Cells are then detected using peroxidase labelled anti-mouse immunoglobulin and an appropriate substrate. Monoclonal antibody was kindly supplied by B. Chesebro, Hamilton, MT. Cultures were infected with approximately 50 focus forming units (FFU) FLV, treated with drugs at 2 hr post infection and then FFU detected after 5 days incubation at 37°C in 5% CO_2, 95% air.

Data in Table 1 indicate that FLV replication could be inhibited in a dose related manner by AZT when 100 pg/ml or greater were used. By contrast, Met-ENK was incapable of inhibiting viral replication when up to 100 μg/ml was used. Thus, for combination therapy the dose of AZT used was 1 ng/ml, since this dose could provide limited (approximately 35%) inhibition of replication of FLV. Subsequently, AZT and Met-ENK were added to Dunni cell cultures simultaneously to determine if a combination effect could be detected. As noted in Table 2, the addition of Met-ENK to AZT had no added benefit related to inhibition of FLV replication. By contrast, when BALB/c spleen cells were treated with Met-ENK and then added to AZT for therapy of FLV-infected Dunni cells, increased inhibition of replication was noted. Whereas AZT alone resulted in a 25% (49.8 vs 65.6 in controls) inhibition, the combination of AZT and Met-ENK treated spleen cells resulted in a reduction of greater than 50% (31.3 vs 65.6) in the number of FFU observed. This response was directly related to the concentration of Met-ENK used. The use of Met-ENK treated spleen cells in the absence of AZT provided no significant abrogation of FLV replication (data not shown).

Table 1. Effects of AZT or methionine enkephalin on Friend leukemia virus replication in *Mus dunni* cells

Group Number	# Focus forming units ± S.D.[a]
Control[b]	32.2 ± 1.9
AZT 50 pg/ml	32.3 ± 2.5
100 pg/ml	28.8 ± 1.0
500 pg/ml	26.3 ± 4.2
1 ng/ml	20.8 ± 2.1*
10 ng/ml	0.0*
100 ng/ml	0.0*
Methionine enkephalin	
10 ng/ml	26.4 ± 4.7
1 μg/ml	30.0 ± 7.9
10 μg/ml	31.0 ± 3.5
50 μg/ml	29.3 ± 1.5
100 μg/ml	32.3 ± 1.5

[a] *Mus dunni* cells are grown to confluence in 24 well cluster plates and then infected with a 1:200 dilution of FLV stock virus (approximately 50 FFU). After 5 days at 37°C in 5% CO_2, 95% air the cultures are stained with immunoperoxidase labelled anti-gp70 monoclonal antibody and foci are counted.
[b] Four replicates are used for each group to determine the mean and standard deviation of the number of FLV induced foci of cell growth.
* Statistically significant at $p<0.05$ using a Student's t test.

Table 2. Effect of AZT and methionine enkephalin combined for treating FLV in cell culture

Group Number	#Focus forming units ± S.D.[a]
Control[b]	59.5 ± 3.5
AZT 1 ng/ml	36.5 ± 5.3*
AZT + Met-ENK 1 μg/ml	36.8 ± 3.2*
AZT + Met-ENK 10 μg/ml	35.3 ± 3.4*
AZT + Met-ENK 50 μg/ml	35.8 ± 2.6*
AZT + Met-ENK 100 μg/ml	39.5 ± 5.2*
Cultures incubated in the presence of 10^6 mouse spleen cells.	
Control[b]	65.6 ± 3.1
AZT 1 ng/ml	49.8 ± 5.3*
AZT + Met-ENK 1 μg/ml	42.3 ± 2.9*
AZT + Met-ENK 10 μg/ml	40.0 ± 3.4*
AZT + Met-ENK 50 μg/ml	34.3 ± 3.6*,**
AZT + Met-ENK 100 μg/ml	31.3 ± 3.0*,**

[a] *Mus dunni* cells are grown to confluence in 24 well cluster plates and then infected with a 1:200 dilution of FLV stock virus (approximately 50 FFU). After 5 days at 37°C in 5% CO_2, 95% air the cultures are stained with immunoperoxidase labelled anti-gp70 monoclonal antibody and foci are counted.
[b] Four replicates are used for each group to determine the mean and standard deviation of the number of FLV induced foci of cell growth.
* Statistically significant at $p<0.05$ using a Student's t test compared to control.
**Statistically significant at $p<0.05$ using a Student's t test compared to AZT alone.

It is interesting to note that preliminary experiments have demonstrated that the Met-ENK effect is inhibited by the opioid receptor antagonist naloxone (data not shown).

3. CONCLUSIONS

The data clearly indicate that a murine retrovirus infection can be established in Dunni cells *in vitro* and that this is inhibitable in a dose related manner by AZT. By contrast Met-ENK demonstrated no direct antiviral effect whether used alone or in combination with AZT. However, when mouse spleen cells were treated with Met-ENK and added to AZT, this therapeutic combination was more beneficial than AZT alone. These results support the concept that Met-ENK is working via an immunostimulatory mechanism in combination with direct antiviral effects of AZT.

The concept of combined antiviral chemotherapy and immune therapy is not new. This approach has been used both in human retrovirus infections and in animal models.[5] Some success have been reported to date but as yet there are no such combined therapies that have gained acceptance for clinical use in AIDS patients. We believe that the AZT and Met-ENK combination has potential for use in HIV infection. This is based on the results of Bihari *et al.*,[2] who showed that Met-ENK can boost helper T cell numbers in AIDS patients and our data,[3] that indicate that Met-ENK can stimulate immunity in mice and inhibit the progression of retroviral disease when combined with AZT.

Met-ENK has been shown to bind to lymphocytes via selective opioid receptors,[6] suggesting that the immunostimulatory effects of this peptide may be receptor mediated. In this regard, we demonstrated that a general opioid receptor antagonist, naloxone, was capable of inhibiting the ability of Met-ENK to stimulate spleen cells to exhibit anti-FLV activity (unpublished observations). The immune mechanisms involved in Met-ENK mediated antiviral activity remain to be determined. It is likely that developing a clearer understanding of the mechanisms involved will contribute greatly to the determination of whether or not the combination of AZT and Met-ENK can be applied to retrovirus infections in humans.

REFERENCES

1. Wybran J, Schandene L, Van Vooren J-P, Vandermoten G, Lattine D, Sonnet J, De Bruyere M, Taelman H, and Plotnikoff NP. Immunologic properties of methionine-enkephalin, and therapeutic implications in AIDS, ARC, and Cancer. Ann. NY Acad. Sci. 496: 108-114, 1987.
2. Bihari B, Plotnikoff NP, Freeman KD, Cort S, Dowling J, Diuguid C, Smith B, Altmann E, and Gum S. Methionine enkephalin in the treatment of AIDS related complex, Proc. 7th Intl. Conf. on AIDS, Florence, Italy, 1991.
3. Specter SC, Plotnikoff N, Bradley WG and Goodfellow D. Methionine enkephalin combined with AZT therapy reduce murine retrovirus-induced disease. Int. J. Immunopharmac. 6: 911-917, 1994.
4. Burger RA, Warren RP, Huffman JH, and Sidwell RW. Effect of methionine enkephalin on natural killer cell and cytotoxic T lymphocyte activity in mice infected with influenza A virus. Immunopharm. Immunotoxicol. 17: 323-334, 1995.
5. Specter S and Hadden JW. Immunotherapy for AIDS: Status and prospects. In: AIDS and Other Manifestations of HIV Infection 2nd Ed., Wormser, G. (Ed) Raven Press, New York, pp. 625-630, 1992.
6. Linner KM, Quist HE, and Sharp BM. Met-enkephalin-containing peptides encoded by proenkephalin A mRNA expressed in activated murine thymocytes inhibit thymocyte proliferation. J. Immunol. 154: 5049-5060, 1995.

ON THE EVOLUTION OF OPIOID MECHANISMS AND IMMUNE DEFENSES

Fernando L. Renaud[1] and Enid Z. Tomei[2]

[1] Biology Department
University of Puerto Rico
Río Piedras Campus, San Juan, Puerto Rico
[2] Department of Psychiatry
Emory University School of Medicine
Atlanta, Georgia

1. ABSTRACT

Results from our laboratory suggest that opioid-modulated phagocytosis originated early in evolution and fundamental aspects of this mechanism have been conserved. β-endorphin-like immunoreactivity detected in the ciliate *Tetrahymena* appears to modulate phagocytosis. We have compared the effects of opioids on phagocytosis in *Tetrahymena* and in Fc-mediated phagocytosis by peritoneal murine macrophages. These effects are remarkably similar: a) opioid agonists inhibit phagocytosis by a naloxone-reversible mechanism with effective concentrations in the nanomolar range, b) the effect of acute exposure is dose-dependent and biphasic, c) chronic exposure to morphine results in a state akin to desensitization and tolerance, d) the effect of morphine on tolerant cells may be stimulatory under certain circumstances, e) withdrawal of morphine from tolerant cells may inhibit phagocytosis suggesting that tolerant cells may require morphine to perform this function at a basal level. Pharmacological data suggest that the opioid receptor in *Tetrahymena* is mu-like and may be associated with a G_i-like protein since pertussis toxin pre-treatment will counteract the inhibitory effect of opioids. Our work suggests that the influence of opioids on the immune system originated early in evolution since phagocytosis may be considered the primeval cell defense mechanism.

2. INTRODUCTION

The presence of opioid peptides has been reported in a wide variety of organisms from protozoa to mammals. Nonetheless, information about opioid mechanisms in invertebrates is scarce (1). Interestingly enough, opioids have been reported associated with the modulation of endocytic processes in more primitive organisms, such as pinocytosis in *Amoeba* and phagocytosis in the protozoan ciliate *Tetrahymena* and in a snail (1, 2). This

AIDS, Drugs of Abuse, and the Neuroimmune Axis, Edited by Friedman *et al.*
Plenum Press, New York, 1996

suggests that the connection between opioids and phagocytosis originated early in evolution, prior to the origin of metazoa. Since phagocytosis may be considered the primeval cell defense mechanism, it may be implied that the association between opioids and the immune system arose early in evolution.

We have chosen to focus our attention on two model systems that show a remarkable parallelism in their opioid mechanisms in spite of their evolutionary distance: the free-living ciliate *Tetrahymena* and murine peritoneal macrophages. *Tetrahymena* has been reported to produce a wide variety of hormones, including peptide hormones such as insulin and β-endorphin (3). Furthermore, there is evidence that the endogenous peptide may play a role in the modulation of chemotaxis and phagocytosis (2). The *Tetrahymena* opioid receptor has been characterized partially by means of both biochemical and pharmacological techniques (2,4). Pharmacological evidence suggests that this receptor is mu-like, since morphine is the most potent and effective ligand in the modulation of phagocytosis (4).

Phagocytosis has also been reported to be affected by morphine in murine peritoneal macrophages (5). Recently we have demostrated that chronic exposure to morphine results in the development of a state akin to desensitization/tolerance (6). We describe here some previously unreported aspects of the opioid mechanism in macrophages; and compare these features with those of the *Tetrahymena* opioid mechanism.

3. MATERIALS AND METHODS

3.1 *Tetrahymena* Cell Cultures and Phagocytosis Assay

Tetrahymena cells were cultured as previously described (4). The phagocytosis assay was performed as reported elsewhere(4); in brief, cells were washed with buffer and resuspended in the presence of tantalum particles of 3μm diameter, samples were taken at different time intervals, fixed and the % phagocytosis scored by microscopical examination. In the case of acute exposures, morphine (Sigma) in the appropiate concentration was added to the buffer in which the assay is taking place prior to, or simultaneously with, the addition of tantalum particles.

3.2 Culturing of Peritoneal Macrophages and Phagocytosis Assay

Macrophage cultures and the phagocytosis assay were performed as described previously (6). In brief, thioglycollate-elicited cells were cultured in RPMI supplemented with fetal bovine serum. For acute exposure, macrophages were pre-incubated at 37 °C for 30 min with morphine concentrations ranging from 10^{-9} to 10^{-6}M. Following addition of opsonized SRBC (sheep red bloood cells), phagocytosis was allowed to proceed for 20 minutes at 37 °C. Uningested cells were lysed by hypotonic shock followed by glutaraldehyde fixation and staining. One hundred cells were counted by microscopy per triplicate well; % inhibition was calculated as described below.

3.3 Statistical Analysis

The data obtained in these experiments was analysed for significancy by the student's t-test. Data points are presented as the standard deviation of the mean and at least six replicates were included per sample. Results were expressed in terms of either % inhibition (the difference in % phagocytosis between control and experimental cells divided by % phagocytosis of control cells and multiplied by 100) or % phagocytosis of control cells (a % phagocytosis equal to that of control cells is 100%).

4. RESULTS

4.1 Effect of Morphine Concentration on Phagocytosis after Acute Exposure

The outcome of phagocytosis in *Tetrahymena* after incubating with different morphine concentrations is illustrated in Fig. 1. When cells were pre-incubated with the drug prior to the initiation of phagocytosis a biphasic effect was observed with a maximal inhibitory effect of around 22% at 30 nM morphine. However, when the pre-incubation period is omitted a sustained inhibition is observed, with a maximal inhibitory effect of around 50%; these effects have been reported previously to be naloxone-reversible (4). A similar biphasic effect was obtained when morphine was added to murine peritoneal macrophages (Fig. 2), with maximal inibitory effect of around 25-30% at 50-100 nM morphine. Likewise, this inhibition was naloxone-reversible (Fig. 2).

4.2 Effect of Chronic Exposure to Morphine and Drug Withdrawal on Phagocytosis

Exposure of *Tetrahymena* cells to 30 nM morphine for 16 hrs results in a significant stimulation of phagocytosis when compared to opiate-naive cells (Fig. 3). However, removal of morphine from the medium resulted in significant inhibition of phagocytosis as compared

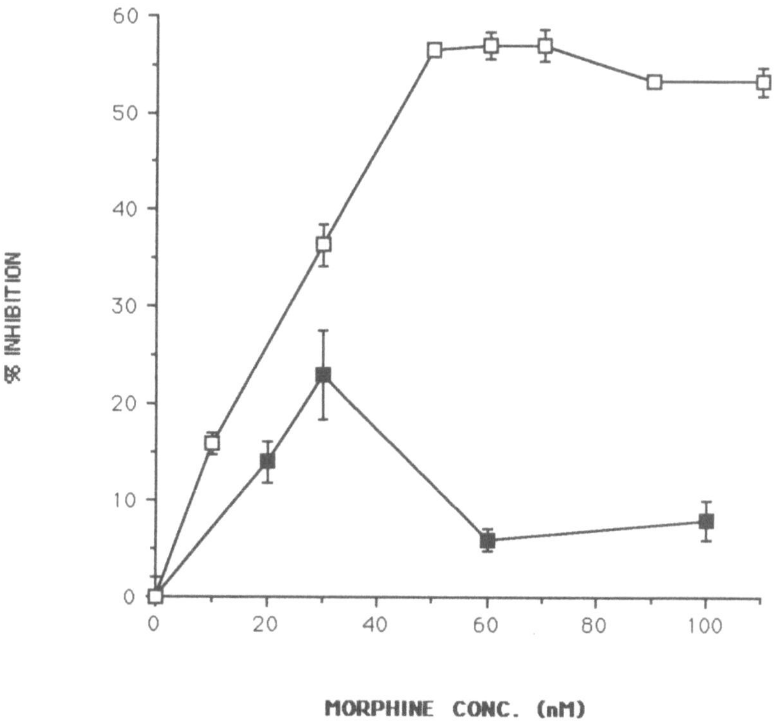

Figure 1. Effect of morphine on phagocytosis in *Tetrahymena* when cells are pre-incubated for 3 min with the drug before the assay (filled squares) and when the pre-incubation period is omitted (open squares); % inhibition was calculated as described in text . In this and in all following figures data are expressed as mean ± SD. (Figure taken from Chiesa et al., 1993).

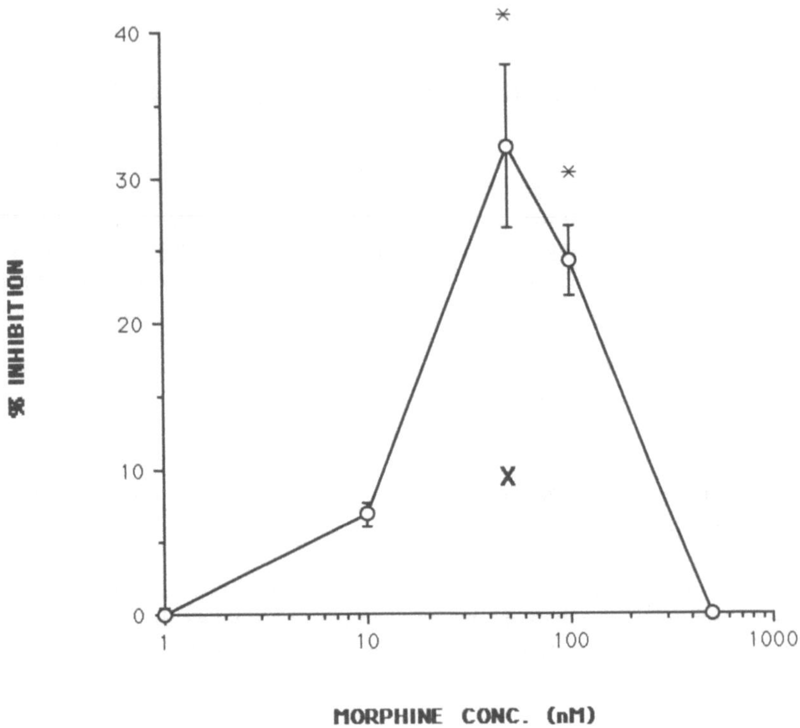

Figure 2. Effect of morphine concentration on inhibition of phagocytosis of sheep red blood cells (SRBC) by murine peritoneal macrophages. The X indicates the % inhibition observed in the presence of both 50 nM morphine and 50 nM naloxone. * $p < 0.01$ when compared to control cells, n = 12.

to control cells (Fig. 3). Comparable results have been obtained with macrophages: a 10 hr exposure to morphine results in a significant stimulation of phagocytosis when compared to control cells (Fig. 3). On the other hand, opioid withdrawal for 5 hrs from cells treated with morphine for 8 hrs results in significant inhibition of the phagocytosis process when compared to control cells (Fig. 3). Nevertheless, withdrawal for only 1hr had no effect.

5. DISCUSSION

The data shown here point to a remarkable parallelism in the opioid mechanisms in *Tetrahymena* and macrophages. For instance, under some conditions acute exposure to nanomolar concentrations of morphine inhibits phagocytosis in both types of cells in a biphasic, dose-dependent manner. The reason for the biphasic nature of the curve is unknown at the moment, although the sustained inhibition observed in the case of *Tetrahymena* when the 3 min pre-incubation period is omitted suggests that a rapid desensitization is taking place during the pre-incubation period at the higher drug concentrations. This is further supported by the fact that if the pre-incubation period is extended for 10 min, an inhibitory concentration of morphine has no effect on phagocytosis in *Tetrahymena*, suggesting that tachyphyllaxis may be taking place (7). It remains to be seen if a shorter pre-incubation period will result in sustained inhibition of phagocytosis by peritoneal macrophages. That these effects are mediated in both cell types of cell by an opioid receptor is suggested by the

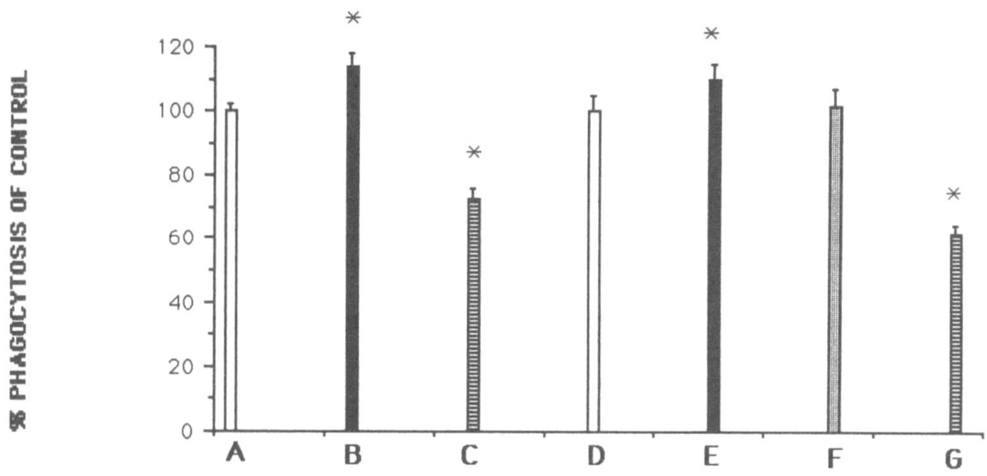

Figure 3. Effect of chronic opioid exposure and withdrawal on phagocytosis by *Tetrahymena* and murine peritoneal macrophages. Data in this figure is a composite from several independent experiments. A= *Tetrahymena* control cells, B= *Tetrahymena* exposed for 16 hrs to 30 nM morphine prior to the phagocytosis assay; C= *Tetrahymena* cells exposed for 16 hrs to 30 nM morphine, but washed three times prior to the phagocytosis assay which was conducted in the absence of morphine; D= macrophage control cells; E= macrophages exposed for 10 hrs in the presence of 100 nM morphine prior to the phagocytosis assay; F= macrophages exposed for 8 hrs in the presence of 100 nm morphine, followed by washing and incubation in drug-free medium for 1 hr prior to phagocytosis of SRBC; G= macrophages exposed for 8 hrs in the presence of 100 nM morphine, followed by washing and incubation in drug-free medium for 5 hrs prior to phagocytosis of SRBC. *$p \leq 0.05$ when compared to control cells.

naloxone-reversibility of the inhibition by morphine. Reversibility by naloxone has been used in previous work to measure the pA_2 for naloxone of the *Tetrahymena* opioid receptor and the data suggest that this receptor is mu-like in terms of this parameter (4). This differs from data presented by other workers that have suggested that delta receptors predominate in lower invertebrates (8); the resolution of this controversy awaits the cloning and sequencing of the *Tetrahymena* opioid receptor. A μ-subtype has also been reported in rat macrophages by molecular biology techniques (9), but interestingly enough it seems to be expressed in only a subset of the macrophage population, which might explain the partial nature of the inhibition obtained in our work, if a similar partial expression of this receptor is found in mouse macrophages.

Another point of similarity in the *Tetrahymena* and macrophage opioid mechanisms is that under some conditions chronic exposure to morphine may result in a stimulatory effect rather than inhibitory. Analogous stimulatory effects by morphine in tolerant tissues have been reported in other systems, such as the guinea pig myenteric plexus, where the investigators explain differential effects of morphine on the basis of distinct G-proteins associated with the opioid receptor under various conditions (10). It is unknown if such an explanation is applicable to the systems under study in this paper, albeit G-proteins undoubtedly play a role in the modulation of phagocytosis in both *Tetrahymena* and macrophages. For example, pertussis toxin has been reported to block the inhibitory effect of morphine in *Tetrahymena* (2), and G-proteins have been detected by immunoblots in this organism (11).

Another intriguing observation is the fact that morphine withdrawal from putatively tolerant cells, results in an inhibitory effect similar in magnitude to that caused by acute exposure. Again a comparable observation was made in the guinea pig ileum and was attributed to coupling of the opioid receptor with a G_s in the tolerant state (10); thus, morphine withdrawal would turn off the activation of a stimulatory pathway. At the moment we do not know why morphine withdrawal-induced inhibition of phagocytosis is manifested immediately in *Tetrahymena* and guinea pig ileum, wheras it requires several hrs for its manifestation in macrophages. A more detailed study of this phenomenon is required to answer this question. Nevertheless, these observations may have interesting clinical implications because of the pivotal role that macrophages play in immune defenses. It may be that subjects that use drugs on a continuous basis are in a homeostatic equilibrium that allows their immune sytem to function with an efficiency similar to that of opiate naive individuals. Under these conditions, opiate withdrawal may create a disturbance on macrophage functions that may putatively impair their ability to fight infections. Opiate withdrawal has been postulated to be a factor in immune dysfuction (12). It would be of great interest to determine if other macrophage functions, such as oxidative burst and cytokine production are similarly affected by opioid tolerance and withdrawal. If so, this would be of great clinical relevance, not only for understanding health problems in drug users, but also when administering opioids in a clinical setting.

The data presented in this paper demonstrates that a remarkable parallelism exists in the opioid mechanisms in cells from two phylogenetically distant organisms, *Tetrahymena* and murine peritoneal macrophages. In both these types of cell morphine modulates phagocytosis and other functions (2, 6). Since association between opioids and endocytic processes has also been reported in several invertebrates (1, 2), this suggests that the modulation of endocytosis by opioids originated early in evolution. Phagocytosis is undoubtedly among the most primitive cell defense mechanisms since it is present even in organisms that lack the capacity to generate antibodies. Therefore the association between opioids and cell defense mechanisms appears may have taken place early in evolution, prior to the origin of metazoa, and seems to have been conserved.

6. ACKNOWLEDGEMENTS

The authors are grateful for permission to use a figure from the Society of Protozoologists. This work was supported by Department of Education grant P120A40059, NIH-MBRS grant S06 GM08102 and NSF grantMCB-9105024.

7. REFERENCES

1. F. L. Renaud, R. Chiesa, F. Rodríguez and N. Tomassini, Studies on the opioid mechanism in *Tetrahymena*, *in*: Cell surface-associated receptors and their ligands in invertebrates and protists. G.Csaba, Ed., Springer-Verlag, Heidelberg (in press).
2. F.L. Renaud, R. Chiesa, J.M. De Jesús, A. López, J. Miranda and N. Tomassini, Hormones and signal transduction in protozoa, Comp Biochem Physiol 100A: 41-45D (1991).
3. LeRoith, S. Liotta, J. Roth, J. Shiloach, M.E. Lewis, C.B. Pert and D.T. Krieger, Corticotropin and β-endorphin-like materials are native to unicellular organisms. Proc Natl Acad Sci USA 79: 2086-2090 (1982).
4. R. Chiesa, W.I. Silva and F.L. Renaud, F. L., Pharmacological characterization of an opioid receptor in the ciliate *Tetrahymena*. J Euk Microbiol 40: 800-804 (1993).
5. M. Rojavin, I. Szabo, J.L. Bussiere, T.J. Rogers, M.W. Adler and T.K. Eisenstein, Morphine treatment in vitro or in vivo decreases phagocytic functions of murine macrophages, Life Sci. 53: 997-1006 (1993).
6. A. M. Casellas, H. Guardiola and F. L. Renaud, F.L., Inhibition by opioids of phagocytosis in peritoneal macrophages, Neuropeptides 18: 35-40 (1991).
7. A. Salamán, M. Román, F.L. Renaud and W.I. Silva, Effect of chronic opioid treatment on phagocytosis in *Tetrahymena*. Neuropeptides 16: 115-120 (1990).

8. B. Zipser, J.B. O'Neill, M.R. Ruff, C.C. Smith, W.J. Higgins and C.B. Pert, The opiate receptor: a single 110 kDa recognition molecule appears to be conserved in *Tetrahymena*, leech and rat. Brain Res. 463: 296-304 (1988).
9. M. Sedqi, S. Roy, S. Ramakrishnan, R. Elde and H.H. Loh, Complementary DNA cloning of a μ-opioid receptor from rat peritoneal macrophages, Biochem. Biophys. Res. Com. 209: 563-574 (1995).
10. L. Wang and A. R. Gintzler, Morphine tolerance and physical dependence: reversal of opioid inhibition to enhancement of cAMP formation, J. Neurochem. 64: 1102-1106 (1995).
11. F.L. Renaud, I. Colón, J. Lebrón, N. Ortiz, F. Rodríguez and C. Cadilla, A novel opiod mechanism seems to modulate phagocytosis in *Tetrahymena*, J Euk Microbiol 42: 205-207 (1994).
12. H.N. Bhargava, P.T. Thomas, S. Thorat and R.V. House, Effects of morphine tolerance and abstinence on cellular immune function, Brain Res. 642: 1-10 (1994).

11

PURIFICATION AND CHARACTERIZATION OF A SECRETED T CELL β-ENDORPHIN ENDOPEPTIDASE*

Afshin Safavi,[1] Bonnie C. Miller,[2] Louis B. Hersh,[1] and G. Larry Cottam[2†]

[1] Department of Biochemistry
University of Kentucky
Lexington, Kentucky 40536-0084
[2] Department of Biochemistry
University of Texas Southwestern Medical Center at Dallas
Dallas, Texas 75235-9038

SUMMARY

Primary murine $CD4^+$ and $CD8^+$ T cells and the EL-4 thymoma cell line secrete a metal-dependent, thiol endopeptidase that hydrolyzes β-endorphin at essentially equivalent rates at one of either of two peptide bonds (leu^{17}-phe^{18} or phe^{18}-lys^{19}) yielding β-endorphin$_{1-17}$ (γ-endorphin) or β-endorphin$_{1-18}$ and their corresponding C-terminal fragments β-endorphin$_{18-31}$ and β-endorphin$_{19-31}$. This endopeptidase was purified to homogeneity from EL-4 cell conditioned medium (>1,000 fold, 26% yield, a single band of ≈110 kDa via SDS-PAGE). The enzyme also cleaves dynorphin A_{1-17} and dynorphin B_{1-13}, but not Leu-enkephalin, dynorphin A_{1-9}, γ-endorphin, or β-endorphin$_{18-31}$. The endopeptidase is expressed constitutively in EL-4 cells and upon anti-CD3 activation of $CD4^+$ and $CD8^+$ T cells. Based on cleavage sites identified in a number of opioid peptide substrates, it can be concluded that the enzyme exhibits a complex specificity with a preference for cleaving on the amino side of hydrophobic or basic residues of larger peptide substrates. The presence of such an extracellularly acting peptidase clearly could be important in attenuating or

---

* Abbreviations used. PMSF = phenylmethylsulfonyl fluoride; PCMB = para-chloromercuribenzoic Acid; DTNB = 5,5'-dithio-bis(2-Nitrobenzoic Acid); EDTA = ethylenediaminetetraacetic acid; EGTA = ethylene glycol-bis (β-aminoethyl ether) N,N,N',N' tetraacetic acid; GEMSA = guanidino ethylmercaptosuccinic acid, cFP = N-1-(R,S)-carboxy-3-phenyl-propyl, pAB = para aminobenzoate, LDH = lactate dehydrogenase, SDS-PAGE = sodium dodecysulfate polyacrylamide gel electrophoresis, GRF = growth hormone releasing factor, $C_{12}E_8$ = N-dodecyl octaethylene glycol monoether.

† Send correspondence regarding this manuscript to: Dr. G. Larry Cottam, Department of Biochemistry, The University of Texas Southwestern Medical Center at Dallas, 5323 Harry Hines Blvd., Dallas, Texas 75235-9038. Voice: (214) 648-3332; Fax: (214) 648-8856; e-mail: Cottam@utsw.swmed.edu.

modifying the biological activity of opioid peptides in their role as extracellular chemical signals between cells.

INTRODUCTION

In vivo many peptide hormones, neuromodulators, and growth factors function as chemical signals that serve to communicate between cells or systems such as the neurological and immune systems. Membrane bound ectoenzymes or soluble peptidases present outside cells that perform extracellular processing of these peptide signals may have a key role in extracellular regulation of peptidergic signaling. We recently reported that anti-CD3 antibody activated murine $CD4^+$ and $CD8^+$ spleen T cells and the EL-4 thymoma cell line metabolize β-endorphin to β-endorphin$_{1-17}$ (γ-endorphin), β-endorphin$_{1-18}$, and their corresponding C-terminal peptides, and that the endopeptidase catalyzing this reaction might be secreted (Miller et al, 1994, 1995). Here we report the purification and characterization of the secreted endopeptidase that hydrolyzes β-endorphin from EL-4 cells. This peptidase, which also is expressed by activated primary T cells, may have an important regulatory role in modulating the effects of β-endorphin in the immune system.

MATERIALS AND METHODS

Chemicals. Human β-endorphin$_{1-31}$, γ-endorphin, dynorphins A $(_{1-5})$, $(_{1-6})$, $(_{1-7})$, $(_{1-8})$, $(_{1-9})$, $(_{1-10})$, $(_{1-13})$, $(_{1-17})$, $(_{3-8})$, and α -neo-endorphin, were purchased from Bachem (CA). GEMSA was obtained from Calbiochem. Cyclosporin A was from Sandoz Pharmaceuticals (East Hanover, NJ). N-dodecyl octaethylene glycol monoether ($C_{12}E_8$) was a generous gift from Quantum Chemical Corp. All other reagents and peptides were purchased from Sigma Chemical Co. (St. Louis, MO) unless otherwise specified.

β-Endorphin Endopeptidase Activity. β-endorphin endopeptidase activity was assayed by HPLC using either the disappearance of β-endorphin or the appearance of γ-endorphin. Reaction mixtures (100 μl total volume) containing β-endorphin (30 mM), NaCl (50 mM), Tris-HCl, (80 mM, pH 7.5) were initiated by addition of enzyme and incubation at 37° C. Reactions were terminated at timed intervals by the addition of 5% trifluoroacetic acid and heating for 2 min at 100° C. Peptide products were separated on a Vydac C-4 reverse phase column using a linear gradient of 5 to 75% acetonitrile in 0.10% trifluoroacetic acid with a flow rate of 1 ml/min for 1hr, detected by absorbance at 214 nm, and quantitated from integrated peak area. Standard curves were constructed using authentic standards of β-endorphin and γ-endorphin.

Cell Culture and Endopeptidase Purification. EL-4 cells were cultured (0.25 x 10^6 cells per ml) in RPMI 1640 supplemented with 5% fetal bovine serum at 37° C, using a humidified incubator containing 10% CO_2 in the gas phase. To prepare conditioned medium used for the purification of the β-endorphin endopeptidase, EL 4 cells (2 x 10^{10}) were harvested by centrifugation and washed with Hank's balanced salt solution supplemented with 45 mM sodium phosphate buffer, pH 7.4, (HBSS), then resuspended in HBSS (5x10^6 cell per ml) and incubation for 2 to 3 days. Conditioned medium was separated from the cell pellet by centrifugation and the b-endorphin endopeptidase activity in both the conditioned medium and the cell pellet were determined. Cell viability was determined by trypan blue exclusion. The conditioned medium was concentrated and desalted (40 mM Tris-HCl, pH 7.5) with an Amicon concentrator using a YM 30 membrane and centrifuged (40,000 g for

20 min) to remove denatured proteins and cell debris before absorption on a 15 ml Accell Plus QMA anion exchange column. The β-endorphin endopeptidase activity was eluted with a linear gradient of NaCl (0 to 0.4 M) in 40 mM Tris-HCl buffer, pH 7.5. The endopeptidase activity was then separated using a 35 ml Toyopearl Butyl-650S column (ToSoHAAS) and a linear gradient of ammonium sulfate (20 to 0%). The final purification step was to fractionate the β-endorphin endopeptidase activity by size using a Sephadex-200 gel-filtration column (40 mM Tris-HCl buffer, pH 7.5).

Substrate Specificity, Kinetics and Identification of Bond Cleavages. Reaction mixtures containing the peptide substrate (100 mM), NaCl (50 mM), Tris-HCl (80 mM, pH 7.5), and the purified enzyme in a total volume of 100 μl were incubated (0 to 6 hr) before determining the β-endorphin endopeptidase activity. To identify specific bonds cleaved the peptides produced were collected and their N-terminal sequence determined by automated Edman degradation (Applied Biosystems Model 120A system).

RESULTS

Purification of a β-Endorphin Endopeptidase Secreted from EL-4 Cells

The β-endorphin endopeptidase activity in both the cell free conditioned media and in the El 4 cell pellet was determined. Over 95% of the total β-endorphin endopeptidase activity was in the cell free conditioned media yet all of the lactate dehydrogenase, a cytosolic enzyme, remained in the cell pellet. These observations coupled with the facts that there was no cell loss and trypan blue exclusion assays indicated that >95% of the cells were viable, these results imply that the β-endorphin endopeptidase is secreted. To determine whether the endopeptidase in the EL-4 cell pellet is membrane bound or a soluble enzyme, the cells harvested by centrifugation were sonicated and separated into soluble and membrane fractions by centrifugation with the $C_{12}E_8$ detergent added to solubilize proteins in the membrane fraction prior to performing assays. All of the β-endorphin endopeptidase activity was found in the soluble cell fraction.

The β-endorphin endopeptidase was purified from the conditioned medium using anion-exchange, hydrophobic, and molecular sieve chromatography procedures. Starting with $2x10^{10}$ cells secreting 123 mg of protein in the conditioned medium, 30 μg of purified enzyme was obtained in 26% yield, with an overall purification of approximately 1,000 fold and a final specific activity of 977 nmol of β-endorphin hydrolyzed per min per mg of enzyme protein. This endopeptidase represents ~0.1% of the secreted proteins. The purified enzyme exhibited a single protein band when analyzed by SDS-PAGE, with a molecular weight of 110 kDa.

HPLC analysis of β-endorphin metabolism by the secreted endopeptidase revealed β-endorphin$_{1\text{-}17}$ (γ-endorphin) and β-endorphin$_{1\text{-}18}$ as major metabolites. There was some further metabolism of these products in unfractionated media, however, after the first anion exchange chromatography step, γ-endorphin formation was linear and stable and was used as a measure of enzyme activity. Therefore, the initial activity for the endopeptidase is slightly under-estimated.

Characterization of the Purified β-Endorphin Endopeptidase

Metallo Thiol Endopeptidase. β-Endorphin hydrolysis was completely inhibited by the metal chelators 1,10-phenanthroline and to a lesser extent by EDTA and EGTA (Table 1)

Table 1. Inhibitors of β-endorphin endopeptidase

Inhibitor	Concentration (mM)	% Inhibition
Iodoacetamide	0.1	18
	1.0	82
PMSF	1.0	41
PCMB	0.1	52
DTNB	0.1	22
	1.0	44
Iodoacetate	1.0	26
N-ethylmaleimide	0.01	31
	0.05	100
Leupeptin	0.5	18
	1.0	93
EDTA	0.1	59
	1.0	77
EGTA	1.0	29
	10.0	100
1,10-phenanthroline	0.1	39
	1.0	100
Aminophenylmercuric acetate	0.1	100
Amastatin	0.1	0
Pepstatin A	0.2	0
cFP-Ala-Ala-Phe-pAB	0.1	0
Captopril	0.1	0
Phosphoramidon	0.1	0
GEMSA	0.01	0

Purified enzyme was preincubated with the inhibitor 20 min at 37° C in 80 mM Tris-HCl buffer, pH 7.5 and 50 mM NaCl. Reactions were initiated by the addition of β-endorphin. Results are expressed as the percentage of inhibition of the untreated enzyme.

indicating the peptidase is a metallo-enzyme. Consistent with the sensitivity of the enzyme to metal chelating agents was the finding that the enzyme is inhibited by cobalt, copper, nickel, and zinc, but not by barium, calcium, magnesium, or manganese. The enzyme was completely inactivated by 50 μM NEM, and inhibited to a lesser extent by iodoacetamide, iodoacetate, PCMB, and DTNB indicating it contains a reactive thiol group.

β-endorphin hydrolysis by the endopeptidase was not inhibited by amastatin, a specific aminopeptidase inhibitor, GEMSA, a specific carboxypeptidase E inhibitor, cFP-Ala-Ala-Phe-pAB, a specific inhibitor of endopeptidases 24.15 and 24.16, captopril, a specific angiotensin converting enzyme inhibitor, phosphoramidon, a specific neprilysin inhibitor, or pepstatin A, a specific cathepsin D inhibitor.

pH Optimum. With β-endorphin as substrate the endopeptidase showed maximal activity at pH 6.9 for cleavage at both the Leu^{17}-Phe^{18} bond or Phe^{18}-Lys^{19} bond (Fig. 1).

Peptide Substrate Specificity. The specificity of the endopeptidase for other peptides was investigated by determining the V_{max} for various peptide substrates by following their disappearance by reverse-phase HPLC (Table 2). Of the opioid peptides examined, the endopeptidase hydrolyzed β-endorphin at the highest rate and the 17 amino acid peptide dynorphin A at approximately the same rate. Dynorphin B_{1-13} was hydrolyzed at ~3/4 the rate of β-endorphin with dynorphin A_{1-13}, dynorphin A_{1-10}, dynorphin A_{1-8}, and dynorphin A_{1-9} at much slower rates. The cleavage site in opioid peptide substrates was identified by

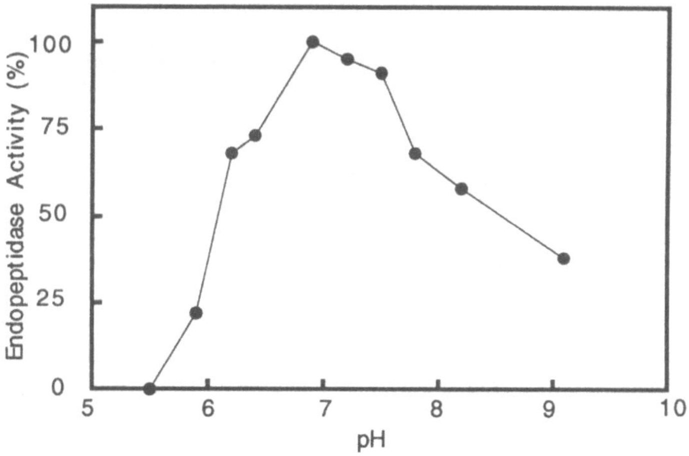

Figure 1. pH Dependence of Purified β-Endorphin Endopeptidase Activity. β-Endorphin endopeptidase activity was assayed as a function of pH using 2-[N-Morpholino]ethane-sulfonic acid (100 mM in the range of pH 5.5 to 6.5) or 1,3-bis[tris(Hydroxymethyl)-methylamino]propane (100 mM from pH 6.3 to 9) and is expressed as a percentage of the maximal activity obtained.

collecting product peaks and determining their sequence by automated Edman degradation (Table 3).

The following peptides were not cleaved at a detectable rate: dynorphin A_{1-5}, Y-G-G-F-L; dynorphin A1-6, Y-G-G-F-L-R; dynorphin A_{1-7}, Y-G-G-F-L-R-R; Phe^7 dynorphin A_{1-7}, Y-G-G-F-L-R-F; dynorphin A_{3-8}, G-F-L-R-R-I; $Met^5Arg^6Phe^7$ Enk, Y-G-G-F-M-R-F; Substance P1-6, R-P-K-P-Q-Q; Substance P_{1-7}, R-P-K-P-Q-Q-F; Leucopyrokinin Fragment, F-T-P-R-L; α-neoendorphin, Y-G-G-F-L-R-K-Y-P-K; β-neoendorphin, Y-G-G-

Table 2. Specific activity of purified β-endorphin endopeptidase using various peptide substrates

Peptide	Specific Activity (nmol/min/mg)
GRF (1-29)	213 ± 25
Dynorphin A (1-17)	167 ± 6
Dynorphin B (1-13)	137 ± 2
Pancreastatin (1-49)	96 ± 18
Dynorphin B (1-9)	94 ± 4
β-endorphin (1-31)	71 ± 13
Insulin B Chain	71 ± 13
Dynorphin A (1-13)	34 ± 1
Dynorphin A (1-10)	34 ± 1
Dynorphin A (1-8)	6 ± 0.2
Dynorphin A (1-9)	3 ± 0.1
$Met^5Arg^{6,7}Val^8Gly^9$ Enk	3 ± 0.1

The indicated peptide substrate (0.1 mM) was incubated (37° C) in a reaction mixture (100 μl total volume) containing purified enzyme (0.1-3 μg), Tris-HCl buffer, (80 mM , pH 7.5), and NaCl (50 mM). At time intervals (0 to 6 hours) samples were removed to determine the rate of substrate disappearance by HPLC.

Table 3. Cleavage sites of opioid peptides by purified β-endorphin endopeptidase

Peptide	Peptide Sequence and Bond cleavages
β-endorphin (1-31)	Y-G-G-F-M-T-S-E-K-S-Q-T-P-L-V-T-**L-F-K**-N-A-I-I-K-N-A-Y-K-K-G-E
Dynorphin A (1-17)	Y-G-G-F-L-R-R-I-R-P-**K-L**-K-W-D-N-E
Dynorphin B (1-13)	Y-G-G-F-L-**R-R**-Q-F-L-V-V-T
Dynorphin B (1-9)	Y-G-G-F-L-**R-R**-Q-F
Dynorphin A (1-13)	Y-G-G-F-L-**R-R**-I-R-P-K-L-K

The indicated substrate (0.1 mM) was incubated at 37° C in reaction mixtures (100-200 μl total volume) containing purified enzyme (0.1-3 μg), Tris-HCl buffer, (80 mM, pH 7.5), and NaCl (80 mM). After 3 to 6 hours the reactions were stopped by addition of TFA and heating. To determine the specific peptide bond cleavage sites, the peptide products produced were separated via RP-HPLC, collected and subjected to N-terminal sequence analysis. Peptide bond cleavage sites are represented by bold letters.

F-L-R-K-Y-P; Bradykinin, R-P-P-G-F-S-P-F-S; Angiotensin $I_{1\text{-}10}$, D-R-V-Y-I-H-P-F-H-L; β-endorphin$_{1\text{-}17}$, Y-G-G-F-M-T-S-E-K-S-Q-T-P-L-V-T-L; β-endorphin$_{18\text{-}31}$, F-K-N-A-I-I-K-N-A-Y-K-K-G-E; ACTH$_{1\text{-}24}$, S-Y-S-M-E-H-F-R-W-G-K-P-V-G-K-K-R-R-P-V-K-V-Y-P; Galanin (Rat), G-W-T-L-N-S-A-G-Y-L-L-G-P-H-A-I-D-N-H-R-S-F-S-D-K-H-G-L-T. In general, dynorphin B peptides were cleaved about 4 fold faster than dynorphin A peptides; compare dynorphin $B_{1\text{-}9}$ and $_{1\text{-}13}$ vs. dynorphin $A_{1\text{-}9}$ and $_{1\text{-}13}$, implying that residues at the carboxy-terminus of the cleavage sites may be of importance. Comparison of the rate of cleavage of dynorphin$_{1\text{-}6}$ and $_{1\text{-}7}$ to that of dynorphin$_{1\text{-}8}$ reveals the importance of the amino acid at the P2' position.

β-endorphin was hydrolyzed by the purified endopeptidase at either one of two bonds Leu^{17}-Phe^{18} or Phe^{18}-Lys^{19} at apparently equivalent rates (Fig. 2) as reported previously with the crude enzyme and confirms that both initial cleavages are catalyzed by one enzyme.

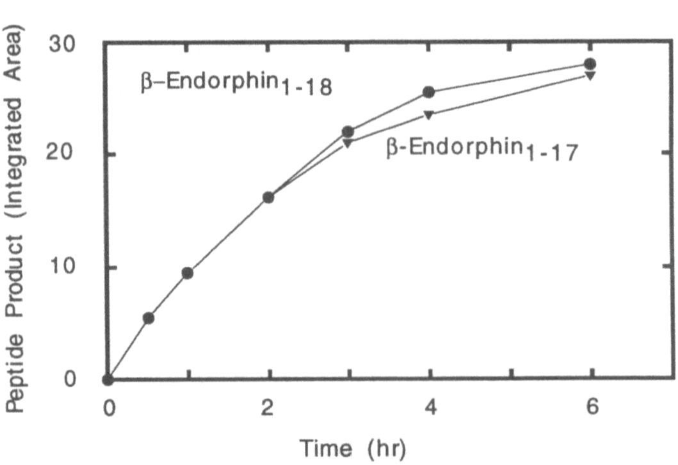

Figure 2. Relative Rates and Stoichiometry of β-Endorphin Metabolite Formation using the Purified Endopeptidase. Reactions were initiated by the addition of purified enzyme (0.1 μg) to reaction mixtures containing β-endorphin (100 μM), Tris-HCl buffer, (80 mM, pH 7.5), and NaCl (50 mM) in a total volume of 100 μl. Incubations were perfomed at 37° C and at the time intervals noted samples were removed and the apparent rate of formation of β-endorphin $_{1\text{-}17}$ and β-endorphin$_{1\text{-}18}$ was determined via HPLC chromatograms.

Dynorphin B_{1-13} was cleaved between Arg^6-Arg^7, and dynorphin A_{1-17} was cleaved between Lys^{11}-Leu^{12}.

The β-endorphin endopeptidase activity is neither inhibited by bestatin, a specific aminopeptidase inhibitor, nor does it have aminopeptidase activity using alanine β-naphthylamide (Hersh, 1981) as substrate. The cleavage of dynorphin A-17 was inhibited ~50 % in the presence of an equimolar concentration of β-endorphin. The extent of enzyme inactivation by heat was the same using pancreastatin (hydrophobic cleavage), β-endorphin (basic and hydrophobic cleavage) and dynorphin B_{1-13} (basic cleavage) as substrates providing additional evidence that all of the reported cleavages are due to a single enzyme activity.

DISCUSSION

β-endorphin$_{1-31}$ is one of several pro-opiomelanocortin derived peptides which are released from cells in the pituitary gland as well as in neurons within the central nervous system (Mains et al, 1977; Krieger et al, 1981). Immune system cells are reported to synthesize and release pro-opiomelanocortin derived peptides also (Westly et al, 1986, Zurawski et al, 1986, Kavelaars et al, 1989, Heijnen et al, 1991, and Prežwlocki et al, 1992). β-Endorphin elicits both opioid and non-opioid receptor dependent responses in immune cells (Sibinga and Goldstein, 1988; Bhargava, 1990; Van den Bergh et al, 1991). The four amino acid N-terminal sequence of β-endorphin is considered essential for binding to opioid receptors while C-terminus sequences are reported to bind to non-opioid receptors (Hazum et al, 1979). β-endorphin and its metabolites, α- and γ-endorphin modulate IL-1 induced IL-2 production (Bessler et al, 1990). Van den Bergh et al, (1994) reported that β-endorphin$_{1-31}$ and β-endorphin$_{18-31}$ enhanced IL-2, IL-4, and IFN-γ production in $CD4^+$ T-cells.

An endopeptidase which hydolyses β-endorphin and that is secreted from EL-4 cells has been purified to homogeneity. The purified endopeptidase hydrolyzes β-endorphin either to β-endorphin $_{1-17}$ (γ-endorphin) or to β-endorphin $_{1-18}$, and their respective C-terminal fragments. The same endopeptidase is expressed by anti-CD3 activated murine $CD4^+$ T cells (Miller et al, 1994; 1995). The enzyme is considered to be a metallo thio endopeptidase because it is inhibited by metal chelators and it is inactivated by N-ethylmaleimide, iodoacetamide, and DTNB. The purified endopeptidase shares some properties with a cytosolic enzyme from rat brain referred to as the gamma-endorphin generating enzyme (Lebouille et al, 1985, 1989). Both enzymes cleave β-endorphin at the Leu^{17}-Phe^{18} and Phe^{18}-Lys^{19} bonds of β-endorphin, and both are inhibited by metal chelators and sulfhydryl reagents.

The purified β-endorphin endopeptidase is capable of cleaving relatively large peptides. In contrast, other peptidases such as neprilysin, endopeptidase 24.15, endopeptidase 24.16, and aminopeptidase N do not efficiently hydrolyze β-endorphin or larger peptides. The substrate bond specificity is complex. In addition to requiring extended substrate, the only consistent peptide bond cleavage pattern observed is cleavage on the amino side of hydrophobic or basic amino acids, however, not all basic and hydrophobic amino acids are recognized. There is also an apparent requirement for an amino acid at the P2' position similar to reports for endopeptidases 24.15 (Butler et al, 1987; Wolz et al, 1991) and meprin (Orlowski et al, 1983; Dando et al, 1993) where the specificity is believed to be influenced by residues not only in P1 and P1', but extends to residues in the P3 and P3' positions.

The possibility that this purified endopeptidase is one of the lysosomal cathepsins can be ruled out by several criteria. Cathepsins B, H, L, N, S, and D all have their optimum pH below 6.0, and molecular weights between 20 to 42 kDa (Barret & McDonald, 1980; Graf et al, 1979). Although cathepsin G has a neutral pH optima, its hydrolysis of β-endorphin produces a totally different spectrum of products as compared to the endopeptidase described here (A. Safavi and L. Hersh, unpublished results).

In summary, a novel thiol-metallo endopeptidase which is secreted from EL-4 cells and which cleaves β-endorphin and other relatively large opioid peptides has been purified and characterized. Whether this enzyme is unique to T-cells and its physiological role are yet to be established.

ACKNOWLEDGMENTS

This research was supported in part by Grants No. DA02243, DA 08801, and DA07062 from the National Institute on Drug Abuse.

REFERENCES

1. Barrett, A. J., and McDonald, J. K. (1980) *Mammalian Proteases*, a Glossary and Bibliography, pp. 267-290, Academic Press, New York.
2. Bessler, H., Sztein, M. B., and Serrate, S. A. (1990) β-endorphin modulation of IL-1 induced IL-2 production. *Immunopharmacology*. 19, 5-14.
3. Bhargava, H.N. (1990) Opioid peptides, receptors, and immune function. *NIDA Research Monograph* 96, 220-223.
4. Butler, P. E., McKay, M. J., Bond, J. S. (1987) Characterization of meprin, a membrane-bound metalloendopeptidase from mouse kidney. *Biochem J.* 241, 229-235.
5. Dando, P. M., Brown, M. A., and Barrett, A. J. (1993) Human thimet oligopeptidase *Biochem. J.* 294, 451-457.
6. Gottlieb, M., and Chavko, M. (1987) Silver staining of native and denatured eucaryotic DNA in agarose gels *Anal. Biochem.* 165, 33-37.
7. Graf, L., Kenessey, A., Patthy, A., Grynbaum, A., Marks, N., and Lajtha A. (1979) Cathepsin D generates gamma-endorphin from beta-endorphin. *Arch. Biochem. Biophys.* 193, 101-109.
8. Hames, B.D. (1981) *Introduction to PAGE, in Gel Electrophoresis of Protein: A Practical Approach*, Hames B.D. and Rickwood D. eds, pp 1-86. IRL Press, London.
9. Hazum, E., Chang, K-J., Cuatrescasas, P. (1979) Specific nonopiate receptors for β-endorphin. *Science* 205, 1033-1035.
10. Heijen, C.J., Kavelaars, A., Ballieux, R.E. (1991) β-endorphin: cytokine and neuropeptide. *Immunological Reviews*., 199, 41-63.
11. Hersh, L. B. (1981) Solubilization and characterization of two rat brain aminopeptidase activities on methionine enkephalin. *Biochemistry*. 20, 2345-2350.
12. Kavelaars, A., Ballieux, R.E., Heijnen, C.J. (1989) The role of IL-1 in the corticotropin-releasing factor and arginine vasopressin induced secretion of immunoreactive β-endorphin by human peripheral blood mononuclear cells. *J. Immunol.* 142, 2238-2342.
13. Krieger, D. T., Yamaguchi, H., and Liotta, A. S. (1981) Human plasma ACTH, lipotropin, and endorphin. *Adv. Biochem. Psychopharmacol.* 28, 541-556.
14. LeBouille, J.L.M., Hendriks, R.W., Soeter, N.M., Burbach, J.P.H. (1989) Properties of a Leu-Phe-cleaving endopeptidase activity putatively involved in β-endorphin metabolism in rat brain. *J. Neurochem.* 52, 1714-1721.
15. Lebouille, J. L. M., Hendriks, R. W., Soeter, N. M., and Burbach, P. H. (1989) Properties of a Leu-phe-cleaving endopeptidase activity putatively involved in β-endorphin metabolism in rat brain. *J. Neurochem*. 52, 1714-1721.
16. Lebouille, J. L. M., Visser, W. H., Hendriks, R. W., Van Nispen, J. W., Greven, H. M., and Burbach, P. H. (1985) Inhibition of gamma-endorphin generating endopeptidase activity or rat brain by peptides: structure activity relationship. *Biochem. and Biophy. Res. Comm.* 133, 897-903.
17. Mains, R. E., Eipper, R. A., and Ling, N. (1977) Common precursor to corticotcopins and endorphins. *Proc. Natl. Acad. Sci.* 74, 3014-3018.
18. Miller, B. C., Thiele, D. L., Rodd, D., Hersh, L. B., and Cottam, G. L. (1994) Active β-endorphin metabolites generated by T-cell ectopeptidases. *Proceedings of the second annual symposium on the*

brain-immune axis and substance abuse. Sharp, B., Risenstein, T. K., Madden, and Friedmann, H. (eds.) Plenum Press, New York.

19. Miller, B.C., Thiele, D,. Hersh, L.B., and Cottam, G.L. (1995) A secreted peptidase involved in T cell β-endorphin metabolism. *Immunopharmacol. in press.*
20. Orlowski, M., Michaud, C., and Chu, T. G. (1983) A soluble metalloendopeptidase from rat brain. Purification of the enzyme and determination of specificity with synthetic and natural peptides. *J. Biochem.* 135, 81-88.
21. Prezwlocki, R., Hassan, A.H.S., Lason, W. Epplen, C., Herz, A., Stein, C. Gene expression and localization of opioid peptides in immune cells of inflamed tissue. Neuroscience 1992: 48: 491-500.
22. Sibinga, N.E.S., Goldstein, A. (1988) Opioid peptides and opioid receptors in cells of the immune system. *Ann. Rev. Immunol.* 6, 219-249.
23. Van den Bergh, P., Rozing, J., Nagelkerken, L. (1991) Opioid peptides as cytokines in T cell activation. *Adv. Neuroimmunol.* 1, 189-203.
24. Van den Bergh, P., Rozing, J. Nagelkerken, L. (1993) Identification of two moieties of β-endorphin with opposing effects on rat T-cell proliferation. *Immunology* 79, 18-23.
25. Van den Bergh, P., Rozing, J., Nagelkerken, L. (1994) Identification of distinct sites of beta-endorphin that stimulate lymphokine production by murine $CD4^+$ T cells. *Lymphokine Cytokine Res.* 13, 63-69.
26. Westly, H.J., Kleiss, A.J., Kelly, K.W., Wong, P.K.Y., Yuen, P-H. (1986) Newcastle disease virus-infected splenocytes express the proopiomelanocortin gene. *J. Exp. Med.* 163, 1589-1594.
27. Wolz, R. L., Harris, R. B., and Bond, J. S. (1991) Mapping the active site of meprin-A with peptide substrates and inhibitors. *Biochemistry.* 30, 8488-8493
28. Zurawski, G., Bebedik, M., Kamb, B.J., Abrams, J.S., Zurawski, S.M., Lee, F.D. (1986) Activation of mouse T-helper cells induces abundant preproenkephalin mRNA synthesis. *Science* 232, 772-775.

12

EFFECTS OF CENTRALLY ADMINISTERED OPIOID AGONISTS ON MACROPHAGE NITRIC OXIDE PRODUCTION AND SPLENIC LYMPHOCYTE PROLIFERATION

Gabrielle M. Schneider and Donald T. Lysle

Department of Psychology
University of North Carolina at Chapel Hill
Chapel Hill, North Carolina

1. INTRODUCTION

In recent years nitric oxide has received a great deal of attention. Although nitric oxide has been well known to environmental scientists for some time, the impact of nitric oxide in the biological sciences is recent and overwhelming. In fact, *Science* named nitric oxide the molecule of the year in 1992, and over 4,000 papers have been published since that time. Nitric oxide has been shown to play a role in a wide variety of biological activities, being produced and utilized in practically every major organ system in the body. Despite the short half life and simplistic chemical structure of nitric oxide, it has become clear that this molecule plays an important role in immune processes.

Nitric oxide is derived from the nitrogen oxidation of L-arginine, via the enzyme nitric oxide synthase (NOS), which yields both nitric oxide and citrulline.[1,2,3] Nitric oxide is unstable; it rapidly complexes with certain iron-containing compounds [4,5] or converts to various other reactive nitrogen intermediates. These intermediates include nitrite (NO_2-) and nitrate (NO_3-), which are more stable products that are formed non-enzymatically upon exposure to oxygen and, unlike nitric oxide, they can be more easily measured.[6,2] Biochemical characterizations of the cloned and/or purified nitric oxide synthases responsible for nitric oxide production in biological systems have been achieved.[3,7] There are two isoforms of nitric oxide synthase present in endothelial cells, platelets and neurons that are calcium/calmodulin-dependent and are constitutively expressed. In contrast, macrophages, neutrophils, Kupffer cells and smooth muscle cells, express an inducible form of nitric oxide synthase which is calcium/calmodulin-independent.[7]

The well established finding that elevations in the production of nitric oxide by macrophages limit the proliferative response of lymphocytes led us to hypothesize that an elevation in nitric oxide production by macrophages might be responsible for the pronounced suppression of lymphocyte proliferation to mitogen induced by acute administration of

AIDS, Drugs of Abuse, and the Neuroimmune Axis, Edited by Friedman *et al.*
Plenum Press, New York, 1996

morphine. To begin our investigation, we examined the effect of morphine on nitric oxide production in splenocyte cultures stimulated with the mitogen, Con-A.[8,9] The results show that acute *in vivo* administration of morphine induces a marked increase in nitrite, the more stable end-product of nitric oxide degradation, in culture supernatants. We found that removal of adherent cells from these cultures eliminates morphine-induced suppression of lymphocyte proliferation, suggesting that nitric oxide production by splenic macrophages present in the adherent cell population is responsible for the suppression. To support this suggestion, we showed that the addition of a competitive inhibitor of oxidative L-arginine metabolism, N^G-mono-methyl-L-arginine (L-NMMA), to cultures of unfractionated spleen cell suspensions dose-dependently attenuates the suppression of lymphocyte proliferation to mitogen induced by morphine, indicating the involvement of alterations in the L-arginine-dependent nitric oxide synthesizing pathway. Furthermore, the attenuation of morphine-induced suppression afforded by addition of L-NMMA to culture is countered by addition of excess L-arginine, the preferred substrate for nitric oxide synthase, providing additional confirmation of the involvement of the L-arginine-dependent nitric oxide synthesizing pathway. In conclusion, our laboratory has the first published studies showing that morphine administration modulates the production of nitric oxide by macrophages, and that this alteration in nitric oxide production is related to changes in T-lymphocyte proliferation.[8,9]

The present research was conducted to further our understanding of the opioid processes involved in the modulation of macrophage nitric oxide production and its effect on lymphocyte proliferation following opioid administration. The first objective was to determine whether nitric oxide production and lymphocyte proliferation are modulated through central mechanisms via intracerebroventricular (ICV) microinjection of opioid compounds. There are two possibilities whereby opioids interact with and influence the immune system. One possibility is that opioids alter immune status by acting directly on the cells of the immune system. Studies conducted *in vitro* have produced evidence which supports a direct effect of opioids on immunocyte function.[10,11,12,13] Therefore, it is possible that immunocyte opioid receptors are involved in immune alterations produced by *in vivo* administration of morphine. The other possibility is that opioids influence immune functioning indirectly via opioid receptors found in the central nervous system. There is substantial evidence supporting the existence of a complex, bidirectional link between the central nervous system and the immune system.[14,15] Recently, experimental evidence has emerged showing that morphine's immunomodulatory effects involve central opioid receptors. It has been shown that administration of opioids to the central nervous system can influence immune status.[16,17,18] In addition, studies from our group have shown that a single ICV microinjection of morphine dose-dependently induces alterations in lymphocyte proliferation to T- and B-cell mitogens and NK cell cytotoxicity.[19] Our studies also have shown that ICV administration of N-methylnaltrexone, a compound that does not cross the blood-brain barrier, dose-dependently antagonizes morphine's immunomodulatory effects, whereas systemic administration of N-methylnaltrexone at doses that do not act centrally were ineffective at blocking morphine's effects.[20] Our research, along with that of other laboratories, provides support for the hypothesis that morphine can alter the immune system via opioid receptors in the central nervous system. The present study will provide further evidence for the hypothesis that immune processes can be modulated through action at opioid receptors in the central nervous system.

The second objective was to determine which central opioid receptor subtype(s) is responsible for the centrally mediated effect on immune status. There are at least three main subtypes of opioid receptors, mu, delta, and kappa, and while morphine has considerable affinity for the mu receptor it can act at the kappa and delta receptor subtypes as well.[21] To determine which central opioid receptor subtype is involved in the modulation of nitric oxide production and lymphocyte proliferation following morphine administration, compounds selective for the particular subtypes of opioid receptor were administered. To investigate the role of the mu receptor subtype [D-Ala^2,N-MePhe^4,Gly-ol^5] enkephalin (DAMGO) was administered; [D-Pen^2,D-Pen^5] enkephalin (DPDPE) was used to determine the role of the delta receptor subtype; and U69,593 was employed to investigate the role of the kappa receptor subtype. These compounds were chosen because they show greater than 100 times the affinity for their target receptor than for other opioid receptor subtypes.[22]

The third objective was to link alterations in nitric oxide production and lymphocyte proliferation which occurs after opioid compounds are centrally administered. To accomplish this a competitive inhibitor of the nitric oxide synthase pathway, L-NMMA, was added to cell cultures. We hypothesize that blocking the production of nitric oxide with L-NMMA will also block the suppression of the proliferative response induced by opioid administration. To verify our findings are due to the stereoselective action of the compound we assessed the effects of the inactive stereoisomer, D-NMMA. The addition of L-NMMA, but not D-NMMA, should interfere with nitric oxide production and thus attenuate suppression of lymphocyte proliferation if nitric oxide production is responsible for the suppression of lymphocyte proliferation following ICV opioid administration.

2. METHODS

2.1 Animals

Male rats of the Lewis strain, 65 days old and 250-300 grams in weight, were purchased from the Charles-River Laboratories. Upon arrival, the subjects were individually caged in a colony room where a reversed day-night (12 hour) cycle was maintained. Food and water were provided ad libitum, and they received a two-week acclimation period prior to the experimental manipulations.

2.2 Drug Administration

Lewis rats were stereotaxically implanted with a cannula into the lateral ventricle and then allowed a one week post operative recovery period. Following the recovery period the rats were given an acute microinjection dose of an opioid agonist. For rats in the DAMGO study, they were divided into four groups (n=5), and received an ICV injection of either deionized water, or DAMGO dissolved in deionized water at a dose of .01, .1 or 1.0 μg in a 5 μl volume. For the studies using DPDPE or U69,593 a dose of 0, 1, 10 or 100 μg in a 5 μl volume of the respective drug was administered.

2.3 Immune Assays

For the assessment of each selective opioid agonist study, the animals were sacrificed 1 hour after ICV administration of the drug and the spleen and the brain were removed. The spleen was dissociated into a single cell suspension that was used in the immune assays. The brain was placed in formalin and later sectioned to verify correct placement of the cannula.

The lymphocyte proliferation assay employed Toxic Shock Syndrome Toxin (TSST-1) to induce proliferation. TSST-1 is commonly referred to as a Superantigen because it involves both macrophages and T-cells and it activates a greater proportion of T-cells than mitogens. The use of TSST-1 in the present study, provides an examination of a more refined immune response than that measured by mitogen-induced stimulation, for it involves both macrophage and T-cells, as well as T-cell receptor recognition.[23,24] In contrast to mitogen, TSST-1 binds to MHC class II molecules on macrophages for presentation to the T-cell

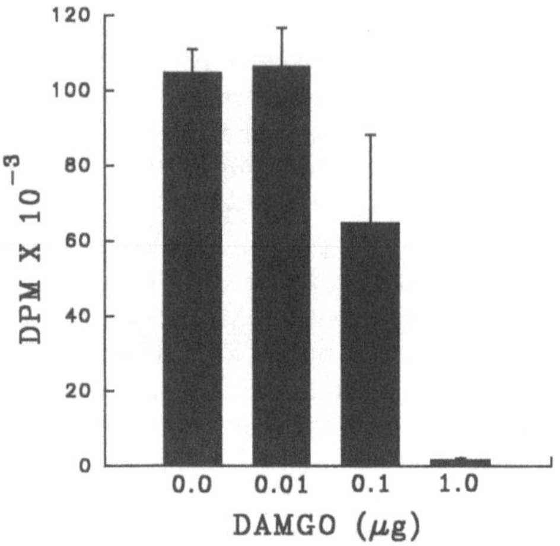

Figure 1. Rats were administered DAMGO ICV at a dose of 0, 0.01, 0.1 or 1.0 μg in a 5 μl volume 1 hour before sacrifice. Cultures of splenocytes were then incubated with 5 μg/ml of TSST-1 for 72 hours. Lymphocyte proliferation was then expressed as the mean (±SEM) of the average triplicate DPM.

receptor.[25] The single cell suspension of splenocytes was incubated with TSST-1 at concentrations of 0, .05, .5, and 5.0 μg/ml. The plates were incubated for 72 hours and were pulsed with ^{3}H-thymidine 18 hours before the end of the 72 hour incubation period. Cell proliferation following stimulation with TSST-1 was determined by measuring ^{3}H-thymidine incorporation.

Greiss reagent was used to determine the concentration of nitrite in the supernatant of TSST-1 stimulated splenocyte cultures. Splenocyte cultures were incubated for 72 hours, and the concentration of nitrite in the supernatant was determined. Fifty microliters of each sample was plated in duplicate in 96 well plates. Absorbances were read at a 550 nm wavelength using a Biotek plate reader and the concentration of nitrite in each sample was calculated on the basis of a standard curve (Figure 1).

3. RESULTS

3.1 ICV Drug Administration

For all concentrations of TSST-1, the microinjection of the mu-selective opioid receptor agonist, DAMGO, showed a dose-dependent effect. Figure 1 shows the results of ICV administration of DAMGO on splenocyte proliferation following stimulation with the optimal concentration (5.0 μg/ml) of TSST-1. The results show that the centrally administered microinjections of DAMGO induce a significant dose-dependent decrease in the proliferative response of splenocytes to TSST-1.

Figure 2 shows the results of ICV administration of DAMGO on nitrite levels in the supernatant of splenocytes following stimulation with 5.0 μg/ml TSST-1. The results show that a centrally administered microinjection of DAMGO induces a significant dose-dependent increase in the production of nitric oxide by splenic macrophages as determined by nitrite levels in the supernatant.

In the studies assessing the effect of the delta-selective opioid receptor agonist, DPDPE, or the kappa-selective opioid receptor agonist, U69,593, there was not a significant dose-dependent alteration in either the proliferative response or the concentration of nitrite in the supernatant (data not shown).

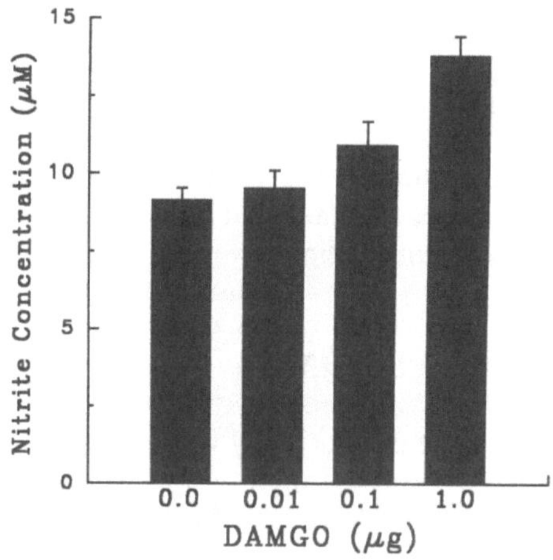

Figure 2. Rats were administered an ICV dose of DAMGO at a dose of 0, 0.01, 0.1 or 1.0 μg in a 5 μl volume 1 hour before sacrifice. Cultures of splenocytes were then incubated with 5 μg/ml of TSST-1 for 72 hours. Levels of nitrite (μM) in the supernatant were measured using Greiss reagent.

3.2 Addition of Nitric Oxide Synthase Inhibitor

To determine whether the DAMGO-induced increase in nitric oxide production is related to the suppression of proliferation to TSST-1, the nitric oxide synthase inhibitor, N^G-mono-methyl-L-arginine (L-NMMA) was added to the splenocyte cultures. These results show that for all doses of DAMGO that induced suppression of proliferation to TSST-1, L-NMMA antagonized this suppression. The top panel of figure 3 shows the results for the splenocytes stimulated with the optimal concentration of TSST-1 (5.0 μg/ml). As expected the animals receiving a 1.0 μg microinjection of DAMGO displayed marked suppression of lymphocyte proliferation compared to the vehicle-treated animals. The top panel of figure 3 illustrates that the addition of L-NMMA antagonizes the suppressive effect of DAMGO on proliferation in a concentration-dependent manner. Over the range of doses of DAMGO

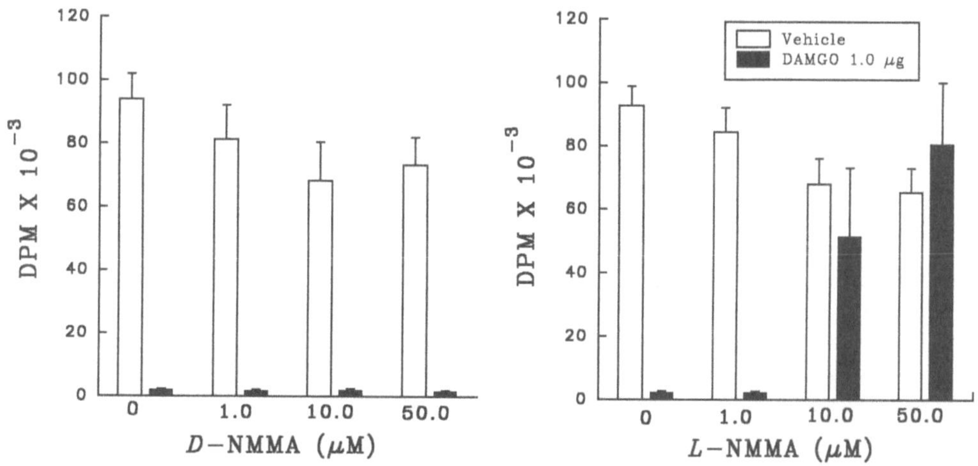

Figure 3. Rats were administered vehicle or a 1.0 μg dose of DAMGO ICV 1 hour before sacrifice. Cultures of splenocytes were then co-incubated with 5 μg/ml of TSST-1 and either 0, 1.0, 10.0 or 50.0 μM of L-NMMA (Left Panel) or D-NMMA (Right Panel). Lymphocyte proliferation was then measured in terms of the mean average triplicate (±SEM) DPM. The results for the vehicle injection are shown in open bars and the results for the 1.0 μg dose of DAMGO are shown in shaded bars.

administered, D-NMMA failed to attenuate the lymphocyte suppression. The bottom panel of figure 3 shows that the addition of the inactive enantiomer, D-NMMA, to the cultures does not reduce the suppressive effect of the administration of 1 μg DAMGO. This demonstrates that the effect of L-NMMA is stereoselective. These findings suggest the mu-opioid receptors in the central nervous system are involved in the regulation of splenic macrophage nitric oxide production and that this alteration in nitric oxide synthase activity influences T-lymphocyte proliferation.

4. DISCUSSION

The present study was conducted to investigate the effects of central administration of selective opioid agonists on splenic nitric oxide production and lymphocyte proliferation. We found that central administration of DAMGO induces dose-dependent increases in nitric oxide production by splenic macrophages and suppression of lymphocyte proliferation to TSST-1 indicating that a centrally administered opioid compound can influence nitric oxide production and lymphocyte proliferation through a centrally mediated pathway. The central administration of both DPDPE and U69,593 did not produce a significant alteration in either nitric oxide production or lymphocyte proliferation. Thus, only the mu selective opioid agonist, DAMGO, significantly altered the production of nitric oxide by splenic macrophages and the proliferation of splenic lymphocytes. These findings indicate that the mu opioid receptor subtype is the opioid receptor subtype involved in the centrally mediated effects of opioids on the immune system.

Although the effects of DAMGO on nitric oxide production and lymphocyte proliferation are dose-dependent suggesting that the mu receptor is involved in the effects, additional studies are required to confirm that these effects are mediated pharmacologically through the mu opioid receptors. In addition, studies using agonists and antagonists selective for the mu receptor subtypes should be completed to elucidate which mu receptor subtype is involved in the alterations of nitric oxide and proliferation.

This study also was completed to verify that the changes in nitric oxide production levels contributed to the changes in lymphocyte proliferation. To accomplish this we used a competitive inhibitor of the arginine dependent pathway in the production of nitric oxide, L-NMMA and its enantiomer, D-NMMA. The L-NMMA compound did attenuate the opioid induced suppression of lymphocyte proliferation in a dose-dependent fashion; however, the stereoisomer, D-NMMA, did not reduce the suppression of lymphocyte proliferation in our DAMGO treated animals. This outcome indicates that it is the disruption of the nitric oxide synthesis pathway, and not simply an ancillary effect of an additional compound that contributes to the attenuation of the opioid induced suppression of lymphocyte proliferation.

The importance of this area of research extends in the directions of opioid pharmacology and basic immunology. As mentioned, nitric oxide has recently been found to be involved in an extremely wide range of biological processes. In addition to numerous other biological systems, nitric oxide plays an important role in the immune system. For example, nitric oxide's role in infectious disease is demonstrated by studies showing that it is involved in the cytostatic activity of macrophages on parasitic growth.[26,27,28] Moreover, mice lacking inducible nitric oxide synthase have markedly reduced resistance to parasitic and bacterial infection.[29,30] The development of autoimmune disease also has been linked to alterations in the expression of nitric oxide, as spontaneous autoimmune disease in MRL-lpr/lpr mice has been shown to be dependent upon enhanced expression of nitric oxide.[31] In addition to the impact of nitric oxide directly upon infectious organisms and immunoreactive tissue, nitric oxide also has important regulatory functions in the immune system. There is evidence strongly supporting a role for nitric oxide in the suppression of antibody formation to tetanus toxoid and sheep red blood cells following immunization with *Salmonella typhimurium*.[32,33] Furthermore, numerous studies have shown that nitric oxide limits the proliferative activity of lymphocytes.[34,35,36]

In conclusion, this study has furthered our understanding of the action of the opioid system, the central nervous system, the immune system, and the role of nitric oxide in the interaction of those systems. It has been demonstrated that opioids modulate the immune system and that they influence the immune system by altering the production of nitric oxide. Given that nitric oxide plays a role in disease processes suggests that opioids can regulate resistance to disease via regulation of nitric oxide; however, it has been shown that nitric oxide can have both a beneficial and detrimental role in our immune defenses. Thus, further research needs to be completed to determine how opioids influence the equilibrium between the facilitative and suppressive effects nitric oxide exerts on immune function.

5. ACKNOWLEDGEMENTS

This work was supported by a grant to Donald T. Lysle from the National Institute of Mental Health (MH46284).

REFERENCES

1. Hibbs, J.B., Tiantor, R.R., & Vavrin, Z. (1987). Macrophage cytotoxicity: Role for L-arginine deaminase and iminonitrogenoxidation of nitrite. *Science, 235*, 473-476.
2. Iyengar, R., Stuehr, D.J., & Marletta, M.A. (1987). Macrophage synthesis of nitrite, nitrate, and N-nitrosamines: precursors and role of the respiratory burst. *Proc. Natl. Acad. Sci. USA 84*, 6369-6373.
3. Marletta, M. A., Yoon, P.S., Iyengar, R., Leaf, C.D., & Wishnok, J.S. (1988). Macrophage oxidation of L-arginine to nitrite and nitrate: nitric oxide is an intermediate. *Biochem., 27*, 8706-8711.
4. Goretski, J., & Hollocher, T.C. (1988). Trapping of nitric oxide produced during denitrification by extracellular hemoglobin. *J. Biol. Chem., 263*, 2316-2323.
5. Pellat, C., Henry, Y., & Drapier, J.C. (1990). IFN-γ-activated macrophages: detection by electron paramagnetic resonance of complexes between L-arginine-derived nitric oxide and non-heme iron proteins. *Biochem. Biophys. Res. Comm., 166*, 119-125.
6. Green, L.C., Wagner, D.A., Glogowski, J., Skipper, P.L.,Wishnok, J.S., & Tannenbaum, S.R. (1982). Analysis of nitrate, nitrite, and [^{15}N]nitrate in biological fluids. *Anal. Biochem., 126*, 131-136.
7. Nathan, C. (1992). Nitric oxide as a secretory product of mammalian cells. *FASEB J. 6*, 3051-3064.
8. Fecho, K., Maslonek, K.A., Coussons-Read, M.E., Dykstra, L.A., & Lysle, D.T. (1994). Macrophage-derived nitric oxide is involved in the depressed Con A-responsiveness of splenic lymphocytes from rats administered morphine in-vivo. *Journal of Immunology, 152*, 5845-5852.
9. Fecho, K., Maslonek, K.A., Dykstra, L.A., & Lysle, D.T. (1995). Mechanisms whereby macrophage-derived nitric oxide is involved in morphine-induced suppression of splenic lymphocyte proliferation. *Journal of Pharmacology and Experimental Therapeutics, 272*, 477-483.
10. Wybran, J., Appelboom, T. Famey, J.P. & Govaerts, A. (1979). Suggestive evidence for receptors for morphine and methionine enkephalin on normal human blood T-lymphocytes. *J. Immunol., 123*, 1068-1070.
11. Eisenstein, T.K., Taub, D.D., Adler, M.W. and Rogers, T.J. (1991). The effect of morphine and DAGO on the proliferative response of murine splenocytes. *Adv. Exp. Med. Biol., 288*, 203-209.
12. Bayer, B.M., Gastonguay, M.R. and Hernandez, M.C. (1992). Distinction between the in vitro and in vivo inhibitory effects of morphine on lymphocyte proliferation based on agonist sensitivity and naltrexone reversibility. *Immunopharmacology, 23*, 117-124.
13. Peterson, P.K., Sharp, B., Gekker, G., & Keane, W.F. (1987). Opioid-mediated suppression of cultured peripheral blood mononuclear cell respiratory burst activity. *J Immunology, 138*, 3907-3912.
14. Ader, R., Felten, D. & Cohen, N. (1990). Interactions between the brain and the immune system. *Annu. Rev. Pharmacol. Toxicol., 30*, 561-602.

15. Felten, D.L., Felten, S.Y., Bellinger, D.L., Carlson, S.L., Ackerman, K.D., Madden, K.S., Olschowki, J.A., & Livnat, S., (1987). Noradrenergic sympathetic neural interactions with the immune system: Structure and function. *Immunological Reviews*, 100, 225-260.
16. Shavit, Y., DePaulis, A., Martin, F. C., Terman, G. W., Pechnick, R. N., Zane, C. J., Gale, R. P. and Liebeskind, J. C. (1986). Involvement of brain opiate receptors in the immune-suppressive effect of morphine. *Proc. Natl. Acad. Sci*, *83*, 7114-7117.
17. Weber, R.J. & Pert, A. (1989). The periaqueductal grey matter mediates opiate-induced immunosuppression. *Science*, *245*, 188-190.
18. Hernandez, M.C., Flores, L.H., Bayer, B.M. (1993). Immunosuppression by morphine is mediated by central pathways. *J. Pharmacol. Exp. Ther.*, *267*, 1336-1341.
19. Lysle, D.T., Hoffman, K.E., & Dykstra, L.A. Evidence for the involvement of the caudal region of the periaqueductal gray in a subset of morphine-induced alterations of immune status. *Journal of Pharmacology and Experimental Therapeutics*, in press.
20. Fecho, K., Maslonek, K.A., Dykstra, L.A. and Lysle, D.T. Assessment of the involvement of the central nervous system and peripheral opioid receptors in the immunomodulatory effects of acute morphine treatment in rats. *J. Pharmacol. Exp. Ther.*, in press.
21. Jaffe, J.H. and Martin, W.R. (1990). Opioid analgesics and antagonists. In A.G. Gilman, T.W. Rall, A.S. Nies, & P. Taylor (Eds.) Goodman and Gilman's The Pharmacological Basis of Therapeutics. pp. 485-521, Pergamon Press: New York.
22. Goldstein, A. (1987). Binding selectivity profiles for ligands of multiple receptor types: Focus on opioid receptors. *Trends in Pharmacol Sci*, *8*, 456-466.
23. Marrack, P. & Kappler, J. (1990). The staphylococcal enterotoxins and their relatives. *Science*, *248*, 705-711.
24. White, H., Herman, A., Pullen, A.M., Kubo, R., Kappler, J.W., & Marrack, P. (1989). The Vß specific superantigen staphylococcal enterotoxin B: Stimulation of mature T cells and clonal deletion in neonatal mice. *Cell*, *56*, 27-35.
25. Leonard, B.A.B., Lee, P.K., Jenkins, M.K., & Schlievert, P.M. (1991). Cell and receptor requirement for streptococcal pyrogenic exotoxin T-cell mitogenicity. *Infection & Immunity*, *59*, 1210.
26. Green, S.J., Meltzer, M.S. Hibbs, J.B, & Nacy, C.A. (1990). Activated macrophages destroy intracellular *Leishmania major* amastigotes by an L-arginine-dependent killing mechanism. *Journal of Immunology*, *144*, 278-283.
27. James, S.L. & Glaven, J. (1989). Macrophage cytotoxicity against schistosomula of *Schistosoma mansoni* involves arginine-dependent production of reactive nitrogen intermediates. *Journal of Immunology*, *143*, 4208-4212.
28. Vincendeau, P., Daulouede, S., Veyret, B., Darde, M.L., Bouteille, B., & Lemesre, J.L. (1992). Nitric oxide-mediated cytostatic activity on *Trypanosoma brucei gambiense and Trypanosoma brucei brucei*. *Experimental Parasitology*, *75*, 353-360.
29. MacMicking, J.D., Nathan, C., Hom, G. Chartrain, N., Fletcher, D.S., Trumbauer, M., Stevens, K., Xie, Q.W., Sokol, K., Hutchinson, N. Chen, H., & Mudgett, J.S. (1995). Altered responses to baterial infection and endotoxic shock in mice lacking inducible nitric oxide syntase. *Cell*, *81*, 641-650.
30. Wei, X.Q., Charles, I.G., Smith, A., Ure, J., Feng, G.J., Huang, F.P., Xu, D., Muller, W., Mocado, S., Liew, F.Y. (1995). Altered immune responses in mice lacking inducible nitric oxide synthase. *Nature*, *375*, 408-411.
31. Weinberg, J.B., Granger, D.L., Pisetsky, D.S., Seldin, M.F., Misuknois, M.A., Mason, S.N., Pippen, A.M., Ruiz, P. Wood, E.R., & Gilkeson., G.S. (1994). The role of nitric oxide in the pathogenesis of spontaneous murine autoimmune disease: Increased nitric oxide production and nitric oxide synthase expression in MRL-lpr/lpr mice, and reduction of spontaneous glomerulonephritis and arthritis by orally administered N^G-monomethyl-Larginine. *Journal of Experimental Medicine*, *179*, 651-660.
32. Al-Ramadi, B.K., Meissler, J.J., Huang, D., Eisenstein, T.K. (1992). Immunosuppression induced by nitric oxide and its inhibition by interleukin-4. *European Journal of Immunology*, *22*, 2249-2254.
33. Eisenstein, T.K., Huang, D. Meissler, J.J., & Al-Ramadi, B. (1994). Macrophage nitric oxide mediates immunosuppression in infectious inflammation. *Immunobiol.*, *191*, 493-502.
34. Albina, J.E. & Henry, W.L. (1991). Suppression of lymphocyte proliferation through the nitric oxide synthesizing pathway. *Journal of Surgical Research, 50*, 403-409.
35. Fu, Y. & Blankenhorn, E.P. (1992). Nitric oxide-induced anti-mitogenic effects in high and low responder strains. *Journal of Immunology*, *148*, 2217-2222.
36. Pascual, D.W., Pascual, V.H., Bost, K.L., McGhee J.R., & Oparil, S. (1992). Nitric oxide mediates immune dysfunction in the spontaneously hypertensive rat. *Hypertension*, 21, 185-194.

13

PRENATAL MORPHINE EXPOSURE INTERACTS WITH ADULT STRESS TO AFFECT TYPE AND NUMBER OF BLOOD LEUCOCYTES

James T. Martin,[1*] Sandra L. Nehlsen-Cannarella,[2] Gary M. Gugelchuk,[1] and Omar Fagoaga[2]

[1] Basic Science Faculty
College of Osteopathic Medicine of the Pacific
Pomona, California 91766
[2] Immunology Center
Loma Linda University Medical Center
Loma Linda, California 92354

INTRODUCTION

Maternal exposure during pregnancy to drugs of abuse often leads to long term effects on physiological regulatory mechanisms in the offspring. The effects of maternal opiate, cocaine or alcohol abuse on offspring gross morphological and behavioral development have been relatively well studied (1); however, there are few studies on how maternal drug abuse affects offspring *immune* function per se (2,3,4). Opiates given during early development affect levels of brain opiate receptors (5) and pain thresholds in adulthood (6,7). One might expect these long-lasting neural effects to show up in altered cellular immune function, since immune cells employ many of the same biochemical messenger systems as the nervous system and since changes in the brain may result in altered signals from the brain to the lymphoid organs. To explore these questions this study examines how morphine administration to mother rats affects hematological parameters in the adult progeny. Because opiate systems are closely associated with adaptive mechanisms for responding to stress, we examined peripheral blood leucocyte distributions under both normal and stressed conditions.

---

* Address correspondence to: James T. Martin, College of Osteopathic Medicine of the Pacific, College Plaza, Pomona, California 91766-1889.

AIDS, Drugs of Abuse, and the Neuroimmune Axis, Edited by Friedman *et al.*
Plenum Press, New York, 1996

METHODS

Animals

Timed pregnant Sprague-Dawley rats were obtained from Simonsen Laboratories at day 12 and implanted, subcutaneously, on day 14 with Alzet Osmotic Minipumps dispensing 0.85 (HIGH), 0.17 (MID), 0.017 (LOW) or 0 (SAL) ug morphine sulfate/hr, or with no implant (CTRL). Litters were culled at birth to 8 or 9 pups and cross-fostered to untreated mothers, weaned at 28 days and raised in unisex groups of 4. The basic experimental Male rats were sacrificed at 8 months of age under pentobarbital anaesthesia, and blood was removed by cardiac puncture.

Stressor

Animals were stressed the afternoon before sacrifice, midway through the lights-on cycle, and again on the morning of sacrifice, 20 minutes before being anesthetized. The stressor was intermittent cold water swim stress. This type of stressor produces an analgesia mediated by opioid systems (8). Animals were placed in 2 degree C water in a deep plastic container where they could not stand or escape. They were left in the water for 10 seconds and then removed for 5 seconds, sucessively, for a total of twelve times.

Hematology

Blood samples were collected in EDTA tubes and analyzed on a Technicon H1 Hematology Analyzer using a tungsten light source for white cell count and using peroxidase staining for a five part differential analysis of cell types.

RESULTS

We were unsuccessful in obtaining offspring from dams receiving 1.7 ug morphine sulfate/hr, and subsequently switched to 0.85 ug/hr as the high dose. As a result, fewer offspring were available at the high dose. Figure 1 indicates that prenatal morphine exposure has no effect on white blood cell count (WBC) in 8 month old male rats under normal conditions. A different picture emerges when the animals have been stressed. Analysis of variance shows that a significant interaction occurs between stress and drug treatment ($F=4.96$, $DF=4$, $p<.002$). Exposure to the high dose of morphine prenatally resulted in an elevation in WBC thirty minutes after onset of the stressor. Those offspring exposed to the middle dose of morphine appear to respond in the opposite fashion with a reduction in WBC in response to stress.

In the rat a relatively high fraction of leucocytes are lymphocytes. Unpublished data from our lab indicate that both sex and age influence the relative fraction of various leucocytes in the blood. Data presented in Fig. 2 and analyzed by ANOVA indicate that prenatal morphine exposure among 8 month old males does not influence the fraction of lymphocytes in the blood. However, intermittent cold water stress reduces the relative number of lymphocytes in the blood ($F=13.95$, $DF=1$, $P<.0005$) and the higher dose morphine groups tend to be more severely influenced by the stress.

Neutrophils make up the largest fraction of leucocytes after lymphocytes. One may calculate absolute number of neutrophils per unit volume of blood from data on the leucocyte count and percent of the WBC's that are neutrophils. In Fig. 3, the effect of prenatal morphine

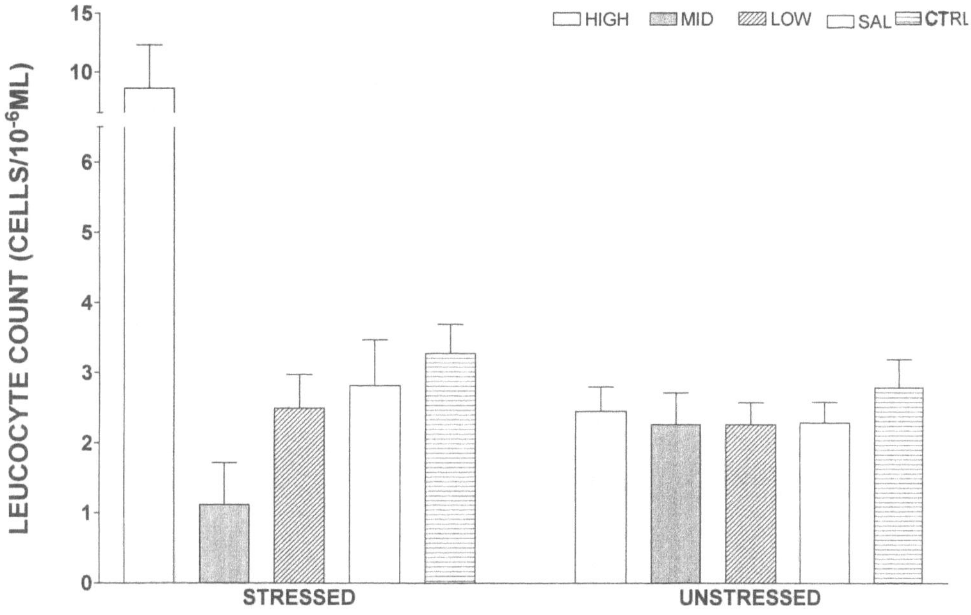

Figure 1. Effect of prenatal exposure to different doses of morphine on blood leucocyte count in stressed and unstressed adult male rats. Values are means +/- S.E.M. (Stressed N_{high}=4, N_{mid}=4, N_{low}=8, N_{sal}=6, N_{ctrl}=13; Unstressed N_{high}=6, N_{mid}=4, N_{low}=9, N_{sal}=11, N_{ctrl}=9).

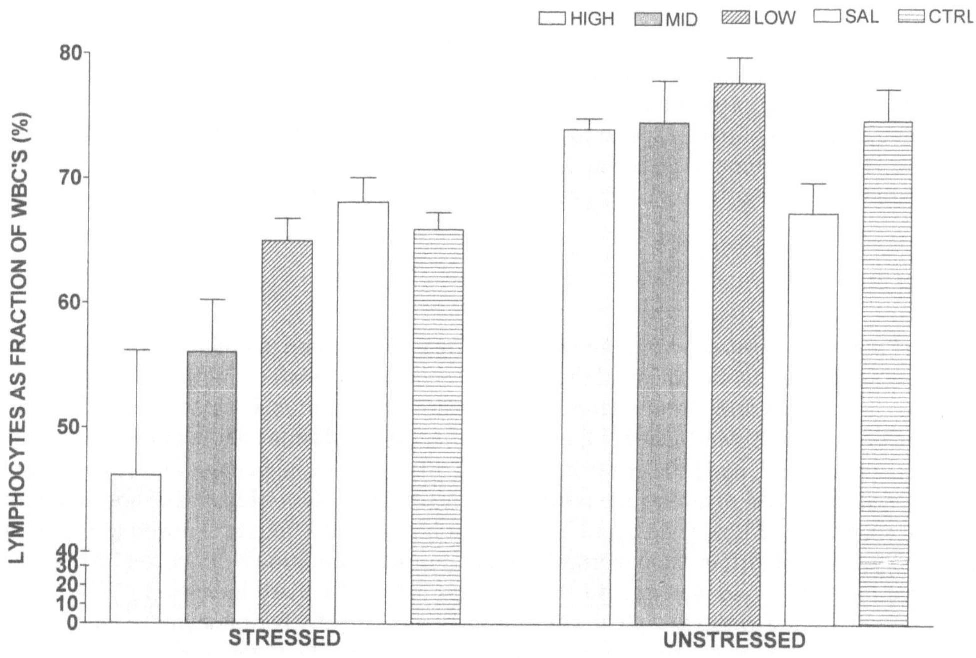

Figure 2. Effect of prenatal exposure to different doses of morphine on lymphocytes as a fraction of blood leucocytes in stressed and unstressed adult male rats. Values are mean percent +/- S.E.M. (Stressed N_{high}=4, N_{mid}=4, N_{low}=8, N_{sal}=6, N_{ctrl}=13 ; Unstressed N_{high}=6, N_{mid}=4, N_{low}=9, N_{sal}=11, N_{ctrl}=9).

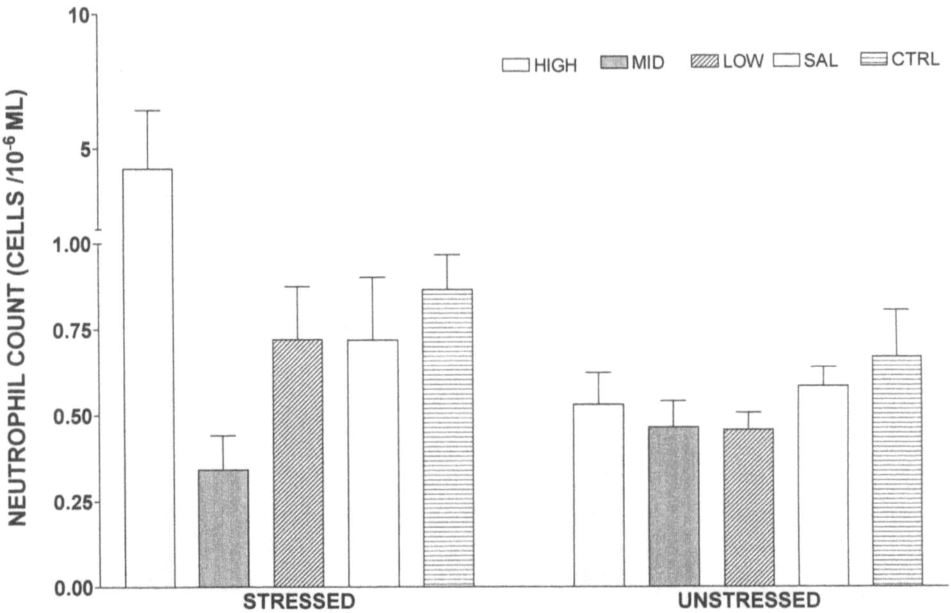

Figure 3. Effect of prenatal exposure to different doses of morpine on absolute number of neutrophils per unit volume blood in stressed and unstressed adult male rats. Values are mean cell number +/- S.E.M. (Stressed N_{high}=4, N_{mid}=4, N_{low}=8, N_{sal}=6, N_{ctrl}=13 ; Unstressed N_{high}=6, N_{mid}=4, N_{low}=9, N_{sal}=11, N_{ctrl}=9).

exposure on blood neutrophil concentration is represented. Intermittent cold water swim stress significantly elevates the number of neutrophils in the blood ($F=11.01$, $DF=1$, $p<.0001$); however, prenatal morphine exposure interacts with the stressor. High dose morphine exposed animals respond to the stressor by increasing the number of neutrophils, but mid level morphine exposed animals do not. In the unstressed condition, morphine exposed animals as a group tend to have lower neutrophil levels than the saline-treated group.

DISCUSSION

Prenatal exposure to morphine and other ligands that bind to opiate receptors induces long lasting effects on physiological regulatory mechanisms in later adulthood. These effects are often not evident until the animal experiences stressful situations or is challenged in some fashion. For example, Martin et al (7) found that maternal infusions of the opiomelanocortin product, alpha-MSH, had little apparent effect on offspring sexual behavior until the animals were tested in a novel or stressful environment. A similar pattern of response appears in the present study. Blood leucocyte count and percent lymphocytes in rats exposed to morphine prenatally did not differ from controls under normal conditions, however, differences emerged following cold water swim stress. Stress induced a sharp increase in WBC in the high dose morphine group as well as a shift from predominately lymphocytes to neutrophils. The mid level morphine group, on the other hand, failed to show the increase in WBC and levels tended instead to decrease. The lowest level morphine group behaved more like the saline pump implanted control. One may entertain several possible explanations for these results. One possibility is that the data in the high morphine group may be skewed by sick individuals, e.g., ill with a lymphoma or other proliferative blood disorder. Since the sample size in this group was very small (N=4), and two of the four animals had very high WBC's, this possibility cannot be excluded. Other data, e.g., body weight and spleen weight, did not indicate that the animals were ill. Moreover, the high dose morphine group had uniformily low percent lymphocytes, suggesting an alternate explanation may be more likely.

Prenatal morphine exposure may be followed by withdrawal at birth which is most likely a major stressor and activator of the hypothalamic-pituitary-adrenal system. Martin (9) has argued that early exposure to elevated opiomelanocortin peptides will produce a more sensitive adult pituitary-adrenal system capable of higher and more sustained secretion of corticosteroids. Since the high morphine group may have experienced the most severe withdrawal, i.e., greatest stress at birth, this group may have a particularly sensitive pituitary adrenal system. Corticosteroids have long been known to affect the regulation of lymphocyte numbers in the blood (10), and Keller et al (11) have shown that stress induced reductions in blood lymphocyte populations in the rat are due to the release of adrenal corticosteroids. In so far as prenatal morphine exposure alters the regulation of adult pituitary adrenal function, it may also modify leucocyte distributions. It seems likely that the drop in lymphocytes is due to their movement out of the vasculature rather than their destruction, since major shifts in blood lymphocyte numbers occur daily in tandem with plasma adrenocortical peaks and troughs (12), and incurring such large losses every day would seem unlikely from a bioenergetic perspective.

Dhabhar et al (12) recently found that restraint stress in rats reduced the blood leucocyte count by 22%. This is in contrast to our findings in which only the middle morphine group showed a tendency for lower WBC. Cold water swim stress results in peripheral vasoconstriction which may have blocked many avenues of escape for the leucocytes. This raises the question of whether there is a selective movement of these cells into certain areas, e.g., skin or lymphoid organs, rather than a generalized movement out of the vasculature. Dhabhar et al (11) also found an increase in neutrophils in the blood of their restraint stressed animals, although their increases were smaller than ours.

Finally, another possibility to explain the differential stress responsiveness of the morphine exposed groups involves a possible dysregulation of opiate ligands or opiate receptors on leucocytes themselves. Immune cells are functionally responsive to corticotropin releasing factor (CRF) (13) and may themselves secrete opiomelanocortins and have opiate receptors (14). It is not clear whether early opiate exposure alters these characteristics.

These mechanisms could all contribute to effects of early opiate exposure on cellular immune parameters, but in the absence of incisive data, further speculation seems unwarranted. Should subsequent studies support a neonatal narcotic withdrawal - stress hypothesis for observed dysregulation of blood leucocyte distributions in the adult, pharmacological approaches to obviate adrenal corticosteroid release in the neonate might be a therapeutic option.

ACKNOWLEDGMENT

This work was supported by grants from the National Institute of Drug Abuse (DA07365) and by grants from the Intramural Research Fund of the College of Osteopathic Medicine of the Pacific.

REFERENCES

1. NIDA Monograph 59 (1985) Current Research on the Consequences of Maternal Drug Abuse. National Clearinghouse for Alcohol and Drug Information, Rockville, MD

2. Sobrian SK, Burton LE, Robinson NL, Ashe WK, James H, Stokes DL, and Turner LM (1990) Neurobehavioral and immunological effects of prenatal cocaine exposure in rat. Pharmacol. Biochem. Behav. 35, 617-629.
3. Gottesfeld Z, Christie R, Felten DL and LeGrue SJ (1990) Prenatal ethanol exposure alters immune capacity and noradrenergic synaptic transmission in lymphoid organs of the adult mouse. Neuroscience 35, 185-194.
4. Culver KW, Ammann AJ, Patridge JC, Wong OF, Wara DW and Cowan MJ (1987) Lymphocyte abnormalities in infants born to drug-abusing mothers. J. Pediatrics 111, 230-235.
5. Tsang D and Ng SC (1980) Effect of antenatal exposure to opiates on the development of opiate receptors in rat brain. Brain Res., 188, 199-206.
6. Kirby ML, DeRossett SE and Holtzman SG (1982) Enhanced analgesic response to morphine in adult rats exposed to morphine prenatally. Pharmacol. Biochem. Behav., 17, 1161-1164.
7. Martin JT, Bradshaw W, Miczek K and Baum MJ (1987) Alpha-melanocyte stimulating hormone infusions during pregnancy in the rat: effects on offspring weight, pain reactivity, and sexual behavior. Psychoneuroendocrinology 12, 439-448.
8. Girardot M-N. and Holloway FA (1984) Cold water stress analgesia in rats: differential effects of naltrexone. Physiol. Behav. 32, 547-555.
9. Martin JT (1978) Embryonic pituitary-adrenal axis, behavior development and domestication in birds. Am. Zool., 18, 489-499.
10. Dougherty TF and White A (1944) Influence of hormones on lymphoid tissue structure and function. The role of the pituitary adrenotrophic hormone in the regulation of the lymphocytes and other cellular elements of the blood. Endocrinology 35, 1-14.
11. Keller SE, Weiss JM, Schleifer SJ, Miller NE and Stein M. (1983) Stress-induced suppression of immunity in adrenalectomized rats. Science 221, 1301-1304.
12. Dhabhar FS, Miller AH, Stein M, McEwen BS and Spencer RL (1994) Diurnal and acute stress-induced changes in distribtion of peripheral blood leukocyte subpopulations. Brain, Behav. Immun. 8, 66-79.
13. Smith EM, Morrill AC, Meyer WJ, Blalock JE (1986) Corticotropin releasing factor induction of leukocyte-derived immunoreactive ACTH and endorphins. Nature 322, 881-882.
14. Sibinga, NES and Goldstein A (1988) Opioid peptides and opioid receptors in cells of the immune system. Ann. Rev. Immunol. 6, 219-249.

14

ENDOGENOUS CANNABINOID LIGANDS

R. Mechoulam,[1] S. Ben Shabat,[1] L. Hanuš,[1] E. Fride,[1] M. Bayewitch,[2] and Z. Vogel[2]

1 Hebrew University
Medical Faculty
Jerusalem 91120, Israel
2 Department of Neurobiology
The Weizmann Institute of Science
Rehovot 76100, Israel

Research on Cannabis commenced early in the 19th century (1). On the chemical side the investigations did not lead very far. By contrast to morphine and cocaine, which were isolated from opium and coca leaves as crystalline salts, the active constituent of Cannabis was quite elusive. It was present in an oily extract which could not be further purified. The first real progress was achieved in the early 1940's by Lord Todd in England and Roger Adams in the US, who independently isolated cannabinol and cannabidiol, both essentially psychoinactive constituents. Synthetic studies led to compounds with Cannabis-like activity, but the active component of the plant was still beyond their reach (1).

The active Cannabis constituent, Δ^9-tetrahydrocannabinol (Δ^9-THC) was isolated, apparently for the first time in pure form, and its structure was elucidated in 1964 by our group in Israel (2). This, rather late, identification brought a renaissance to Cannabis research: most of the natural cannabinoids were isolated from the plant and their structures were elucidated (3); the absolute configuration of this group of compounds was determined and a reasonable scheme of biogenesis was put forward. Total syntheses were achieved for most natural cannabinoids. The basic structure-activity relationships as regards cannabimimetic activity were established, and the metabolic routes were clarified (3).

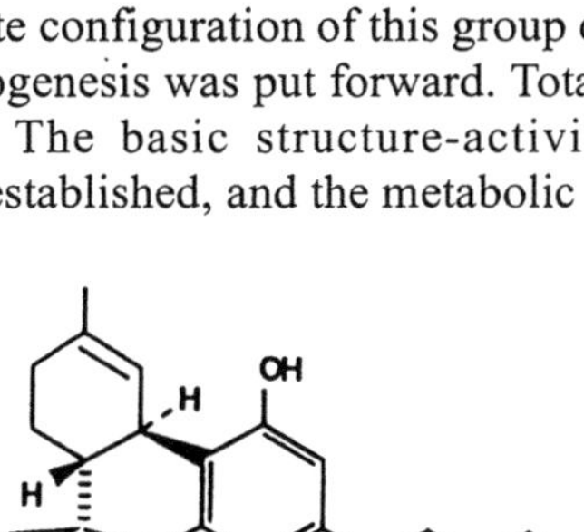

Δ^9-THC (1)

With the clarification of the chemical aspects of Cannabis, interest focused on cannabinoid pharmacology and cellular effects. Although we have learned much on the overt

AIDS, Drugs of Abuse, and the Neuroimmune Axis, Edited by Friedman *et al.*
Plenum Press, New York, 1996

behavioral effects, the neurochemistry, neurophysiology, drug interactions and interactions with membrane components, alterations of macromolecular metabolism, alterations in prostaglandin synthesis and cellular modification as related to specific effects, until recently very little was known on the molecular basis of THC action (4).

Does THC act on a specific receptor or does it produce its actions by a non-specific change in the structure of lipid membranes? An answer, at least a partial one, was to be found in the stereospecificity of THC activity. THC is an asymmetric molecule, i.e. it can exist in two forms (enantiomers) which are mirror images of each other. As receptors are also asymmetric, binding to a receptor will take place only with one of the two asymmetric components. Hence, if a compound has stereospecific action, i.e. if only one of the two possible enantiomers produces the typical activity, it probably has a specific mode of action, possibly through a receptor.

By the mid 1980's work by several groups, including ours, indicated that cannabinoid action was indeed highly stereospecific. Thus, the very potent synthetic cannabinoid HU-210 is several thousand times more active than its synthetic mirror image (HU-211) in many tests in animals, as well as biochemical ones (5). These results prompted several groups to look for a specific receptor in brain and on neuronal cells, which would bind the psychoactive cannabinoids. In 1988 Howlett's group in St. Louis established the presence in rat brain of a specific cannabinoid receptor by the use of a tritium labeled cannabinoid (6). The receptor is found in high concentrations (when compared to other receptors) in the cerebellum, the basal ganglia and other brain areas known to be associated with coordination of movement, memory and emotions. Shortly after the cannabinoid receptor was identified, a group at the US National Institute of Health achieved the cloning of the gene and established the amino acid sequence of the receptor (7). The cannabinoid receptor was shown to be highly specific for binding of compounds with Cannabis-like activity, be they natural or synthetic. None of many known hormones, neurotransmitters or other biologically active compounds of various types were found to bind to the receptor. It was quite unacceptable to most neuroscientists that the brain will waste its resources to synthesize a receptor in order to bind a constituent of a plant. The only reasonable assumption which could be made was that the brain must produce a neuronal mediator, a specific compound (or a family of compounds) which binds to and activates the cannabinoid receptor. The plant cannabinoid, THC, by coincidence happens to bind to the same receptor. In the late 1980's several groups initiated work aimed at the discovery of such a brain constituent.

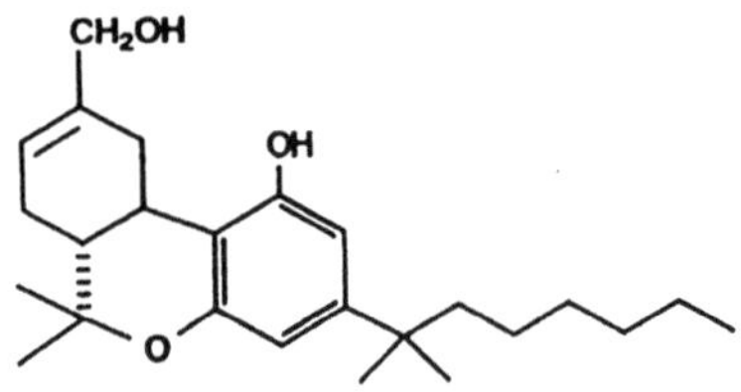

HU-210 (2)

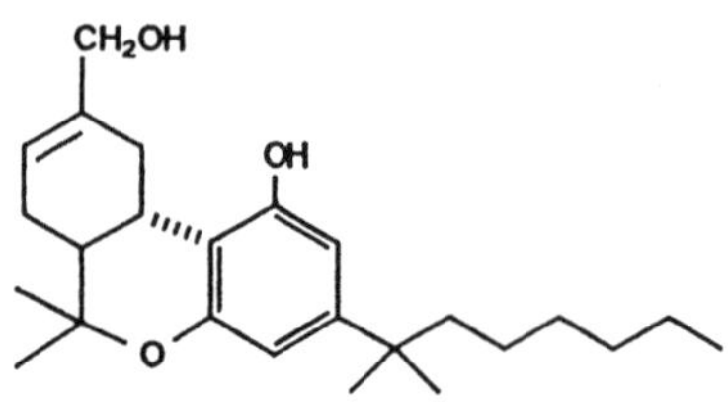

HU-211 (3)

Our group proceeded by preparing a novel, highly psychoactive probe for the cannabinoid receptor, which could be easily labeled with tritium (8). This probe (tritiated HU-243) binds to the receptor and the formed complex was used to assay brain fractions for Cannabis-like activity. A lipid-soluble fraction isolated from pig brain exhibited Cannabis-like activity: on incubation with the receptor, it displaced the radioactive probe. Purification of the constituents of this fraction over many different chromatographic columns ultimately led to the isolation of a single active constituent (9). With advanced physical techniques, such as nuclear magnetic resonance spectroscopy and mass spectrometry, it was possible initially to establish that the endogenous brain constituent was a fatty acid derivative, and then to elucidate its complete structure as arachidonylethanolamide (9). The final proof of the suggested structure was its synthesis from readily available materials. We named this endogenous brain constituent "anandamide" based on the Sanscrit term "ananda", meaning "bliss" and the amide moiety present in the novel compound (9).

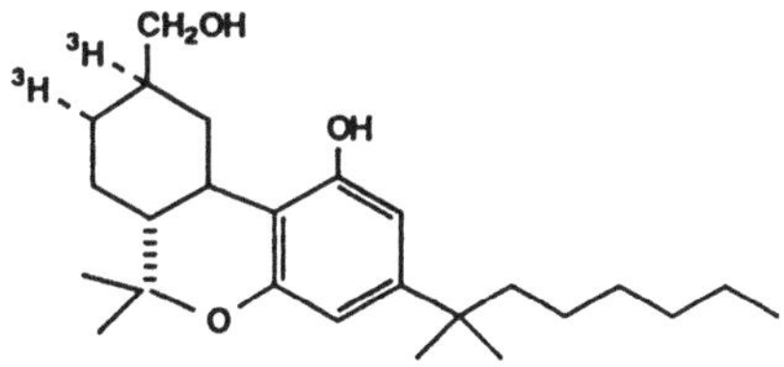

tritium-labelled HU-243 (4)

When tested in animals anandamide paralleled THC as regards analgesia, sedation, motor coordination, and certain biochemical parameters (10,11). Later, using the same techniques two additional compounds, dihomo-γ-linolenylethanolamide and 7,10,13,16-docosatetra- enylethanolamide, structurally closely related to anandamide, were isolated from porcine brain. Both bind to the cannabinoid receptor (12). The brain apparently produces a whole family of anandamide-type compounds.

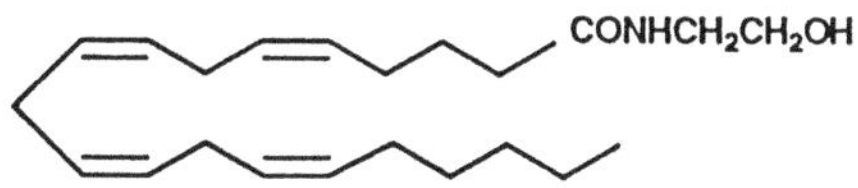

anandamide (5)

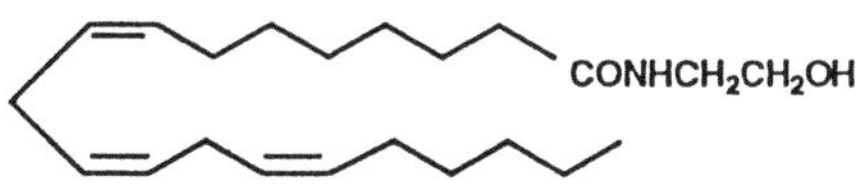

homo-γ-linolenylethanolamide (6)

Anandamide is slightly less potent than Δ^9-THC, the level of potency depending upon the pharmacological measure (11). Anandamide also has a shorter duration of action than Δ^9-THC, which may be due to metabolic factors. Indeed, Deutsch (13) has shown that anandamide is rapidly degraded by an amidase which can be blocked by specific amidase blockers.

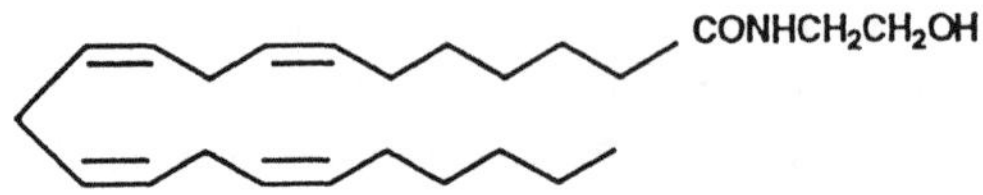

7,10,13,16-docosatetraenylethanolamide (7)

We have reported (14) that anandamide specifically binds to membranes from cells transiently (African green monkey kidney - COS) or stably (Chinese hamster ovary) transfected with an expression plasmid carrying the cannabinoid receptor DNA, but not to membranes from control non-transfected cells. Anandamide also inhibits forskolin-stimulated adenylyl cyclase in transfected cells and in cells that naturally express cannabinoid receptors (N18TG2 neuroblastoma), but not in control non-transfected cells. Weidenfeld et al. (15) have reported that intracerebroventricular injection of anandamide significantly increases the serum levels of ACTH and corticosterone in a dose-dependent manner and causes a pronounced depletion of CRF-41 in the median eminence. THC is known to cause the same activity. Hence, anandamide parallels THC in activating the hypothalamo-pituitary adrenal axis.

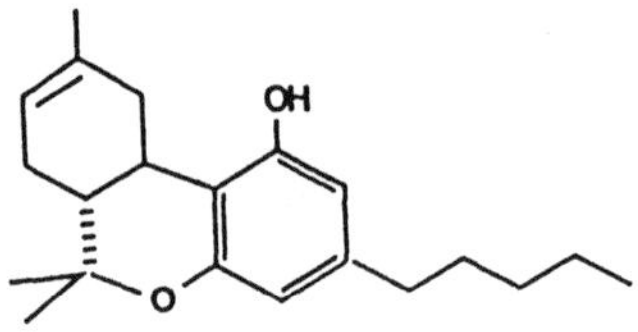

Δ^8-THC (8)

In a recent study we found that the psychoactive delta-8-tetrahydrocannabinol (Δ^8-THC) acts as an efficient antiemetic agent in children undergoing chemotherapeutic treatment. The unexpected absence of cannabimimetic CNS side effects in these young patients made possible the use of high doses of Δ^8-THC (16). We have explained this observation by suggesting that *a*, cannabinoid-induced antiemetic effects are not transmitted through the central CB1 receptors, and that b, the cannabinoid receptor system may not be fully developed in children (17) (hence the lack of cannabimimetic effects). Indeed we have found that in mice the behavioral response of the CB1 receptor is not mature until after the time of weaning (17).

A second cannabinoid receptor (CB2) has been indentified in and cloned from rat spleen (18). CB2 mRNA transcripts have not been found in the brain. CB2 has so far been found only in cells of the immune system. We recently described the identification of a cannabinoid ligand from canine gut which binds to both CB2 and CB1 (19). Its structure was elucidated as 2-arachidonyl glycerol (2-Ara-Gl). 2-Ara-Gl binds to membranes from cells transiently transfected with expression plasmids carrying either CB1 or CB2 DNA. In the presence of forskolin, 2-Ara-Gl inhibits adenylyl cyclase in isolated mouse spleen cells, at the potency level of THC, and on intravenous administration to mice causes the typical tetrad of effects produced by THC: antinociception, immobility, reduction of spontaneous activity and rectal temperature (19).

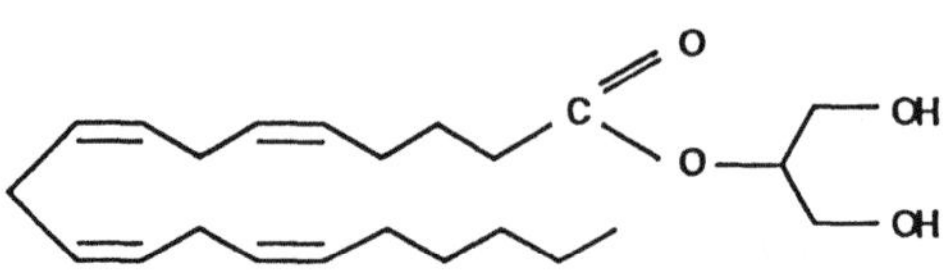

2-arachidonyl glycerol (9)

It should be stressed that anandamide and 2-Ara-Gl are apparently representatives of families of endogenous compounds. We have unpublished data that indicate the presence of yet unidentified brain and peripheral ligands to both CB1 and CB2. This state of knowledge recalls the situation with another group of lipid mediators - the prostaglandins and leukotrienes - as it stood 25 years ago.

What is the physiological role of the cannabinoid receptors and of anandamide and 2-Ara-Gl? We do not yet know. However we can make certain assumptions on the basis of the anatomical distribution of the receptors and of the activity of THC and of the endogenous brain and peripheral cannabinoid ligands.

Presumably, in the brain, the Cannabis agonists act on coordination of movement, via the cannabinoid receptors in the cerebellum and in the basal ganglia, and on memory, via the receptors in the hippocampus (20). Both types of activity are well known effects observed on heavy marihuana intoxication. These processes are very complicated sequences of biological events of which we know very little. The endogenous cannabinoid ligands of the anandamide type may contribute to the clarification of their mechanisms and may even lead to therapeutic advances.

We believe that the role of 2-Ara-Gl is associated with the immune system. THC is known to have immunomodulating properties (21-25) mainly causing suppression of various functions of immune cells. Thus THC in vivo lowers interferon production; in vitro THC modulates the formation of various cytokines.

The presense of CB2 in the spleen and of 2-Ara-Gl in the intestines (both organs with immune functions) strongly suggest that the peripheral cannabinoid receptor system is involved with the immune system. However the picture is still far from clear. Thus Facci et al. (26) have found that palmitoylethanolamide binds to mast cell CB2 and down modulates mast cell activity in vitro. Anandamide was also found to bind to CB2 but, while inactive by itself, it antagonizes the activity of palmitoyl ethanolamide. However we have not observed binding of palmitoylethanolamide to CB2 with Chinese hamster ovary transfected cells. The reasons for these differences have not been established.

Recently Lee et al. showed significant differences between the immunomodulatory activity of anandamide and that of 2-Ara-Gl in mouse splenocytes. 2-Ara-Gl produced a marked and dose-related inhibition of the mixed lymphocyte response, anti-CD3 mAb-induced T-cell and LPS-induced B-cell proliferation. In vitro primary immunoglobulin M antibody-forming cell responses were enhanced by 2-Ara-Gl. Anandamide was inactive in these tests (27). It was concluded that "perhaps centrally produced endogenous cannabinoids are most efficacious at mediating effects on neural tissues, whereas endogenous cannabinoids produced in the periphery exhibit greater efficacy on peripheral targets" (27).

Anandamide has been found to inhibit the proliferation of β lymphocytes, and to cause apoptosis. These cells are known to contain CB1 receptors (28).

A further major biological system in which anandamide or 2-Ara-Gl and the cannabinoid receptors may be involved is fertilization. Schuel et al. (29) have found that sea urchin sperm contains cannabinoid receptors and that anandamide reduces sperm fertilizing capacity by inhibiting the triggering of the sperm fertilization, which is initiated by materials from the egg. This process (the acrosome reaction) is a central one in fertilization, including that of man. The significance of these observations is again far from clear. However these findings may explain earlier observations in humans that cannabinoids impair fertility-related parameters including inhibition of sperm maturation and acrosomal morphogenesis (30).

In conclusion, the identification of two cannabinoid receptors and of numerous endogenous cannabinoid ligands, may not only contribute to our understanding of Cannabis activity, but may also open new routes to elucidation of some basic physiological mechanisms, including the immune system. The interplay between stimulatory and inhibitory messages is a universal feature of cellular regulation. It is quite possible that anandamide, as well as 2-Ara-Gl and related compounds, represent a new mostly inhibitory moiety in biological systems.

ACKNOWLEDGMENTS

This work was supported by National Institute of Drug Abuse Grants DA-6265 (Z.V.) and DA-6481 (R.M.) and by the Israel Science Foundation, administered by the Israel Academy of Sciences and Humanities (Z.V. and R.M.). R.M. is the incumbent of the Lionel Jacobson Professioral Chair in Medicinal Chemistry. Z.V. is the incumbent of the Ruth and Leonard Simon Professorial Chair in Cancer Research.

REFERENCES

1. R. Mechoulam, The Pharmacohistory of Cannabis sativa, in "Cannabinoids as Therapeutic Agents", R. Mechoulam, Ed., CRC Press, 1986, pp. 1-20.
2. Y. Gaoni and R. Mechoulam, Isolation, structure and partial synthesis of an active constituent of hashish, *J. Amer. Chem. Soc.* 86:1646 (1964).
3. R. Mechoulam, N.K. McCallum and S. Burstein, Recent advances in the chemistry and biochemistry of cannabis, *Chem. Revs.* 76:75 (1976).
4. B.R. Martin, Cellular effects of cannabinoids, *Pharmacol. Revs.* 38:45 (1986).
5. R. Mechoulam, W.A. Devane, R. Glaser, Cannabinoid geometry and biological activity, in "Marijuana/Cannabinoids: Neurobiology and Neurophysiology", ed. L. Murphy and A. Bartke. CRC Press, Boca Raton, FL. 1992, pp. 1-33.
6. W.A. Devane, F.A. Dysarz, III, M.R. Johnson, S.L. Melvin and A.C. Howlett, Determination and characterization of a cannabinoid receptor in rat brain, *Mol. Pharmacol.* 34:605 (1988).
7. L.A. Matsuda, S.J. Lolait, M.J. Brownstein, A.C. Young and T.I. Bonner, Structure of a cannabinoid receptor and functional expression of the cloned cDNA, *Nature* 346:561 (1990).
8. W.A. Devane, A. Breuer, T. Sheskin, T.U.C. Järbe, M. Eisen and R. Mechoulam, A novel probe for the cannabinoid receptor, *J. Med. Chem.* 35:2065 (1992).
9. W.A. Devane, L. Hanuš, A. Breuer, R.G. Pertwee, L.A. Stevenson, G. Griffin, D. Gibson, A. Mandelbaum, A. Etinger and R. Mechoulam, Isolation and structure of a brain constituent that binds to the cannabinoid receptor, *Science* 258:1946 (1992).
10. E. Fride and R. Mechoulam, Pharmacological activity of the cannabinoid agonist anandamide, a brain constituent, *Eur. J. Pharmacol.* 231:313 (1993).
11. P.B. Smith, D.R. Compton, S.P. Welch, R.K. Razdan, R. Mechoulam and B.R. Martin, The pharmacological activity of anandamide, a putative endogenous cannabinoid, in mice, *J. Pharmacol. Exp. Ther.* 270:219 (1994).
12. L. Hanuš, A. Gopher, S. Almog and R. Mechoulam, Two new unsaturated fatty acid ethanolamides in brain that bind to the cannabinoid receptor, *J. Med. Chem.* 36:3032 (1993).
13. D.G. Deutsch and S.A. Chin, Enzymatic synthesis and degradation of anandamide, a cannabinoid receptor agonist, *Biochem. Pharmacol.* 46:791 (1993).
14. Z. Vogel, J. Barg, R. Levy, D. Saya, E. Heldman and R. Mechoulam, Anandamide, a brain endogenous compound, interacts specifically with cannabinoid receptors and inhibits adenylate cyclase, *J. Neurochem.* 61:352 (1993).
15. J. Weidenfeld, S. Feldman and R. Mechoulam, The effect of the brain constituent anandamide, a cannabinoid receptor agonist, on the hypothalamo-pituitary-adrenal axis in the rat, *Neuroendocrin.* 59:110 (1994).
16. A. Abrahamov, A. Abrahamov and R. Mechoulam, An efficient new cannabinoid antiemetic in pediatric oncology. *Life Sciences* 56:2097 (1995).
17. E. Fride and R. Mechoulam, Developmental aspects of anandamide: Ontogeny of response and effects of prenatal exposure to anandamide, *Psychoneuroendocrin.* (in press).
18. S. Munro, K.L. Thomas and M. Abu-Shaar, Molecular characterization of a peripheral receptor for cannabinoids, *Nature* 365:61 (1993).
19. R. Mechoulam, S. Ben-Shabat, L. Hanuš, M. Ligumsky, N.E. Kaminski, A.R. Schatz, A. Gopher, S. Almog, B.R. Martin, D.R. Compton, R.G. Pertwee, G. Griffin, M. Bayewitch, J. Barg and Z. Vogel,

Identification of an endogenous 2-monoglyceride, present in canine gut, that binds to cannabinoid receptors, *Biochem. Pharmacol.* 50:83 (1995).
20. M. Herkenham, A.B. Lynn, M.D. Little, M.R. Johnson, L.S. Melvin, B.R. de Costa and K.C. Rice, Cannabinoid receptor localization in brain, *Proc. Natl. Acad. Sci. USA*, 87:1932 (1990).
21. T.W.Klein, C. Newton, W.G. Zhu, Y. Daaka and H. Friedman, Delta-9-tetrahydrocannabinol, cytokines, and immunity to Legionella pneumophila. *Proc. Soc. Exper. Biol. Med.* 209:205 (1995).
22. K.L. McCoy, D. Gainey and G.A. Cabral, Delta-9-tetrahydrocannabinol modulates antigen processing by macrophages. *J. Pharmacol. Exp. Ther.* 273:1216 (1995).
23. H. Friedman, S. Specter and T.W.Klein (eds) in Drugs of Abuse, Immunity and Immunodeficiency. Plenum Press, New York (1991).
24. J.L. Tang, G. Lancz and S. Specter, Delta-9-tetrahydrocannabinol (THC) mediated inhibition of macrophage macromolecular metabolism is antagonized by human serum proteins and by cell surface proteins. *Int. J. Immunopharmacol.* 15:665 (1993).
25. N. Titishov, R. Mechoulam and A.M. Zimmerman, Stereospecific effects of (-) and (+)-7-hydroxy-delta-6-tetrahyrocannabinol-dimethyl-heptyl on the immune system of mice. *Pharmacol.* 39:337 (1989).
26. L. Facci, R. Dal-Toso, S. Romanello, A. Buriani, S.D. Skaper and A. Leon, Mast cells express a peripheral cannabinoid receptor with differential sensitivity to anandamide and palmitoylethanolamide. *Proc. Natl. Acad. Sci. USA.* 92:3376 (1995).
27. M. Lee, K. Hwan Yang and N.E. Kaminski, Effects of putative cannabinoid receptor ligands, anandamide and 2-Arachidonyl-Glycerol, on immune function in B6C3F1 mouse splenocytes, *J. Pharmacol. & Experim. Ther.* 275:529 (1995).
28. H. Schwarz, F.J. Blanco and M. Lotz, Anandamide, an endogenous cannabinoid receptor agonist inhibits lymphocyte proliferation and induces apoptosis, *J. Neuroimmunol.* 55:107 (1994).
29. H. Schuel, E. Goldstein, R. Mechoulam, A.M. Zimmerman and S. Zimmerman, Anandamide (arachidonylethanolamide), a brain cannabinoid receptor agonist, reduces sperm fertilizing capacity in sea urchins by inhibiting the acrosome reaction, *Proc. Natl. Acad. Sci. USA.* 91:7678 (1994).
30. S. Dalterio, F. Badr, A. Bartke and D. Mayfield, Cannabinoids in male mice: effects of fertility and spermatogenesis, *Science* 216:315 (1982).

15

CANNABINOIDS AND IMMUNITY TO *Legionella pneumophila* INFECTION

Thomas W. Klein, Catherine Newton, and Herman Friedman

University of South Florida
Tampa, Florida 33612

INTRODUCTION

Marijuana cannabinoids are known to modulate immune function and to alter host resistance to various infectious agents.[1] Although the mechanism of action of these effects is not understood, cannabinoid receptors (CBRs) are possibly involved because they are believed to be expressed and functional on cells of the immune system.[2,3] Several years ago we reported that Δ^9-tetrahydrocannabinol (THC), a psychoactive cannabinoid, altered both primary and secondary immunity to infection with *Legionella pneumophila* (Lp) when injected into mice.[4,5] The drug altered primary immunity by augmenting the release of acute phase cytokines and thus exacerbating the acute phase response. On the other hand, THC suppressed secondary immunity by decreasing T helper type 1 (Th1) cell activity that normally increases during the development of immunity to Lp. In the present study, we tested for evidence that CBRs are involved in the THC-induced modulation of primary and secondary immunity to Lp. We observed a structure-activity relationship in suppression of primary immunity and an attenuation by pertussis toxin of the cannabinoid effect on Th cell activity. Both of these results are suggestive of CBR involvement in THC modulation of immunity to Lp.

MATERIALS AND METHODS

Primary Infection Studies

A virulent strain of Lp, serogroup 1, was maintained and used as previously described.[4] Briefly, frozen stocks of bacteria were grown on buffered charcoal yeast extract agar (Becton Dickinson, Cockeysville, MD) for 48 hr, harvested into pyrogen-free saline, and the suspension adjusted spectrophotometrically to 8×10^7 cells/ml. THC, as a 98.6% tar, and cannabinol and cannabidiol as powders, were provided by the Research Technology Branch of NIDA (Rockville, MD). Stock solutions of the drugs were dissolved in dimethylsulfoxide (DMSO;Sigma Chemical, St. Louis, MO) and stored under nitrogen gas at -20°C.[5]

AIDS, Drugs of Abuse, and the Neuroimmune Axis, Edited by Friedman *et al.*
Plenum Press, New York, 1996

The synthetic cannabinoid, CP55,940, was kindly provided by Dr. Lawrence Melvin, Pfizer Central Research, Groton, CT. This material was also suspended in DMSO. All drugs were further diluted in DMSO and normal mouse serum prior to injection (5). Female, BALB/c, inbred, mice (Harlan Sprague Dawley, Indianapolis, IN), 8-12 weeks of age, were used for these studies following procedures approved by the Institutional Animal Care and Use Committee of the University. For the experiments, groups of mice (5 per group) were first injected intravenously at day -1 with varying amounts of the different cannabinoids diluted in normal mouse serum, followed on day 0 with an intravenous Lp infection (8×10^6 organisms/mouse), and concluded on day +1 with another i.v. injection of the various cannabinoids. The mortality of the mice was recorded over the next 48 hours, but death usually occurred between 30 minutes and 24 hours.

Cytokine Production by Splenocytes

Single cell, splenocyte suspensions from BALB/c mice were prepared, washed, and cultured (3×10^6 cells/ml) in 24-well tissue culture plates (Costar, Cambridge, MA) with pokeweed mitogen (PWM, Sigma Chemical, St. Louis, MO) and/or THC. The mitogen concentration was 10 μg/ml and the THC was 3 or 5 μg/ml. DMSO (0.05%) was also included as drug diluent control in some of the cultures. For pertussis toxin treatment, splenocyte cultures were preincubated for 18 hours with toxin (50 or 100 ng/ml, Sigma Chemical) and then treated as above with THC and/or mitogen. Culture supernatants were harvested 72 hours after mitogen treatment and assayed for various cytokines by ELISA.

IFNγ, IL4, and IL10 ELISAs

Various cytokines in culture supernatants were measured by sandwich ELISAs as previously described.[5] For IFNγ and IL4, capture antibodies and biotinylated secondary antibodies to mouse IFN and IL4 were purchased from Pharmingen, San Diego, CA. Recombinant cytokines for standard curve analysis were also purchased from Pharmingen. For measuring IL10, a commercial kit was used (Intertest-10X, Genzyme, Cambridge, MA). Here, microwells are supplied with capture, anti-mouse, IL10 antibodies already attached. Biotinylated secondary antibodies and recombinant IL10 are also supplied for use in the kit.

RESULTS

Previously we reported[4] that THC injection coincident with primary infection with Lp caused a shock and collapse type of mortality. For example, mice injected with THC 8 mg/kg) 24 hr before and 24 hr after a sublethal infection began to die within 30 min following the second drug injection. As reported, the death resembled cytokine-mediated shock (i.e septic shock) in both kinetics and symptoms and we hypothesized that THC treatment was in some way increasing the mobilization of acute phase cytokines and this was promoting a septic shock-like death. We established that THC injection, indeed, augmented the mobilization of TNF, IL6, and IL1 in serum and that this was responsible for acute mortality.[4] Although the molecular mechanisms responsible for these findings were not presented, we speculated that changes in the mobilization of arachidonic acid metabolites might have contributed to the increased mobilization of acute phase cytokines and shock. CBRs on immune cells could contribute to this and have recently been implicated in the release of arachidonic acid from macrophages.[6]

Pharmacologists frequently use structure-activity studies to show a relationship between various biological effects and a particular ligand-receptor system. To examine for

Table 1. Effects of cannabinoids on Lp infection

Cannabinoid	Dose	Deaths	Percent Death
THC	4 mg/kg	0 / 4	0 %
THC	6 mg/kg	14 / 27	52 %
Cannabinol	8 mg/kg	0 / 16	0 %
Cannabinol	16 mg/kg	3 / 8	37.5 %
Cannabidiol	16 mg/kg	2 / 16	12.5 %
CP55,940	6 mg/kg	2 / 4	50 %
Lp	NA	0 / 24	0 %

a structure-activity relationship in the shock response, we tested the relative potencies of various cannabinoids and found that the analogues shown to have high potency in other tests (e.g., CP55,940 and THC) also had the highest potency in the shock test. For these studies, groups of mice were injected with varying doses of THC, CP55,940, cannabinol, cannabidiol, or DMSO on day -1 and then infected with Lp. On day +1 after infection, the mice were injected a second time with the various cannabinoids or DMSO. Table 1 shows mortality results from these studies and it can be seen that THC and CP55,940 at the dose of 6 mg/kg induced a 50% mortality which is higher than the 12 and 37% mortalities seen with much higher doses of less active cannabinoids such as cannabinol and cannabidiol. The mice injected with Lp only showed 0% mortality (Table 1) and this was not changed by DMSO injection. Thus, it appeared that cannabinoids with potent cannabimimetic activity in other potency tests were also the most active in the shock assay.

Secondary immunity to Lp infection is due to the expansion of the Th1 population of cells and as noted above we reported that THC injection attenuated secondary immunity by suppressing this expansion.[5] The development of Th1 and Th2 can be studied *in vitro* as well as *in vivo.*[7] For example, stimulation of normal splenocyte cultures with mitogens induces the development of both IFNγ secreting cells (i.e. Th1) as well as cells secreting IL4 and IL10 (i.e. Th2). To test whether THC could alter the development of Th1 and 2 cells *in vitro*, normal splenocytes were cultured with mitogen and also treated with THC or DMSO. Supernatants were collected from these cultures at 72 hours and the level of IFNγ, IL4, and IL10 measured by ELISA as evidence of Th1 and 2 activity. Figure 1 shows that cultures treated with mitogen only (the 0 group) produced all three cytokines indicating, as expected, that both Th1 and Th2 activities were increased after 72 hours. Figure 1, also shows that THC decreases IFNγ but increases IL4 and 10 suggesting that Th1 cells are decreased by drug treatment while Th2 cells are increased. These results suggested that THC can alter Th subpopulations *in vitro* in a way similar to the alteration observed *in vivo*.

Cannabinoid receptors are members of the G protein-coupled receptor family of proteins[8] and are coupled to the G_i complex.[9] Because of this, a number of cannabinoid activities are attenuated by treatment with pertussis toxin which inactivates G_i and suppresses receptor activity.[10] To examine for an indication of receptor activity in the THC-induced decrease in IFNγ and increase in IL4/10, splenocyte cultures were pretreated with pertussis toxin (50 or 100 ng/ml) for 18 hours prior to stimulating with mitogen and THC. Supernatants were collected at 72 hours and cytokines were measured by ELISA as shown in Figure 2. It is seen that pertussis toxin had no effect on the baseline level of IFNγ and IL4 in cultures stimulated with mitogen only (0 group, open and striped bars). Furthermore, THC treatment only (5 μg/ml, open bars) increased IL4 activity but decreased IFNγ activity. However, of interest, is the finding that the combination of pertussis toxin with THC (5 μg/ml, striped bars) attenuates the THC effect in that both the increase in IL4 and the decrease in IFN were diminished (Fig. 2).

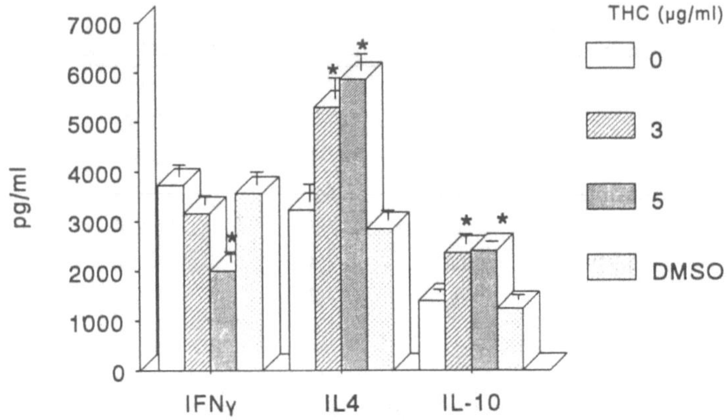

Figure 1. THC treatment of splenocytes decreases mitogen induced IFNγ production but increases IL4 and IL10 production. Splenocytes were prepared from normal BALB\c mice and cultured with THC, DMSO, or medium only plus the mitogen, pokeweed mitogen, for 72 hours. Culture supernatants were then harvested and the concentrations of IFNγ, IL4, and IL10 determined by ELISA (see Materials and Methods section).

DISCUSSION AND CONCLUSIONS

The drug effects reported in this study are seemingly disparate in that they involve on the one hand an effect on the mobilization of acute phase cytokines and increase in the acute phase response while on the other hand they involve an effect on the development of Th cells. However, some common links at the molecular level are possible such as drug effects on arachidonate metabolite mobilization[4,5] which are known to regulate acute phase cytokine production and release and also Th cell development.

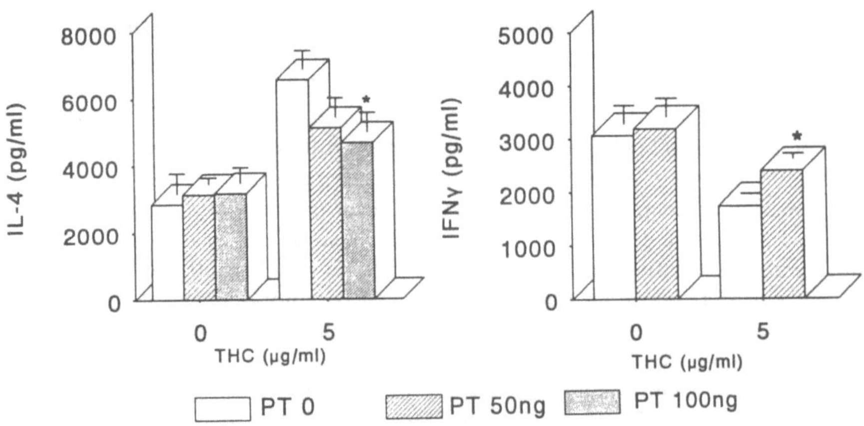

Figure 2. Pertussis toxin treatment attenuates the THC effect on cytokine production. Splenocytes were prepared from normal BALB\c mice and cultured for 18 hours with pertussis toxin (50 and 100 ng/ml) or medium only (i.e. PT 0). The cells were then cultured with THC (5 µg/ml) or DMSO (0 THC) and pokeweed mitogen for 72 hours in the continuing presence of pertussis toxin. Supernatants were collected and the concentrations of IFNγ and IL4 determined by ELISA (see Materials and Methods section).

In addition to these possibilities, CBRs might also be involved. Kaminski was the first to report these receptors are not only present but also functional on cells of the immune system.[2] He showed, among other things, a modest structure-activity relationship in an *in vitro* antibody forming assay with mouse splenocytes. The active analogues (e.g. THC, CP55,940, HU-210) were more potent in suppressing antibody production than were the inactive ones. A similar structure-activity relationship with cannabinoids was recently reported[11] comparing the *in vitro* binding potency of [^{3}H]CP55,940 with *in vivo* potency in mouse behavioral tests. This suggested that receptor binding is sufficient to mediate many of the known behavioral effects of cannabinoids thus supporting a link between CBRs and psychoactivity. To test for such a link in the shock assay, we treated mice, in the present study, with CP55,940 and THC (active analogues) and with cannabinol and cannabidiol (inactive) and observed that the former compounds (i.e. CP55,940 and THC) were more potent than either cannabinol or cannabidiol (Table 1). This suggested a structure-activity relationship and that CBRs were involved in the shock response. During septic shock, cytokines are produced by a variety of tissues and act upon various shock organs to cause collapse and death.[12] It is apparent that CB1 and CB2 mRNA is detected in a variety of tissues[13,14,15] and therefore the receptors might be widely distributed and able to participate in the shock syndrome. More precise information is needed on CB1 and 2 distribution and function in various tissues as well as *in vitro* paradigms for studying drug effects on cytokine production and action to determine the exact function of CBRs in bacterial-induced shock and collapse.

Besides the use of structure-activity studies, other approaches have been used to link CBR activity to biological activity. For example, recently it was reported that pertussis toxin treatment attenuated the cannabinoid-induced suppression of lymphoproliferation and antibody formation.[16] This suggested that a G_i coupled receptor such as CBR was involved in the drug-induced modulation of immunity. We adopted the same approach in the present study and examined the effect of pertussis toxin on the production of Th1 and 2 cytokines *in vitro*. We observed (Fig. 2) that toxin treatment attenuated the cannabinoid effect, especially the one involving IL4 production, suggesting CBRs were involved. cAMP signalling has been implicated in lymphocyte activation and agents which modulate intracellular cAMP have been shown to modulate lymphocyte activity.[17] There is currently some confusion concerning the role of cAMP in Th1 and Th2 development. Some studies suggest that increasing cAMP suppresses mainly Th1 activity[18] while other reports suggest that cAMP also suppresses Th2.[19] Our results suggest that THC treatment might be attenuating the PWM-induced rise in cAMP leading to a decrease in Th1 development but increase in Th2 and that when G_i is blocked by pertussis toxin treatment the THC effect on Th cells is lessened. Studies are currently in progress to determine the activity of prostaglandins and dibutyryl cAMP in modulating the PWM-induced Th activity and also in modulating the effects of cannabinoids in this system. It is possible that THC is affecting Th cell development by means of either a CBR-independent mechanism involving arachidonic acid release or a CBR-dependent mechanism coupled to G_i. Either mechanism could engage the cAMP pathway which although not clearly defined appears to be involved in activation and differentiation of Th cells.[20]

SUMMARY

In this report, we reviewed previous work showing that cannabinoid injection into mice can alter immunity to infection with *Legionella pneumophila*. In addition, we present new evidence that CBRs are involved in the drug effects. THC injection into mice one day before and one day after a primary, sublethal infection with Lp resulted in animal mortality within 30 min following the second drug injection. This death resembled cytokine-mediated shock (i.e septic shock), in both kinetics and symptoms, and indeed THC treatment was increasing the mobilization of acute phase cytokines. To test for a role of CBRs in the shock response, we looked for a structure-activity relationship by testing the relative potencies of various cannabinoids. We found that the analogues shown to have high potency in other tests (e.g. CP55,940 and THC) also had the highest potency in the shock test, while lower potency compounds (e.g. cannabinol and cannabidiol) were less effective. Thus, it appeared that cannabinoids with potent cannabimimetic activity were also potent in the shock assay implicating CBR involvement. We also reviewed drug effects on the development of CMI to a secondary infection and reported that drug treatment caused a shift in the normal development of Th1 and Th2 helper cells. The role of CBR in this shift was examined by studying the effect of pertussis toxin on the drug-induced changes in Th1 and 2 development. The results showed that pretreatment of splenocytes with toxin attenuated the THC effect on Th1 and Th2 cytokine production suggesting that CBR- and G_i- linked mechanisms were involved. These studies suggest that CBRs are involved in the cannabinoid-induced modulation of the cytokine and Th cell networks. However, more work is needed to define which tissues are the targets of the drug effects and which receptor subtypes are mediating the immune modulation.

ACKNOWLEDGMENT

This work supported by grant # DA03646 from the National Institute on Drug Abuse.

REFERENCES

1. Friedman, H., Shivers, S., and Klein, T.W., Drugs of abuse and the immune system. In: Dean, J.H., Luster, M. I., Munson, A.E., and Kimber, I. (eds.), Immunotoxicology and Immunopharmacology, Second Edition, pp. 303-322, Raven Press, New York, 1994.
2. Kaminski, N.E., Abood, M.E., Kessler, F.K., Martin, B.R., and Schatz, A.R. Identification of a functionally relevant cannabinoid receptor on mouse spleen cells that is involved in cannabinoid-mediated immune modulation. Mol. Pharm. 42:736-742, 1992.
3. Daaka, Y., Friedman, H., and Klein, T.W. Cannabinoid receptor proteins are increased in Jurkat, human T-cell line after mitogen activation. J. Pharmacol. Exp. Ther. 276: 1996 (in press).
4. Klein, T.W., Newton, C., Widen, R., and Friedman, H. Δ^9-tetrahydrocannabinol injection induces cytokine-mediated mortality of mice infected with Legionella pneumophila. J. Pharmacol. Exp. Ther. 267:635-640, 1993.
5. Newton, C.A., Klein, T.W., and Friedman, H. Secondary immunity to *Legionella pneumophila* and Th1 activity are suppressed by delta-9-tetrahydrocannabinol injection. Infect. Immun. 62:4015-4020, 1994.
6. Burstein, S., Budrow, J., Debatis, M., Hunter, S.A., and Subramanian, A. Phopholipase participation in cannabinoid-induced release of free arachidonic acid. Biochem. Pharmacol. 48:1253-1264, 1994.
7. Clerici, M. and Shearer, G.M. A Th1 to Th2 switch is a critical step in the etiology of HIV infection. Immunol. Today 14: 107-111, 1993.
8. Matsuda, L.A., Lolait, S.J., Brownstein, M.J., Young, A.C., and Bonner, T.I. Structure of a cannabinoid receptor and functional expression of the cloned cDNA. Nature 346:561-546, 1990.
9. Howlett, A.C. Inhibition of neuroblastoma adenylate cyclase by cannabinoid and nantradol compounds. Life Sci. 35:1803-1810, 1984.
10. Howlett, A.C., Qualy, J.M., and Khachatrian, L.L. Involvement of G_i in the inhibition of adenylate cyclase by cannabimimetic drugs. Mol. Pharm. 29: 307-313, 1986.
11. Compton, D.R., Rice, K.C., De Costa, B.R., Razdan, R.K., Melvin, L.S., Johnson, M.R., and Martin, B.R. Cannabinoid structure-activity relationships: correlation of receptor binding and *in vivo* activities. J. Pharmacol. Exp. Ther. 265:218-226, 1993.
12. Tracey, K.J. and Lowry, S.F. The role of cytokine mediators in septic shock. Adv. Surg. 23: 21-56, 1990.

13. Munro, S. Thomas, K.L., and Abu-Shaar, M. Molecular characterization of a peripheral receptor for cannabinoids. Nature 365: 61-65, 1993.
14. Shire, D., Carillon, C., Kaghad, M., Calandra, B., Rinaldi-Carmona, M., Le Fur, G., Caput, D., and Ferrara, P. An amino-terminal variant of the central cannabinoid receptor resulting from alternative splicing. J. Biol. Chem. 270: 3726-3731, 1995.
15. Galieque, S., Mary, S., Marchand, J., Dussossoy, D, Carriere, D., Carayon, P., Bouaboula, M., Shire, D., Le Fur, G., and Casellas, P. Expression of central and peripheral cannabinoid receptors in human immune tissues and leukocyte subpopulations. Eur. J. Biochem. 232: 54-61, 1995.
16. Kaminski, N., Koh, W.S., Yang, K.H., Lee, M., and Kessler, F.K. Suppression of the humoral immune response by cannabinoids is partially mediated through inhibition of adenylate cyclase by a pertussis toxin-sensitive G-protein coupled mechanism. Biochem. Pharm. 48:1899-1908, 1994.
17. Kammer, G.M. The adenylate cyclase-cAMP-protein kinase A pathway and regulation of the immune response. Immunol. Today 9:222-229, 1988.
18. Betz, M. and Fox, B.S. Prostaglandin E_2 inhibits production of Th1 lymphokines but not of Th2 lymphokines. J. Immunol. 146: 108-113, 1991.
19. Parker, C.W., Huber, M.G., and Godt, S.M. Modulation of IL4 production in murine spleen cells by prostaglandins. Cell. Immunol. 160: 278-285, 1995.
20. Stam, W.B., Van Oosterhout, A.J.M., and Nijkamp, F.P. Minireview:Pharmacologic modulation of Th1- and Th2-associated lymphokine production. Life Sci. 53:1921-1934, 1993.

CANNABINOIDS AND INTERLEUKIN-6 ENHANCE THE RESPONSE TO NMDA IN DEVELOPING CNS NEURONS

D. L. Gruol,* J. G. Netzeband, Z. Qiu, I. L. Campbell, and K. L. Parsons

Department Neuropharmacology
The Scripps Research Institute, La Jolla, California 92037

INTRODUCTION

Maternal cannabinoid use during pregnancy is harmful to the central nervous system (CNS) of the developing infant[12]. Cannabinoids pass easily from the mother to the fetus, where they can access neuronal receptors in the developing CNS. Cannabinoid receptors are known to be expressed by CNS neurons, although their role in normal brain functions has yet to be defined. It is likely that these receptors mediate some form of intercellular signaling, since biochemicals endogenous to the CNS (e.g., anandamide) [5] have been shown to act at CNS cannabinoid receptors.[4] Cannabinoid receptors are expressed during the main period of morphological and physiological development of the CNS,[11] a correlation that may reflect a role in the developmental process. Hyperactivation of these receptors by maternal cannabinoid use could lead to a disruption of the normal signaling pattern and, consequently, altered development and permanent changes in CNS function.

Effects of cannabinoids on the developing CNS may be particularly damaging when combined with other neurotoxic insults such as those occurring with human immunodeficiency virus (HIV) infection. HIV infection during early development produces a variety of neurologic disorders, that are thought to be caused directly or indirectly by viral infection of the CNS.[8] HIV infection presumably interferes with one or more of the processes involved in normal CNS development, although the toxic factors and their sites and mechanisms of action are still under investigation. HIV infection in the CNS occurs predominantly in the macrophage or microglial cells and only rarely in the neuronal or glial population.[8] One postulated mechanism of HIV-induced neuropathology is that the infected macrophages/microglia release cytokines that are toxic and impair or alter neuronal or glial cell function.[8] The cytokine interleukin-6 (IL-6) is known to be elevated in the CNS of HIV infected individuals[7] and may be a mediator of CNS

* Correspondence to: Dr. Donna Gruol, Department of Neuropharmacology, CVN 11, The Scripps Research Institute, 10666 North Torrey Pines Road, La Jolla, CA 92037, Phone: (619) 784-7060; Fax: (619) 784-7393; email: gruol@riscsm.scripps.edu.

damage and dysfunction in HIV-infected individuals. Consistent with this possibility, overexpression of IL-6 in the CNS of transgenic mice causes extensive CNS pathology that becomes more evident with maturation, especially in the cerebellar region of the CNS.[1]

The combination of HIV infection and drug use is likely to have complex and perhaps widespread effects on the constantly changing substratum of the developing CNS. However, few studies have addressed this issue. As a first approach to this problem, we are assessing the actions of IL-6 and cannabinoids, alone and in combination, on the physiological properties of developing CNS neurons. For these studies we are using a model system, primary cultures of cerebellar granule neurons obtained from rats and transgenic mice. The cerebellar granule neurons express both IL-6[6] and cannabinoid receptors,[2] making them an ideal CNS preparation to examine the neuronal actions and interactions of these agents. The current studies focus on IL-6 and cannabinoids effects on calcium signaling elicited by stimulation with N-methyl-D-aspartate (NMDA), an agonist at the NMDA subtype of glutamate receptor. Glutamate is the main excitatory transmitter in the CNS and is thought to play a critical role in neuronal development, particularly through NMDA receptors.[10] Calcium signaling linked to NMDA receptors is a major pathway for calcium to enter the cell, where it serves as an important second messenger.

METHODS

Granule neuron cultures were prepared from 8 day postnatal rat pups or 10 day postnatal transgenic mouse pups according to our standard methods.[13] Briefly, granule neurons were dissociated by enzymatic treatment and plated on coverglasses (~10^6 cell/ml) in medium containing DMEM/F12 plus 10% horse serum and supplemented with 30 mM glucose, 2 mM glutamine, 25 mM KCl, and 25 μM penicillin-streptomycin. Brief treatment with FUDR (20 μg/ml) minimized the number of non-neuronal cells in the cultures. Half of the cultures were treated chronically with IL-6 (5 ng/ml; 500 units/ml), which was added to the culture medium 1 day after plating and supplemented on days 4 and 7. The culture medium was replaced with physiological saline before measurements were made.

Intracellular calcium was measured in individual granule neurons using standard microscopic fura-2 digital imaging and previously published methods.[13] Real-time digitized

---

Figure 1. Chronic treatment with IL-6 selectively enhances the response of cerebellar granule neurons to the glutamate receptor agonist NMDA. **A,B.** Phase contrast micrographs of cultured rat granule neurons (some marked with arrows) in control cultures at 1 (A) and 7 (B) days *in vitro* (DIV). When placed in culture the granule neurons are typically rounded in shape. During the first day in culture they attach to the substrate, start to extend processes, and initiate migration. By 7 DIV neuronal clusters with thick interconnecting fiber tracts have formed. These developmental changes were similar in control and IL-6 treated cultures and paralleled developmental changes known to occur *in vivo*. The cultured granule neurons are ~10 μm in diameter. **C,D.** Calcium signals elicited in control and IL-6 treated granule neurons by brief application (at the arrows) of NMDA, an agonist at the NMDA subtype of glutamate receptor, and domoate, an agonist at the kainate/AMPA subtype of glutamate receptor. The responses are from 4 different neurons, 2 from control cultures and 2 from IL-6 treated cultures. Agonists were applied (by a 1 sec micropressure pulse) from a drug pipette containing 200 μM NMDA (**C**) or 5 μM domoate (**D**) dissolved in bath saline. For studies with NMDA, Mg^{2+}-free (to remove the Mg^{2+} block of the NMDA channel that occurs at normal resting membrane potentials) physiological saline with 5 μM glycine (an essential a co-agonist at the NMDA receptor) was used. For studies with domoate, physiological saline was used. **E,F.** Mean values (±SEM) for the peak amplitude of the calcium signal to NMDA and domoate in a population of neurons studied at 6 DIV and 8 DIV. Resting calcium levels were subtracted from peak values on an individual cell basis. At both culture ages chronic treatment with IL-6 significantly enhanced the calcium signals to NMDA. IL-6 had no effect on the calcium signals to domoate at 6 DIV but significantly depressed them at 8 DIV. * = significant difference from the respective control value. For all studies, statistical significance was determined by ANOVA followed by the Fisher post-hoc test for multiple comparisons. $P<0.05$ was considered indicative of a statistically significant difference.

display, image acquisition, and calcium measurements were made with MCID imaging software (Imaging Research Inc.). Calcium levels in the somata of approximately 5-10 cells were measured in each microscopic field. Several fields were examined in each culture dish and data combined according to treatment.

RESULTS

Chronic treatment of cultured rat granule neurons with IL-6 during development in culture significantly enhanced the calcium response to NMDA.[13] Representative results are shown in Figure 1. This effect of IL-6 was specific for the response to NMDA, as calcium

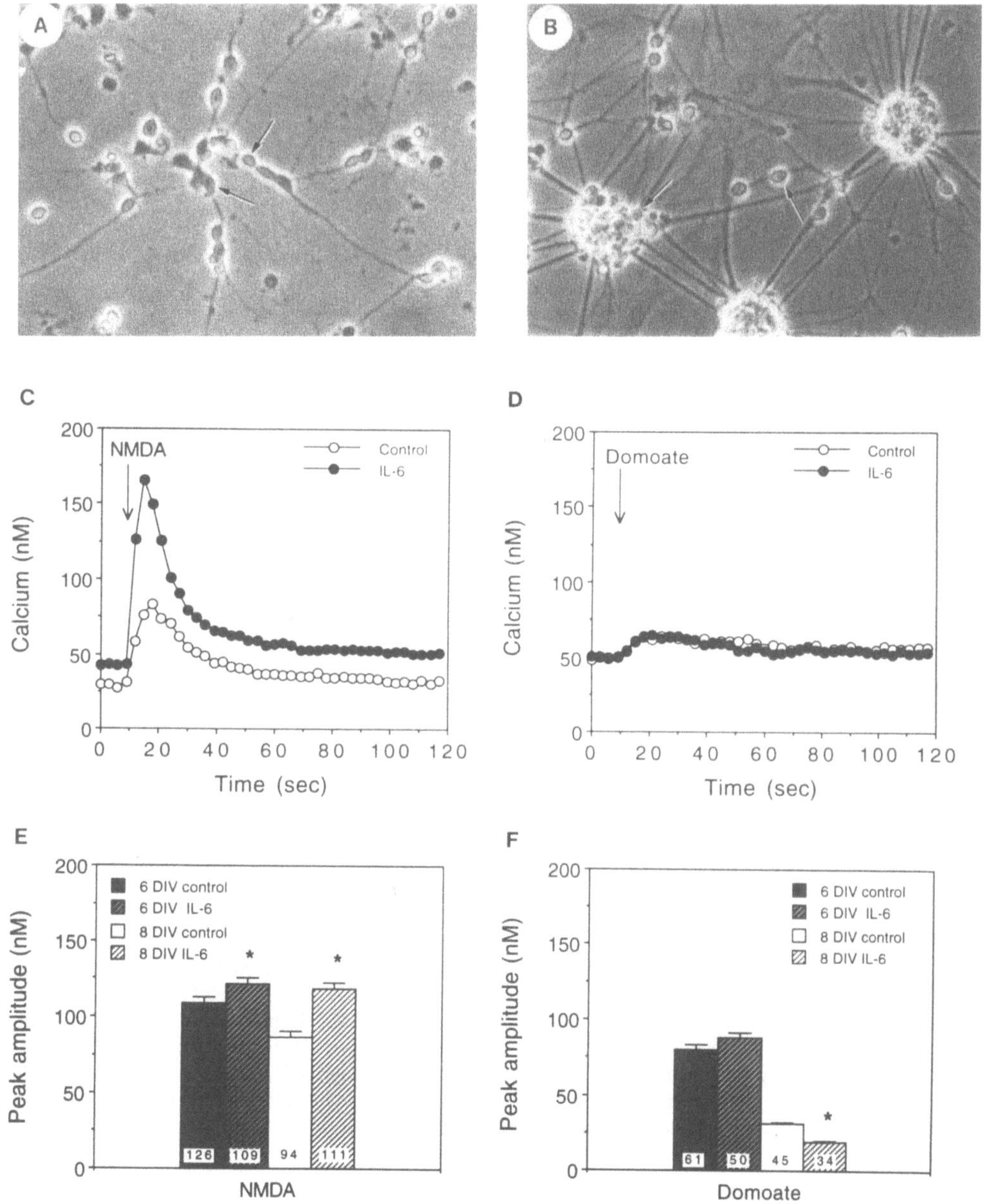

signals to domoate, an agonist at the kainate/AMPA subtype of glutamate receptor, were not enhanced by IL-6 treatment. Chronic treatment with IL-6 was required for this effect; acute exposure (~30 min; by bath addition) to IL-6 did not influence the calcium signals to NMDA.[13]

Cultured granule neurons obtained from 10 day postnatal transgenic mouse pups that overexpress IL-6 in their CNS[1] also showed an enhanced response to NMDA. Representative results from these studies are shown in Figure 2. IL-6 production in these mice was targeted to astrocytes,[1] a cell type that is closely associated with neurons. The neurons from the transgenic mice were exposed to IL-6 in vivo up to the day of culture, and possibly during the culture period, since a small number of astrocytes are present in the cultures and may continue to produce IL-6 in culture.

The cannabinoid receptor agonists WIN 55,212-2 (10 to 100 nM) and R-1 Methanandamide (10 to 100 nM) when applied acutely (~10-20 min; via bath addition) to control or chronic IL-6 treated cultured rat granule neurons also significantly enhanced the calcium signal to NMDA in a dose-dependent manner. Resting calcium levels were increased as well. In the chronic IL-6 treated neurons, the cannabinoid induced enhancement of the calcium signal to NMDA added to the enhancement produced by chronic IL-6. Representative results are shown in Figure 3. SR141716A, a cannabinoid receptor antagonist, blocked the actions of WIN and Methanandamide on the calcium signal to NMDA (data not shown), suggesting the involvement of the CNS cannabinoid receptor. However, these experiments were complicated by agonist activity of the antagonist.

DISCUSSION

Results from the current studies show that calcium signaling to NMDA stimulation is significantly enhanced by exposure to cannabinoids and IL-6 in developing CNS neurons.

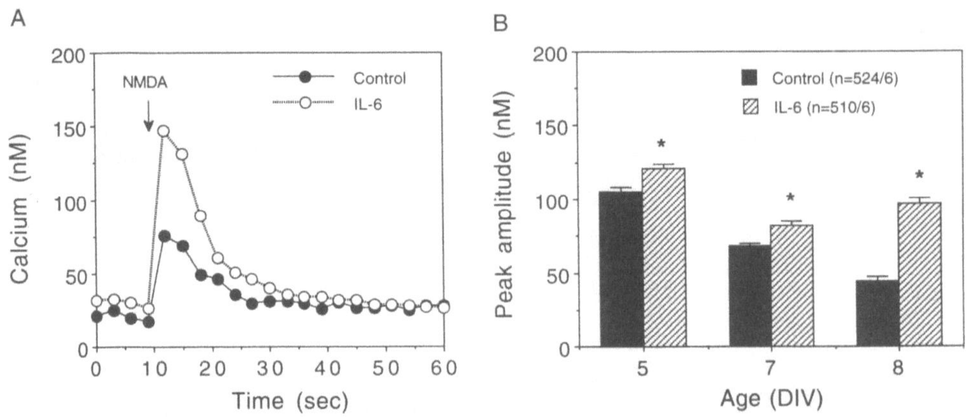

Figure 2. Cultured granule neurons from transgenic mice that overexpress interleukin-6 in the CNS show an enhanced response to NMDA. **A.** Calcium signals elicited by NMDA in granule neurons from a control and IL-6 transgenic mouse (IL-6) and maintained in culture for 8 days. NMDA was applied by a brief micropressure pulse (at the arrow) as described in Figure 1. **B.** Mean values (±SEM) for the peak amplitude (resting values subtracted) of the calcium signals to NMDA in neurons from control (Control) and IL-6 transgenic pups (IL-6) maintained in culture for 5, 7 and 8 days. At all culture ages, the response to NMDA was significantly larger in the granule neurons from the transgenic animals. Numbers in parenthesis are the number of cells tested/number of culture dishes tested. The data are from 2 culture sets. * = significant difference from the respective control value.

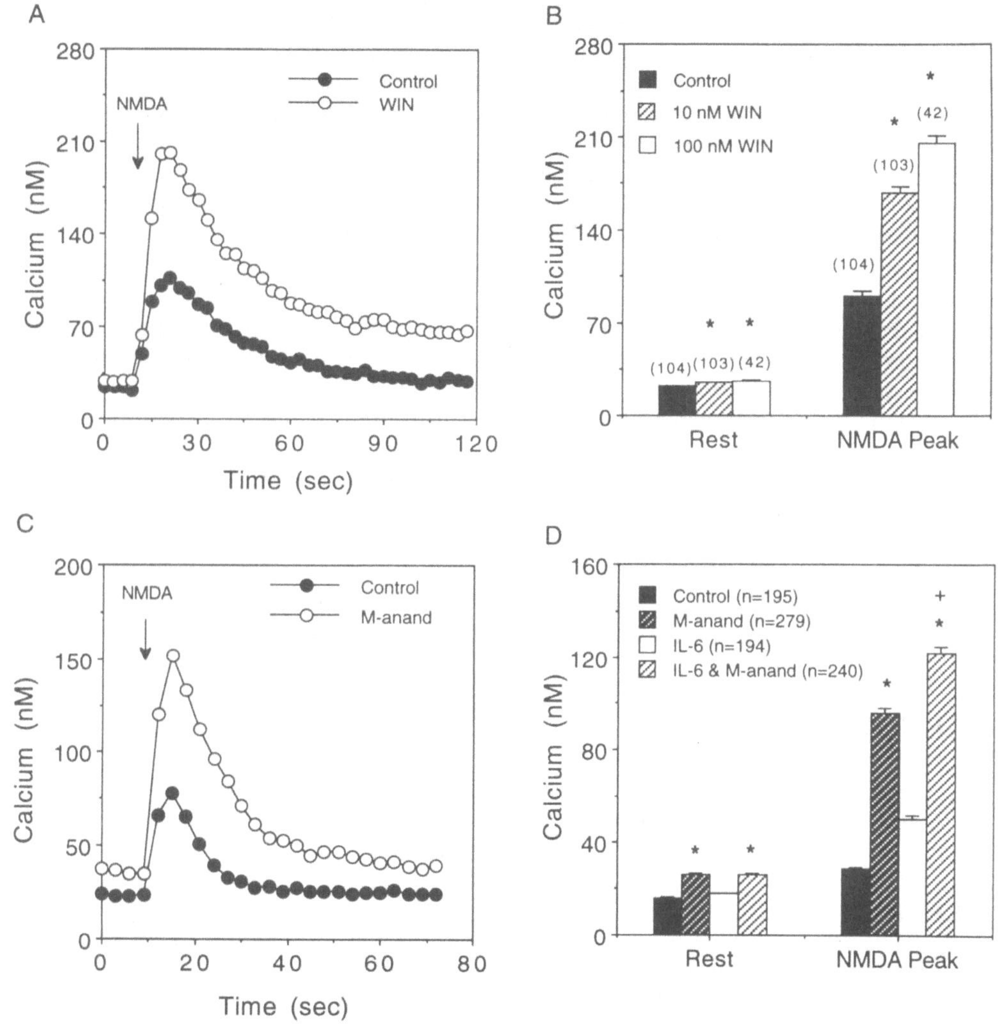

Figure 3. Acute exposure to cannabinoid receptor agonists enhances the calcium signal to NMDA in control and IL-6 treated rat granule neurons. **A.** Calcium signals elicited by NMDA in granule neurons under control conditions and after addition of the synthetic cannabinoid receptor agonist WIN 55,212-2 (10 nM; WIN) to the bath. Recordings are from 2 different neurons in the same culture dish (6 days in culture). NMDA was applied by a brief micropressure pulse (at the arrow) as described in Figure 1. **B**. Mean values (±SEM) for the peak amplitude (resting values subtracted) of the calcium signals to NMDA in neurons in control cultures and cultures exposed to 10 or 100 nM WIN (6 day cultures). WIN significantly enhanced the calcium signals to NMDA in a dose-dependent manner. WIN also enhanced resting calcium levels. Numbers in parenthesis are the number of cells tested/number of culture dishes. **C.** Calcium signals elicited by NMDA in granule neurons under control conditions and after addition of the synthetic cannabinoid receptor agonist R-1 Methanandamide (30 nM; M-anand) to the bath. Recordings are from 2 different neurons in the same culture dish (6 days in culture). NMDA was applied by a brief micropressure pulse (at the arrow) as described in Figure 1. **D**. Mean values (±SEM) for the peak amplitude (resting values subtracted) of the calcium signals to NMDA in neurons from control and chronic IL-6 treated cultures (6 day cultures) with and without bath exposure to R-1 Methanandamide (30 nM). The response to NMDA was enhanced by R-1 Methanandamide in both control and chronic IL-6 treated neurons. Numbers in parenthesis are the number of cells studied. * = significant difference from the respective control value (i.e., no M-anand present); + = significantly different from M-anand treated cultures. Calcium signals to NMDA were significantly larger in IL-6 treated cultures compared to controls (significance not indicated by an asterisk).

IL-6's effects required chronic treatment, whereas the effects of cannabinoids were observed with acute exposure. Chronic treatment was used to simulate IL-6 exposure in the CNS of HIV-infected infants; acute exposure to cannabinoids was used to simulate maternal drug use. Combined treatment with cannabinoids and IL-6 resulted in a larger calcium signal to NMDA in the cultured neurons than observed with either agent alone. These results suggest that maternal cannabinoid use could enhance the detrimental effects of IL-6 on the CNS of her HIV-infected infant. Similar IL-6/cannabinoid interactions may occur in the CNS of HIV-infected adults; further studies will be required to test this possibility.

Cannabinoids are known to alter the physiological properties of CNS neurons,[2] but studies of their actions on calcium signaling to NMDA stimulation have not been reported previously. Our results suggests that calcium signaling linked to NMDA receptor activation may be an important pathway for both cannabinoid and IL-6 effects on the CNS. Alterations in the response to NMDA by IL-6 and cannabinoids alone or in combination could lead to widespread CNS effects, which are likely to be detrimental. Disruption of pathways linked to NMDA receptors has been shown to produce neuronal damage and to contribute to CNS disease.[10] Excessive stimulation of NMDA receptors can result in cell death, an effect that is thought to involve increases in intracellular calcium.[3] Moreover, calcium signaling pathways and the response to NMDA have been proposed to be involved in the neurotoxicity of HIV infection in the CNS.[9] Our results suggest that cannabinoid use could increase this neurotoxicity, through cannabinoid actions on NMDA receptor mediated calcium signaling, and thereby enhance the disruptive effects of HIV infection on the CNS.

ACKNOWLEDGMENT

Supported in part by MH47680, AA07456 and ARC6420. We thank Floriska Chizer for secretarial help and Jodi Caguioa and Dan Sweeney for technical assistance.

REFERENCES

1. Campbell, I.L., Abraham, C.R., Masliah, E., Kemper, P., Inglis, J.D., Oldstone, M.B. and Mucke, L., Neurologic disease induced in transgenic mice by cerebral overexpression of interleukin- 6, *Proc. Natl. Acad. Sci.*, 90 (1993) 10061-10065.
2. Childers, S.R., Pacheco, M.A., Bennett, B.A., Edwards, T.A., Hampson, R.E., Mu, J. and Deadwyler, S.A., Cannabinoid receptors: G-protein-mediated signal transduction mechanisms, *Biochem. Soc. Symp.*, 59 (1993) 27-50.
3. Choi, D.W., Excitotoxic cell death, *J. Neurobiol.*, 23 (1992) 1261-1276.
4. Devane, W.A., Hanus, L., Breuer, A., Pertwee, R.G., Stevenson, L.A., Griffin, G., Gibson, D., Mandelbaum, A., Etinger, A. and Mechoulam, R., Isolation and structure of a brain constituent that binds to the cannabinoid receptor, *Science*, 258 (1992) 1946-1949.
5. Di Marzo, V., Fontana, A., Cadas, H., Schinelli, S., Cimino, G., Schwartz, J.C. and Piomelli, D., Formation and inactivation of endogenous cannabinoid anandamide in central neurons, *Nature*, 372 (1994) 686-691.
6. Gadient, R.A. and Otten, U., Expression of interleukin-6 (IL-6) and interleukin-6 receptor (IL-6R) mRNAs in rat brain during postnatal development, *Brain Res.*, 637 (1994) 10-14.
7. Gallo, P., Frei, K., Rordorf, C., Lazdins, J., Tavolato, B. and Fontana, A., Human immunodeficiency type 1 (HIV-1) infection of the central nervous system: an evaluation of cytokines in cerebrospinal fluid, *J. Neuroimmunol.*, 23 (1989) 109-116.
8. Johnson, R.T., McArthur, J.C. and Narayan, O., The neurobiology of human immunodeficiency virus infections, *FASEB J.*, 2 (1988) 2970-2981.
9. Lipton, S.A., Models of neuronal injury in AIDS: another role for the NMDA receptor? *TINS*, 15 (1992) 75-79.
10. McDonald, J.W. and Johnston, M.V., Physiological and pathophysiological roles of excitatory amino acids during central nervous system development, *Brain Res.Rev.* 15 (1990) 41-70.

11. McLaughlin, C.R., Martin, B.R., Compton, D.R. and Abood, M.E., Cannabinoid receptors in developing rats: detection of mRNA and receptor binding, *Drug & Alcohol Dependence*, 36 (1994) 27-31.
12. Navarro, M., Rubio, P. and Rodriguez deFonseca, F., Behavioral consequences of maternal exposure to natural cannabinoids in rats, *Psychopharmacology*, 107 (1995) (In Press).
13. Qiu, Z., Parsons, K.L. and Gruol, D.L., Interleukin-6 selectively enhances the intracellular calcium response to NMDA in developing CNS neurons, *J. Neurosci.*, 15 (1995) 6688-6699.

17

CANNABINOID RECEPTOR EXPRESSION IN IMMUNE CELLS

D. A. Dove Pettit, D. L. Anders, M. P. Harrison, and G. A. Cabral

Department of Microbiology and Immunology
Medical College of Virginia/Virginia Commonwealth University
Richmond, Virginia

1. INTRODUCTION

It is now recognized that cannabinoids exert their effects both by receptor and non-receptor-mediated mechanisms. The cannabinoid receptor family consists of two G protein-coupled receptors, the first of these, designated as CB1, is limited primarily to neural tissue while the second, designated as CB2, is found primarily within immune cells at peripheral sites.[1-3] Recently, an amine-terminal splice variant of CB1, designated CB1a, was identified in a human lung cDNA library,[4] but protein expression of this splice variant has not been demonstrated in tissue. Evidence for the presence of cannabinoid receptors on immune cells has been obtained using reverse transcription-polymerase chain reaction (RT-PCR) and radioligand binding assay as barometers of receptor message and protein expression, respectively.[5] The identification and quantitation of receptor protein based on binding of radiolabeled ligand does not allow for differentiation between the expression of CB1 and CB2, since these receptors share similar ligand binding profiles. On the other hand, RT-PCR, while not allowing for assessment of receptor protein levels, is a highly sensitive and discriminatory measure of cannabinoid receptor type-specific gene expression. Nevertheless, this technique suffers from several potential deficiencies especially when used to study intron-less genes such as those for CB1 and CB2 where genomic DNA (gDNA) amplification products would have the same size as products derived from cDNA. Furthermore, there are difficulties in quantitative standardization which could compromise interpretation of results.

To circumvent these problems we have developed monospecific polyclonal antiserum to an amine terminal immunodominant epitope of CB1 which is highly conserved between human, mouse, and rat. In addition, we have utilized a novel highly-sensitive and semi-quantitative technique, mutagenic reverse transcription-PCR (MRT-PCR),[6] to discriminate the expression of CB1 and CB2 mRNA in immune and neural cells. We have applied these probes to the definition of CB1 expression in rat brain, rat spleen, and immune cell types of human, mouse, and rat origin. Identification of cannabinoid receptor subtype expression on immune cells, especially B lymphocytes and macrophages, suggests that these proteins may play a

AIDS, Drugs of Abuse, and the Neuroimmune Axis, Edited by Friedman *et al.*
Plenum Press, New York, 1996

role in the functional activities attributed to these cell types. Therefore, it is important to use these newly developed techniques to determine whether co-expression of receptor subtypes occurs within immune cells, whether differential expression of cannabinoid receptors takes place in the course of immune cell maturation and/or activation state, and if receptor-ligand interaction results in the downregulation of CB1 or CB2 by means of intracellular sequestration of formed complexes and/or regulation of receptor gene expression.

2. METHODS

2.1 Cells and Culture

Human T-lymphoblast CCRF-CEM (CCL 119), T-lymphoblast Molt-4 (CRL 1582), myeloblast KG-1 (CCL 246), histiocytic lymphoma U-937 (CRL 1593), promyelocyte HL-60 (CCL 240), and monocyte THP-1 (TIB 202) cells and murine myelomonocyte WEHI-3 (TIB 68) and lymphoblast $P388D_1$ (TIB 63) cells were obtained from the American Type Culture Collection (ATCC, Rockville, MD). Murine mast/basophil mastocytoma PT18 cells[7] were a gift of Dr. Thomas Huff of the Department of Microbiology and Immunology at this institution. Cells (except for PT18) were grown and maintained in RPMI 1640 medium supplemented with 10% heat-inactivated fetal calf serum (FCS; Bio Whittaker, Walkersville, MD), 1% L-glutamine, 1% non-essential amino acids, 1% minimal essential medium vitamins, 100 U/ml Penicillin, 100 μg/ml Streptomycin, 25 mM HEPES [4-(2-Hydroxyethyl) 1-piperazine ethanesulfonic acid], and 1.5% sodium bicarbonate at 37°C in a humidified 5% CO_2 atmosphere. PT18 cells were grown and maintained as above with the exception that 5% heat-inactivated FCS, 5% horse serum, 10 μg/ml Gentamycin, 1 mM sodium pyruvate, 1 mM oxalacetic acid, 40 μM 2-mercaptoethanol, and 20% (v/v) WEHI-3 cell-conditioned medium also were added to the culture medium. Total cell counts were performed using a hemocytometer.

2.2 Mutagenic Reverse Transcription-Polymerase Chain Reaction (MRT-PCR)

Total RNA from tissue or cultured cells was used for assessment of cannabinoid receptor message. Since the rat, human, and mouse CB1 share greater than 97% homology, the reverse transcription (RT) primer and the PCR primers were designed to amplify mRNA of rat, human, and mouse origin. The following RT primer was synthesized to be complementary to CB1 mRNA and to contain a single base mismatch which would allow for the introduction of a unique *Msp*I site in reverse-transcribed CB1 mRNA: 5′GGCCTGTGAA TGGATATGTA CCTGTCGATG GCTGTGAGGA AC***C***GGCTGCC CAC3′. The ***C*** designates the base mutation generating the unique *Msp*I restriction site. The sequence for the RT primer extends from base 613 to 665 of rat CB1 cDNA, where +1 corresponds to the A of the initiation codon for methionine. For PCR amplification of CB1, 5′ATGAA GTCGA TCCTA GATGG3′ and 5′GGCCT GTGAA TGGAT ATGTA3′ were employed as the 5′ PCR sense primer (bases 1 - 20) and 3′ anti-sense primer (bases 646 - 665), respectively. The 20 base 3′ anti-sense primer is identical to the 5′ terminus of the RT primer, allowing for the amplification of the point mutation generated in the cDNA during reverse transcription. The size of the amplicon for rat, human, and mouse CB1 is approximately 665 base pairs (bp). The amplicon derived from mRNA (cDNA) can be digested with *Msp*I to generate two fragments of approximately 623 and 42 bp; whereas, the product generated from gDNA remains undigested (i.e., 665 bp). For assessment of expression of human CB2 message,

5′TCATAGTCAC GCTGCCAATC TTCAGCAGGA AGACAGCCTT GG***G***ATCCACA CCAT3′ was employed as the 3′ RT primer which extends from base 293 to 346 of human CB2 cDNA sequence, where +1 corresponds to the A of the initiation codon for methionine. A point mutation was synthesized into the RT primer, corresponding to base 304, thus converting an ***A*** to ***G***. This base change generates an unique *Bam*HI restriction site. For PCR amplification, 5′ATGGA GGAAT GCTGG GTGAC A3′ and 5′TCATA GTCAC GCTGC CAATC T3′ were employed as the 5′ sense primer (bases 1 to 21) and 3′ anti-sense primer (bases 326 to 346), respectively. The 21 base 3′ primer has the same 5′ terminus as the RT primer, but flanks the engineered restriction site. This allows for the discrimination of amplicons generated from cDNA rather than gDNA. The expected amplicon for human CB2 is 346 bp. *Bam*HI digestion of amplification products derived from cDNA would result in the generation of a 304 bp and 42 bp fragment. Amplicons derived from gDNA cannot be digested with *Bam*HI (346 bp).

The reverse transcription step for MRT-PCR was performed by mixing 10 fmol of the appropriate RT primer with 2 μg of total RNA in RT buffer (1mM Tris-HCl, pH 8.3, 50 mM KCl, 4 mM $MgCl_2$, 1 mM dithiothreitol, 1 mM each dNTP, 10 μl total volume). All solutions were prepared in DEPC-treated water. The reaction mixture was heated to 75°C (5 min), cooled to 42°C, and MuLV reverse transcriptase (10 units in 0.5 μl) plus RNase inhibitor (5 units in 0.5 μl) was added. The reaction mixture, then, was incubated at 42°C for 60 min.

For PCR amplification, 100 ng of each of the appropriate PCR primers were added to the RT reaction mixture. Samples were incubated at 95°C (5 min) and cooled to 4°C, and, then, the following was added: 2 μl 25 mM $MgCl_2$, 4 μl 10X PCR buffer, 31.5 μl MilliQ water, and 0.5 μl (2.5 U/100 μl) AmpliTaq DNA polymerase (Perkin Elmer, Foster City, CA). The preparation was subjected to 30 cycles consisting of denaturation at 94°C (1 min), annealing at 53°C (1 min), and extension at 72°C (1 min). A final extension at 72°C for 10 min was performed. The reaction, then, was cooled to 4°C.

The PCR reaction products (10 μl) were digested with the appropriate restriction enzyme (20 units *Msp*I for CB1, 20 units *Bam*HI for CB2) for 20 hr at 37°C. The digested products were separated using 3% agarose gels and Southern blot analysis was performed to confirm the specificity of the amplicon. Briefly, products were transferred by capillary action onto Qiabrane nylon membranes (Qiagen, Chatsworth, CA) with transfer buffer (0.4M NaOH, 1M NaCl) and neutralized 5 min in 5X SSC (0.75M NaCl, 0.075M sodium citrate, pH7.0). Blotted DNA was cross-linked to the membranes with a UV Stratalinker (Stratagene, La Jolla, CA). The membranes were prehybridized for 4 hr at room temperature in 1X prehybridization buffer (10% formamide, 0.1%(w/v) BSA, 0.1% (w/v) Ficoll 400, 0.1% (w/v) polyvinylpyrrolidone, 0.1% (w/v) sodium dodecyl sulfate, 25 mM Na_2HPO_4, 25 mM NaH_2PO_4, 0.75M NaCl, 0.075M sodium citrate, 250 μg/ml yeast total RNA, pH 6.5). The blots, then, were probed with an end-labeled oligonucleotide[8] (specific activity of 10^8dpm/μg) that was selected to hybridize within the MRT-PCR-amplified domain of either CB1 (5′CGCTA TCTTT GCGGT GGAAC ACGTG3′, corresponding to bases 535 - 559 of rat CB1 cDNA) or CB2 (5′CACAG CAACA GCTGT CTTCT3′, corresponding to bases 95 - 114 of the human CB2 cDNA), thereby imparting specificity to the detection of amplification products. The blots were incubated in hybridization buffer (prehybridization buffer supplemented with the appropriate end-labeled oligonucleotide (1 X 10^6 cpm/ml) and 10% dextran sulfate) overnight at 37°C. Following the hybrizations, blots were washed at 37°C for 5 min (4X), in 2X SSC (0.3M NaCl, 0.03M sodium citrate) followed by one 40 min 2X SSC wash at 37°C. The blots were air-dried and exposed to Kodak XAR film for 48 hr at -80°C.

In all cases oligonucleotide sequences were designed based on differences in homology between CB1 and CB2. The GAP and BESTFIT Programs on the Genetics Computer

Group (GCG) software (University of Wisconsin, Madison, WI) were used to align CB1 and CB2 sequences and to identify potential regions of homology.

2.3 Production of Anti-CB1 Polypeptide Antiserum

Antiserum and affinity-purified antibody were produced to an immunodominant epitope of human CB1 (hCB1) which is conserved for rat and mouse CB1. This epitope sequence (NKSLSSFKENEENIQC) corresponds to amino acids 83 - 98 at the extracellular amine terminus of hCB1. The peptide was synthesized using solid-phase F-moc chemistry and was HPLC-purified to greater than 90% using a Vydac C18 reverse-phase column. The peptide mass was verified by MALDI-TOF mass spectrometry. For immunization, the peptide was coupled via a cysteine thiol to keyhole limpet hemocyanin (KLH) or to bovine serum albumin (BSA) using m-maleimidobenzoyl-N-hydroxysuccinimide ester (MBS; Bioaffinity Systems, Inc., Roscoe, IL). The albumin conjugate was used as an antigen source for assaying antibody titer by enzyme-linked immunosorbent assay (ELISA). New Zealand white rabbits were immunized with antigen in complete Freund's adjuvant and boosted with incomplete adjuvant at 14, 28, and 48 days. Production bleeds were collected at days 52, 56, and 60, screened by ELISA, and the serum affinity-purified using peptide coupled to a thiol-reactive gel (Quality Controlled Biochemicals, Inc., Hopkinton, MA).

2.4 Immunocytochemistry

Rat brain and spleen were embedded in Polyfin (Triangle Biomedical Sciences, Durham, NC), snap-frozen, and stored at -80°C. Sections (8-10 μm-thick) were cut in a Minotome Microtome/Cryostat (Damon/IEC Division, Needham, MA), mounted onto glass slides, and blocked (1 hr, room temperature) with SuperBlock Blocking Buffer in PBS (SBB, Pierce, Rockford, IL). Slides, then, were incubated (1 hr, room temperature) with affinity-purified rabbit anti-CB1 antibody (40 ng/μl in SBB, Quality Controlled Biochemicals) or pre-immunization antiserum from the same animal. Samples were washed (3X) with Phospate Buffered Saline (PBS: 0.01M Sodium phosphate, 0.15M NaCl, pH 7.2) and incubated 1 hr (room temperature) with horseradish peroxidase-conjugated goat anti-rabbit IgG (BioRad, Richmond, CA; 1:32) in SBB. The slides, then, were washed (3X) in PBS and incubated (20 min) in Hanker-Yates solution (Polysciences, Inc., Warrington, PA) as previously described.[9] The histochemical staining reaction was terminated by washing the slides in 0.1M Tris buffer (pH 7.6). Slides, then, were rinsed with deionized distilled water, air-dried, and mounted in Aqua-Mount (Lerner Laboratories, Pittsburgh, PA). Slides were examined with an Olympus BHA light microscope with OM-1 camera attachment (Optical Elements Corporation, Washington, DC).

3. RESULTS

3.1 Mutagenic Reverse Transcription-Polymerase Chain Reaction (MRT-PCR)

MRT-PCR was applied to define the expression of CB1 and CB2 mRNA in rat brain and spleen and in various cell types. Identification of PCR-amplified cDNA from CB1 mRNA was accomplished by recognition of a cleavage product of 623 bp which was generated following digestion with *Msp*I (Figure 1A). CB1 message, as expected, was detected in rat brain. Message for this receptor was detected also in rat lung (data not shown), human T-lymphoblast Molt-4 cells, human THP-1 monocytes (data not shown), and rat thymus T lymphocytes. CB1 message was detected in relatively high levels in THP-1 cells, moderate levels in Molt-4 cells, and relatively low levels in rat thymus T lymphocytes. Message for CB1 was not detected in rat liver (data not shown), human T-lymphoblast CEM cells, human U-937 histiocytic lymphoma cells (data not shown), human promyelocytic leukemia HL-60 cells (data not shown), human myeloblast KG-1 cells, murine mastocytoma PT18 cells, or murine myelomonocyte WEHI-3 cells. Identification of PCR-amplified cDNA from CB2 mRNA was achieved by observation of a cleavage product of 304 bp which was generated following digestion with *Bam*HI (Figure 1B). HL-60 cells, as expected, and U-937 cells were shown to exclusively express CB2 mRNA. The HL-60 cells expressed relatively high levels of CB2 mRNA when compared with that expressed in U-937 cells.

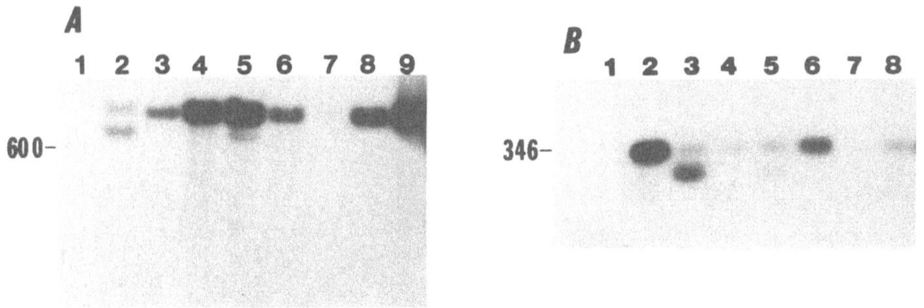

Figure 1. Mutational reverse transcription polymerase chain reaction (MRT-PCR) for definition of CB1 and CB2 mRNA expression in various tissues and cell types. (A). Analysis of CB1 mRNA Expression. Total RNA was subjected to reverse transcription using an oligonucleotide primer containing a single base mismatch generating a unique *Msp*I restriction site. The reverse transcription products then were amplified by PCR using a pair of highly conserved oligonucleotide primers specific for human, rat, and mouse CB1 sequences. The PCR amplification products were digested with *Msp*I and subjected to electrophoretic separation through a 3% agarose gel. The DNA was transferred to a nylon membrane and hybridized to a ^{32}P end-labeled oligonucleotide specific for CB1. Lane 1: 100 bp ladder (Gibco/BRL). The 600 bp marker position is designated at the left margin. Lane 2: total rat brain RNA subjected to MRT-PCR and *Msp*I digestion. Note the presence of undigested 665 bp and digested 623 bp products. For this analysis, one-tenth the amount of MRT-PCR digested product was subjected to agarose gel electrophoresis when compared with other samples since brain is enriched for CB1 message. Total RNA from brain was used as a positive control for CB1 mRNA. Lane 3: total rat brain RNA subjected to MRT-PCR and not subjected to *Msp*I digestion. Lanes 4-9: total RNA from human T-lymphoblast CEM, human T-lymphoblast Molt-4, rat thymus T lymphocyte, murine mastocytoma PT18, murine myelomonocyte WEHI-3, and human myeloblast KG-1 cells. The presence of cleavage product of 623 bp in the lanes for rat brain (lane 2) and Molt-4 (lane 5) indicates expression of CB1 mRNA. In addition, low level expression was detected for rat thymus T-lymphocytes (lane 6). (B). Analysis of CB2 mRNA expression. Total RNA was subjected to reverse transcription using an oligonucleotide primer containing a single base mismatch generating a unique *Bam*HI restriction site. The reverse transcription products then were amplified by PCR using a pair of oligonucleotide primers specific for human CB2 (hCB2). The PCR amplification products were digested by *Bam*HI and subjected to electrophoretic separation through a 3% agarose gel. The DNA was transferred to a nylon membrane and hybridized to a ^{32}P end-labeled oligonucleotide specific for hCB2. Lane 1: 100 bp ladder. The extrapolated position corresponding to 346 bp undigested CB2 product is designated at the left margin. Lanes 2 and 3: human promyelocyte HL-60 cell total RNA subjected to MRT-PCR and either not digested with *Bam*HI (lane 2) or digested with *Bam*HI (lane 3). Lanes 4-7: total RNA from human monocyte THP-1 cells, human premonocyte U-937 cells, rat brain, and murine lymphoblast P388D$_1$ cells subjected to MRT-PCR and *Bam*HI digestion. The total RNA from murine P388D$_1$ cells is devoid of any band as expected since the human oligonucleotide primers selected for MRT-PCR do not hybridize with mouse sequence. Lane 8: CB1 cDNA subjected to MRT-PCR and *Bam*HI digestion. Note the expression of CB2 mRNA (i.e., 304 bp product) in HL-60 (lane 3) and U-937 (lane 5) cells.

3.2 Immunocytochemistry

Affinity-purified antibody to an immunodominant epitope within the rat CB1 amine terminus was used in an indirect immunoperoxidase staining procedure to screen frozen cryostat sections of rat brain and spleen for CB1 protein. The anti-CB1 antibody was shown to immunochemically stain rat brain cryostat sections (Figures 2A and 3) in a pattern which was similar to that obtained from autoradiograms of rat brain slices incubated with the radiolabeled cannabinoid ligand [^{3}H]CP55,940.[10] The molecular layer of the cerebellum (Cer) was intensely stained while the granular layer, although positive, was less intensely stained (Figures 2A and 3C). Intense staining was observed also in the hippocampus (Hi, Figures 2A and 3A), dentate gyrus, interpeduncular nucleus, and for the substantia nigra pars reticulata (SNr). The cortex (Cx), while positive, was less intense than the previously mentioned areas of the brain (Figures 2A and 3B). The staining, in various areas of the unfixed brain, was distributed in a punctate pattern suggestive of a specific compartmental localization within or on neural cells. In contrast, minimal staining for CB1 was observed

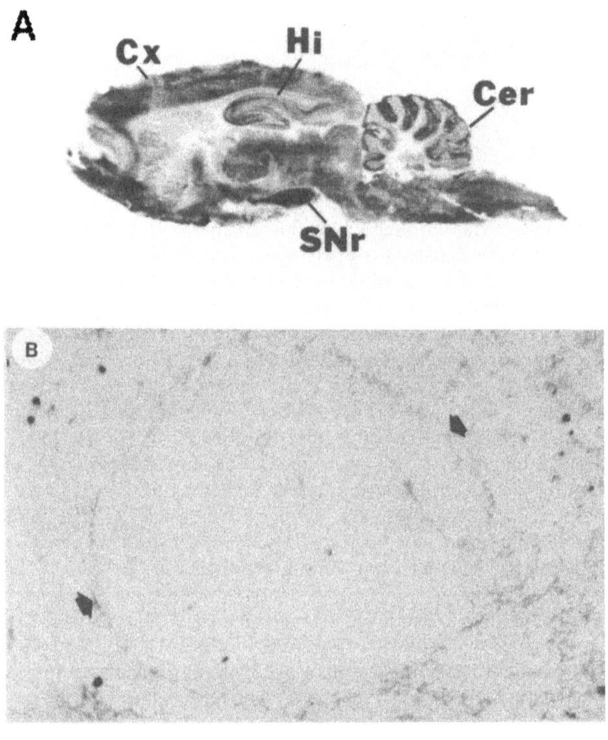

Figure 2. Immunoperoxidase staining of rat brain and spleen for localization of CB1. Fresh frozen rat brain cryostat sections (10 μm) were incubated with affinity-purified rabbit anti-CB1 antibody followed by incubation with horseradish peroxidase-conjugated goat anti-rabbit IgG (heavy and light chains) and developed with Hanker-Yates reagent. (A). Rat Brain (X5). The immunoperoxidase staining pattern is similar to that reported using [^{3}H]CP55,940 ligand binding and autoradiography[10]. Positively stained regions include: Cer: cerebellum; Cx: cerebral cortex; Hi: hippocampus; SNr: substantia nigra pars reticulata. (B). Rat spleen section showing the periarteriolar lymphoid sheath (PALS). Areas within the PALS comprising the T cell area, the mantle zone of the germinal center, and the germinal center are negative. Light immunoperoxidase staining (arrows) was observed in the marginal zone circumscribing the PALS. (X360).

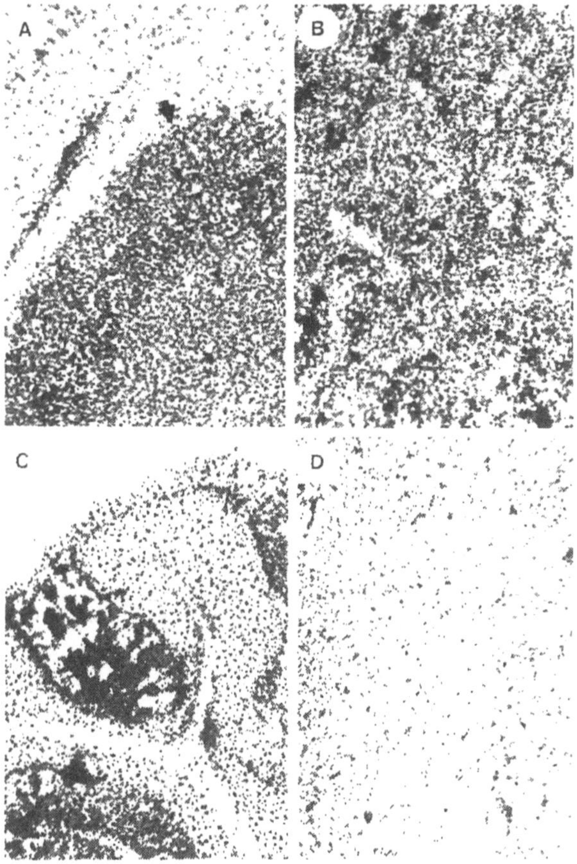

Figure 3. Immunoperoxidase localization of CB1 in select areas of rat brain. Panels A and C represent hippocampal (arrow) and cerebellar areas of the brain stained with affinity-purified anti-CB1 antibody. Panels B and D represent cerebral areas of the brain stained with affinity-purified anti-CB1 antibody or pre-immunization antiserum, respectively. The brain distribution of immunoperoxidase staining is similar to that reported using [^{3}H]CP55,940 ligand binding and autoradiography.[10] Note, however, that the staining within a given area is in a punctate pattern suggestive of a defined compartmental distribution within, or on, individual cells. (A,B, D: X200; C:X400).

in rat spleen (Figure 2B). The red pulp area was devoid of staining. In addition, with the exception of the marginal zone, which exhibited light staining, staining was not discerned within the white pulp area which comprises the periarteriolar lymphoid sheath (PALS). Areas within the PALS, comprising the T cell area, the mantle zone of the germinal center, and the germinal center, exhibited no staining for CB1.

4. DISCUSSION

There is a large body of data which indicate that THC, the major psychoactive component in marijuana, alters cellular activities including those of macrophages. However, the mechanism by which THC affects cell functions, such as the expression of effector molecules, remains to be defined. At relatively high concentrations (i.e., 10^{-5}M and 10^{-6}M) THC may have a direct effect on macrophage function by altering the membrane structure, since THC is a highly lipophilic compound.[11] Such effects may be biologically relevant in terms of direct exposure for lung alveolar macrophages as a consequence of smoking marijuana. However, stereospecificity and structural requirements for biological activity indicate that the cannabinoids also can act via a specific receptor.[12-17] Localization of cannabinoid receptors has been accomplished using binding studies performed with [^{3}H]CP-55,940 and slide mounted sections of rat brain and pituitary.[10] These studies demonstrated that cannabinoid receptor expression occurs in cortical, basal ganglia, and cerebellar structures.[10] The serendipitous discovery of CB1 cDNA (SKR6) in a rat cerebral cDNA library has facilitated the further characterization of CB1 expression at the molecular level.[1] Functional assays performed with Chinese hamster ovary (CHO) K1 cells stably transfected with the SKR6 clone demonstrated inhibition of forskolin-stimulated accumulation of cAMP upon stimulation with THC or a potent analog, CP-55,940.[1] Furthermore, transfection of CHO cells and L cell fibroblasts with CB1 has demonstrated that cannabinoid agonists stimulate both receptor- and non-receptor-mediated signal transduction pathways and that transfected CHO cells show the same rank order of potency for cannabinoid analogs as observed in P2 membrane preparations of rat brain.[18] Collectively, these studies have indicated the expression of a central cannabinoid receptor, CB1, linked to a spectrum of cellular functional activities. Recently, Shire *et al.*[4] have postulated the existence of an amine-terminal splice variant of CB1 which they have designated CB1a. The functional relevance of this putative receptor is unclear.

Although the presence of a high affinity cannabinoid receptor has been difficult to detect in leukocytes,[1,5,19,20] a peripheral cannabinoid receptor cDNA, CB2, has been cloned from the human macrophage cell line, HL-60.[2] Kaminski *et al.*,[5] on the other hand, have reported the expression of CB1 in splenocytes. Recently, Galiègue *et al.*[3] used an antibody to a CB2 cannabinoid receptor domain fusion construct to demonstrate positive staining in human lymph node areas enriched for B-lymphocytes. Nevertheless, whether macrophages and splenocytes exclusively express CB1 versus CB2, co-express both receptors, or differentially express either receptor as a function of cell maturation and/or activation state remains to be defined.

A difficulty in resolving these issues has been the unavailability of specific and highly-sensitive probes for the unequivocal discrimination of CB1 versus CB2 mRNA and protein expression. Studies to date have employed RT-PCR for amplification of cannabinoid receptor mRNA as a barometer of cannabinoid receptor expression. RT-PCR, while highly sensitive, may yield results which are difficult to interpret as a result of spurious amplification of residual or contaminating genomic DNA in the sample. Furthermore, RT-PCR does not allow for direct assessment of cannabinoid receptor expression since mRNA levels detected may not correspond to levels of receptor protein. In the present study, we have attempted to resolve these issues by applying a highly sensitive MRT-PCR procedure modified for the unequivocal discrimination of CB1 versus CB2 mRNA. In addition, we have employed immunocytochemical staining using anti-CB1 affinity-purified antibody to an immunodominant amine-terminal domain of CB1 to examine brain and spleen for CB1 protein distribution.

The MRT-PCR involved an RT primer designed to contain a single nucleotide substitution such that a unique *Msp*I or *Bam*HI restriction site was generated within the cDNA from CB1 or CB2 mRNA, respectively. PCR amplification and digestion with the appropriate restriction enzyme would, thus, impart the ability to discriminate between the amplification of contaminating or residual gDNA and cDNA. Amplicons derived from cDNA, rather than gDNA, are sensitive to digestion with the appropriate restriction enzyme. Using this technique, message for CB1 was detected in rat brain, lung, and thymus T lymphocytes and in human T-lymphoblast Molt-4 and THP-1 macrophage-like cells. Lower levels of CB1 message were detected in thymus T lymphocytes and Molt-4 cells when compared with that expressed in rat brain (Figure 1A). It is possible that the message detected in rat lung, rat thymus T cells, and Molt-4 cells represents amplification product of mRNA derived from residual neural extensions in these tissues. However, THP-1 macrophage-like cells were shown to express relatively high levels of CB1 message when compared with the other cell types examined. Message for CB1 was not detected in rat liver, in human T-lymphoblast CEM, U-937 histiocytic lymphoma, promyelocytic leukemia HL-60, and myeloblast KG-1 cells, and in murine mastocytoma PT18 or myelomonocyte WEHI-3 cells (Figure 1A). It is unlikely that the lack of CB1 mRNA expression in murine cells is due to inappropriate conditions for primer hybridization to mouse sequence during MRT-PCR since these primers have been used to identify CB1 mRNA expression in mouse nueroblastoma cells, N18TG2 (data not shown). Furthermore, the lack of a signal from contaminating CB1 gDNA in PT18 is surprising since the samples were not pre-treated with DNAse. The total RNA derived from PT18 cells has been determined to be of good quality (agarose gel electrophoresis followed by ethidium bromide staining). However, we cannot rule out, at this time, the possibility that this sample contains a substance which may interfere with the MRT-PCR reaction. It is important to note that although our CB1 MRT-PCR primers would have the ability to amplify CB1a cDNA, no amplification product for this putative subtype was observed in any of our reactions. MRT-PCR was applied, also, to the definition of CB2 message expression (Figure 1B). CB2 message was detected in relatively high levels in HL-60 macrophage-like cells and at low levels in U-937 cells. The amplicon present in our analysis of CB1 cDNA using the CB2 MRT-PCR primers, suggests that our MRT-PCR reaction was contaminated with CB2 gDNA. This event demonstrates the utility of MRT-PCR, for if we were using traditional RT-PCR, we would not have been able to determine that the amplicon was derived from contaminating DNA. Collectively, our data suggest that THP-1 cells exclusively express CB1, whereas CB2 is exclusively expressed in HL-60 and U-937 cells.

In addition to the use of MRT-PCR for discrimination of CB1 versus CB2 mRNA expression, we have employed immunochemical staining using an affinity-purified anti-CB1 antibody to enable precise characterization of CB1 protein expression. The specificity of the anti-CB1 antibody has been demonstrated in that Western immunoblot analysis reveals an immunoreactive protein species with the relative molecular weight of approximately 69 kD, which is consistent with the expected size of a glycosylated CB1 protein (Manuscript in preparation). In addition, anti-CB1 antiserum generated to amino acid residues 1 - 78 of CB1 (a kind gift of Dr. Kenneth Mackie) also detects upon Western immunoblotting a protein band of comparable relative molecular weight. Lastly, immunocytochemistry of rat brain sections revealed a staining pattern which parallels that obtained from autoradiography of whole rat brain incubated with [^{3}H]CP55,940, a high-affinity ligand of the cannabinoid receptor.[10] Intense positive staining was observed in the cerebral cortex, hippocampus, dentate gyrus, substantia nigra, interpeduncular nucleus and cerebellum. In contrast, minimal staining was observed in rat spleen with low levels of staining occurring in the marginal zone of the periarteriolar lymphoid sheath (PALS). The marginal zone is known to be populated with macrophages. These cells characteristically exhibit endogenous peroxidase activities due to the presence of peroxisomes and of cytochrome *c* in mitochondria. Studies are in progress using methanol/nitroferricyanide or phenylhydrazine treatment to inhibit potential endogenous peroxidatic activities. This will allow for verification of the specificity of the staining observed in the marginal zone.

The data obtained in the present study indicate that CB1 protein is expressed in neural tissue but is essentially absent from spleen. Furthermore, these observations taken in context with reports that CB2 is expressed in spleen, confirm that CB1 is compartmentalized to neural tissue. In addition, CB1 and CB2 message was found to be expressed selectively at relatively high levels in human THP-1 and HL-60 macrophage-like cells, respectively. These results indicate that these macrophage-like cells may serve as ideal *in vitro* models for defining the role of cannabinoid receptor expression in the mediation of macrophage functions. Finally, the MRT-PCR and immunocytochemical procedures which we have employed may prove ideal for further defining expression of cannabinoid receptor mRNA and protein. Furthermore, the CB1 epitope utilized for the production of anti-CB1 antibody was selected on the basis of sequence conservation and antigenicity. The anti-CB1 antibody generated can be applied to the definition of the intracellular kinetics of CB1 synthesis, post-translational modification, and compartmentation of CB1 protein in tissues and cells of human, mouse, and rat origin.

5. SUMMARY

A novel highly-sensitive and semi-quantitative technique, mutagenic RT-PCR (MRT-PCR) was used to discriminate the expression of neural cannabinoid receptor (CB1) mRNA versus that of peripheral cannabinoid receptor (CB2) mRNA in immune and neural cells. Human pre-monocytic THP-1 cells were shown to exclusively express CB1 message. Conversely, human pre-monocytic HL-60 cells and U-937 (histocytic lymphoma) cells exclusively expressed CB2 message. Anti-CB1 affinity-purified antibody generated to an immunodominant epitope within the amine terminus of CB1 detected CB1 protein in rat brain in a pattern which paralleled that previously reported in autoradiographic studies which utilized whole brain sections and [^{3}H]CP55,940, a high-affinity cannabinoid ligand. Minimal immunocytochemical staining was detected in rat spleen. Collectively, these results, taken in context of reports which indicate CB2 distribution in peripheral tissues, indicate that CB1 is compartmentalized to neural tissue while CB2 is localized in immune cells.

6. ACKNOWLEDGMENT

Supported by National Institute on Drug Abuse/NIH awards DA05832, DA09158, and T32 DA07027.

7. REFERENCES

1. Matsuda, L.A., Lolait, S.J., Brownstein, M.J., Young, A.C., and Bonner, T.I. 1990. Structure of a cannabinoid receptor and functional expression of the cloned cDNA. Nature. *346*:561-564.
2. Munro, S., Thomas, K.L., and Muna, A-S. 1993. Molecular characterization of a peripheral receptor for cannabinoids. Nature. *365*:61-65.
3. Galiègue, S., Mary, S., Marchand, J., Dussosoy, D., Carrière, D., Crayon, P., Bouaboula, M., Shire, D., Le Fur, G., and Casellas, P. 1995. Expression of central and peripheral cannabinoid receptors in human immune tissues and leukocyte subpopulations. Eur. J. Biochem. *232*:54-61.
4. Shire, D., Carillon, C., Kaghad, M., Calandra, B., Rinaldi-Carmona, M., Le Fur, G., Caput, D., and Ferrara, P. 1995. An amino-terminal variant of the central cannabinoid receptor resulting from alternative splicing. J. Biol. Chem. *270*:3726-3731.
5. Kaminski, N. E., Abood, M. E., Kessler, F. K., Martin, B. R., and Schatz, A. R. 1992. Identification of a functionally relevant cannabinoid receptor on mouse spleen cells that is involved in cannabinoid-mediated immune modulation. Mol. Pharmacol. *42*:736-742.
6. Taniguchi, S., Watanabe, T., Nakao, A., Seki, G., Uwatoko, S., and Kurokawa, K. 1994. Detection and quantitation of EP_3 prostaglandin E_2 receptor mRNA along mouse nephron segments by RT-PCR. Am. J. Physiology. *266*:c1453-c1458.
7. Vanderhoek, J. Y., Tare, N. S., Bailey, J. M., Goldstein, A. L., and Pluznik, D. H. 1982. New role for 15-hydroxyeicosatetraenoic acid. Activator of leukotriene biosynthesis in PT-18 mast/basophil cells. J. Biol. Chem. *257*:12191-12195.
8. Chaconas, G., and van de Sande, J. H. 1980. 5′-^{32}P labeling of RNA and DNA restriction fragments. Methods Enzymol. *65*:75-88.
9. Hanker, J. S., Yates, P.E., Metz, C.B., and Rustioni, A. 1977. A new specific sensitive and non-carcinogenic reagent for the demonstration of horseradish peroxidase. Histochem. J. *9*:789-792.
10. Herkenham, M., Lynn, A. B., Little, M. D., Johnson, M. R., Melvin, L. S., De Costa, B. R., and Rice, K. R. 1990. Cannabinoid receptor localization in brain. Proc. Natl. Acad. Sci., USA. *87*:1932-1936.

11. Wing, D.R., Leuschner, J.T.A., Brent, G.A., Harvey, D.J., and Paton, W.D.M. 1985. Quantitation of in vivo membrane-associated delta-1-tetrahydrocannabinol and its effect on membrane fluidity. In: Harvey, D.J. (ed.). Marihuana '84: Proceedings of the Oxford Symposium on Cannabis. p. 85. IRL Press, Oxford.
12. Martin, B.R., Balster, R.L., Tazdan, R.K., Harris, L.S., and Dewey, W.L. 1981. Behavioral comparisons of the stereoisomers of tetrahydrocannabinols. Life Sci. *29*:565-574.
13. Johnson, M.R. and Melvin, L.S. 1986. The discovery of nonclassical cannabinoid analgetics. In: R. Mechoulam (ed.), *Cannabinoids as Therapeutic Agents.* pp.121-145. CRC Press, Boca Raton, FL.
14. Howlett, A.C. 1987. Cannabinoid inhibition of adenylate cyclase: relative activities of marihuana constituents and metabolites. Neuropharmacology. *26(5)*:507-512.
15. Little, P.J., Compton, D.R., Johnson, R.R., Melvin, LS., and Martin, B.R.. 1988. Pharmacology and stereoselectivity of structurally novel cannabinoids in mice. J. Pharmacol. Exp. Ther. *247*:1046-1051.
16. Pertwee, R., Griffin, G., Fernando, S., Li, X., Hill, A., and Makriyannis, A. 1995. AM630, A competitive cannabinoid receptor antagonist. Life Sci. *56*:1949-1955.
17. Bidaut-Russell, M., Devane, A.D., and Howlett, A. C.. 1990. Cannabinoid receptors and modulation of cyclic AMP accumulation in the rat brain. J. Neurochemistry. *55*:21-26.
18. Felder, C.C., Velutz, J.S., Williams, H.L., Briley, E.M., and Matsuda, L.A. 1992. Cannabinoid agonists stimulate both receptor and non-receptor-mediated signal transduction pathways in cells transfected with and expressing cannabinoid receptor clones. Mol. Pharmacol. *42*:838-845.
19. Bouaboula, M., Rinaldi, M., Carayon, P., Carillon, C., Delpech, B., Shire, D., Le Fur, G., and Casellas, P. 1993. Cannabinoid-receptor expression in human leukocytes. Eur. J. Biochem. *214*:173-180.
20. Devane, W. A., Dysarz III, F.A., Johnson, M.R., Melvin, L.S., and Howlett, A.C. 1988. Determination and characterization of a cannabinoid receptor in rat brain. Mol. Pharmacol. *34*:605-613.

18

CANNABINOIDS AND IMMUNITY TO VIRUSES

Steven Specter

Department of Medical Microbiology and Immunology
University of South Florida College of Medicine
12901 N. Bruce B. Downs Blvd.
Tampa, Florida 33612

1. INTRODUCTION

The ability of marijuana to alter the course of viral infections was initially reported by Juel-Jensen in 1972.[1]. In this report, the author associated marijuana smoking with more frequent recurrences of herpes simplex virus (HSV) infections. This anecdotal report was made concerning only a few patients but was the impetus for examining the relationships among cannabinoids, immunity and progression of viral infections. The ability of cannabinoids, especially delta-9-tetrahydrocannabinol (THC), to alter immune functions is well described and has been reviewed.[2] A summary of these findings is listed in Table 1.

1.1 Experimental Studies of Cannabinoids and Herpes Simplex Virus

A series of experimental studies have shed light on some of the mechanisms involved in the interaction of cannabinoids and viral infections (Table 2). The initial report of experimental studies that examined the effects of cannabinoids and viral infection used a mouse model of HSV infection. Morahan and coworkers reported that delta-9-tetrahydrocannabinol (THC) increased susceptibility to HSV infection.[3] Subsequently, studies by Cabral et al. indicated that vaginal infection of guinea pigs with HSV was also exacerbated by exposure to THC.[4] Cabral and coworkers later showed that THC diminished the production of interferon α/β in mice during HSV infection, decreased cytotoxic T lymphocyte responses to HSV infected cells, and lowered macrophage "extrinsic" (not interferon) anti-viral activity.[5-7]

It is interesting to note that Lancz and coworkers reported that supra-pharmacologic concentrations of THC (50 - 100 μg/ml) were able to inhibit the replication of HSV in vitro when the virus was directly exposed to the cannabinoid.[8,9] While these concentrations are supra-pharmacologic, they suggest that THC can directly damage HSV. The authors suggested that THC at lower concentrations might alter the pathogenicity of the virus either via

AIDS, Drugs of Abuse, and the Neuroimmune Axis, Edited by Friedman *et al.*
Plenum Press, New York, 1996

Table 1. Modulation of host responses by THC

Non specific	
	Macrophage phagocytosis ↓
	Natural killer cell function ↓
	IL-1 activity → or ↑
	TNFα production →
	TNFα activity ↓
	IFN activity ↓
	IL-2 activity ↓
	IL-2 receptor expression ↓
Specific	
	Antibody formation ↓
	T lymphocyte blast transformation ↓
	Cytotoxic T cell activity ↓
	anti-bacterial resistance ↓
	anti-viral resistance ↓

→ = unaltered; ↑ = increased; ↓ = decreased

mutagenesis or by chemical interaction. No studies have been reported as follow-up to this initial observation.

2. MURINE RETROVIRUS AND THC

Studies in this laboratory have examined the ability of THC to influence immune responses and virus infection in a murine retrovirus infection, Friend leukemia virus (FLV)[11].

2.1 Suppression of Immunity by THC

Genetically susceptible BALB/c mice develop a profound immune suppression within 7 days of infection with FLV. This progresses so that by 21-28 days post infection immunity is about 10% normal for most cellular and humoral immune parameters. Studies were performed combining FLV infection in vivo with addition in vitro of THC to spleen cell culture from infected mice (Table 3). At 28 days post infection, when THC was added, we were able to demonstrate nearly 100% suppression of phytohemagglutinin induced lymphocyte blastogenesis, interleukin 2 secretion, natural killer (NK) cell activity and tumor necrosis factor alpha activity. Thus, the data suggest that THC has an additive, although minor, effect when added to the suppression caused by this retrovirus. It should be noted, however, that when FLV induced suppression was only 20-30% at 7 days post infection the addition of THC had no additional suppressive effect (data not shown). Thus, it seems that

Table 2. Time line for cannabinoids and virus infections

1972	Association of frequency of HSV recurrence and marijuana smoking[1]
1979	Decreased resistance to HSV in mice following exposure to THC[3]
1985	Decreased resistance to HSV in guinea pigs following exposure to THC[4]
1986	Decreased interferon α/β related to increased HSV susceptibility after THC treatment in mice[5]
1991	Inhibition of HSV replication by treatment of virus with high dose THC[8]
1991	Increased susceptibility to HSV in murine retrovirus-infected mice exposed to THC[10]
1992	Macrophage extrinsic anti-viral activity (not IFN related) inhibited by THC[6]
1993	Decreased CTL activity to HSV infected cells by THC[7]

Table 3. Suppression of immunity by FLV and THC

Response	Percent of Control Response			
	Non-infected		FLV-infected[a]	
	-THC	+THC[b]	-THC	+THC[b]
PHA	100	2	3	0
Cytotoxicity (NK)	100	72	6	0
IL-2 production	100	12	2	0.6
TNF production	100	56	36	8

[a]Mice were infected with 550 focus forming units FLV 28 days prior to harvesting spleen for *in vitro* assay.
[b]Spleen cell cultures were treated with 7.5-10 μg THC/ml. Number represents the mean of 3 experiments.

the THC immune suppressive effects were only significant for a severely weakened immune response.

2.2 Enhanced Mortality Due to THC in Mice with Concurrent FLV and HSV Infection

The *in vitro* experiments were followed by examination of both THC and HSV infection of mice previously infected with FLV to determine whether they would serve as cofactors in the progression of FLV disease[10]. Mice were infected with 550 infectious doses of FLV that would infect 50% of mice (ID_{50}) by intraperitoneal injection and then were left untreated, treated with THC only, HSV only, or THC and HSV (Table 4). The infected control mice all were dead within 5 weeks post infection and this was not altered in mice given 2 mg THC intraperitoneally 5 days post FLV infection. By contrast mice that were co-infected with FLV and HSV (10^3 plaque forming units or 1 LD_{20} given intraperitoneally 7 days post FLV infection) died between 30 and 48 days post FLV infection. Interestingly, mice given THC 5 days post FLV and HSV 7 days post FLV either died at 10-15 days due to HSV infection or survived to day 40. By contrast mice that were injected with THC both 2 days before and after HSV infection had a significantly more rapid death due to the retrovirus infection, with all mice dying between 20 and 26 days post infection. Thus, mice given two cofactors, THC and HSV, died an average of 9 days earlier from their FLV infection than mice given either cofactor alone.

Table 4. Concurrent HSV infection and exposure to THC hastens mortality due to murine retrovirus infection

Treatment Group	Mean Day of Death ± S.D.
FLV alone[a]	33.0 ± 2.0
FLV + HSV[b]	40.5 ± 7.6
FLV + THC (d5)[c]	33.4 ± 4.3
FLV + THC (d5) + HSV (d7)[d]	40.0
FLV + THC (d5) + HSV (d7) + THC (d9)	23.8 ± 3.0[e]

[a]Mice were infected intraperitoneally on day 0 with 550 ID_{50} FLV.
[b]Mice were infected intraperitoneally on day 7 with 10^3 PFU HSV.
[c]Mice were given 2 mg THC intraperitoneally either at day 5 or days 5 and 9.
[d]Mice were given both THC and HSV as described above.
[e]Statistically significant when compared to all other groups using a Wilcoxon rank sum test at $p < 0.05$.

3. CONCLUSIONS

The data indicate that THC can be a cofactor in enhancing the progression of a murine retroviral infection. However, this was only seen when a multifactorial system was utilized and was dependent on the use of drug during concurrent infection with HSV. Thus, it appears that any role THC may have as a cofactor by depressing immunity in retroviral infection may be dependent on the presence of other cofactors such as herpesvirus infections and may be related to the timing of drug exposure. The need for care in setting up the timing of drug exposure and intercurrent infections may be a good indication that the epidemiology of drugs of abuse as cofactors in AIDS is difficult to assess. This may be confounded by such factors as drug dose, timing and what other cofactors may be involved in what is likely to be a multifactorial disease process.

REFERENCES

1. Juel-Jensen, B.E. Cannabis and recurrent herpes simplex. Brit. Med. J. 4: 296, 1972.
2. Friedman, H., Klein, T. and Specter, S. Immunosuppression by marijuana and components. In: Psychoneuroimmunology, 2nd Edition, Ader, R., Cohen, N. and Felten, D. (Eds), Academic Press, Orlando, 1991 pp. 931-953.
3. Morahan, P.S., Klykken, P.C., Smith, S.H., Harris, L.S. and Munson, A.E. Effects of cannabinoids on host resistance to *Listeria monocytogenes* and herpes simplex virus. Infect. Immun. 23: 670-674, 1979.
4. Cabral, G.A., Mishkin, E.M. and Holsapple, M.P. Delta-9-tetrahydrocannabinol decreases host resistance to herpes simplex virus type 2 vaginal infection in the guinea pig. In: Marijuana 84. Proc. Oxford Symp. on Cannabis, IRL Press, 1985, pp. 431-438.
5. Cabral, G.A., Lockmuller, J.C. and Mishkin, E.M. Delta-9-tetrahydrocannabinol decreases alpha/beta interferon response to herpes simplex virus type 2 in the B6C3F1 mouse. Proc. Soc. Exp. Biol. Med. 181: 305-311, 1986.
6. Cabral, G.A., and Vasquez, R. Delta-9-tetrahydrocannabinol suppresses macrophage extrinsic antiherpesvirus activity. Proc. Soc. Exp. Biol. Med. 199: 255-263, 1992.
7. Cabral, G.A., Dove-Pettit, D.A. and Fischer-Stenger, K. Marijuana and host resistance to herpesvirus infection. In: Drugs of Abuse, Immunity and AIDS Friedman, H., Klein, T.W. and Specter, S. (Eds.) Adv. Exp. Med. Biol. 335: 95-106, 1993.
8. Lancz, G., Specter, S. and Brown, H.K. Suppressive effects of delta-9-tetrahydrocannabinol on herpes simplex virus infectivity in vitro. Proc. Soc. Exp. Biol. Med. 196: 401-404, 1991.
9. Lancz, G., Specter, S., Brown, H.K., Hackney, J.F. and Friedman, H. Interaction of delta-9-tetrahydrocannabinol with herpes simplex virus and cultural conditions associated with drug-induced anti-cellular effects. In: Drugs of Abuse, Immunity and Immunodeficiency, Friedman, H., Specter, S. and Klein, T (Eds.), Adv. Exp. Med. Biol. 288: 287-304, 1991.
10. Specter, S., Lancz, G., Westrich, G. and Friedman, H. Combined immunosuppressive activities of delta-9-tetrahydrocannabinol and murine retrovirus. In: Drugs of Abuse, Immunity and Immunodeficiency, Friedman, H., Specter, S. and Klein, T (Eds.), Adv. Exp. Med. Biol. 288: 135-142, 1991.
11. Specter, S., Lancz, G., Westrich, G. and Friedman, H. Delta-9-tetrahydrocannabinol augments murine retroviral induced immunosuppression and opportunistic infection. Int. J. Immunopharmac. 13: 411-417, 1991.

19

ALTERATION OF MACROPHAGE FUNCTIONS BY COCAINE

S. S. Lefkowitz,[1] A. Vaz,[1] J. Lincoln,[2] T. Cain,[2] D. J. Brown,[2] and D. L. Lefkowitz[2]

[1] Department of Microbiology and Immunology
Texas Tech University Health Sciences Center
Lubbock Texas 79430
[2] Department of Biological Sciences
Texas Tech University
Lubbock Texas 79409

1. INTRODUCTION

Studies elucidating the effects of cocaine on immune cells and immune function are relatively recent. Although immunomodulation by cocaine has been reported by a number of investigators, it is not consistently associated with immunosuppression. A review summarized many of the earlier studies of cocaine on the immune system (1). Another study (2) describes a number of immune abnormalities in mice exposed to cocaine including an enhancement of neutrophil phagocytosis, a reduction of T-cell responses to the mitogen phytohemagglutinin, and cytotoxic activity of immune spleen cells. Other reports have described alteration of spleen cell subsets following injection with cocaine (3,4). A number of reports have described a reduction or alteration in the production of certain cytokines (5-7). In a series of publications, Peterson et al. (8-10) have reported an enhancement of HIV replication in cultures of human monocytes via the induction of transforming growth factor β (TGFβ) and tumor necrosis factor (TNFα). An increase in p24, one of the internal viral proteins, was used to quantify viral replication. A recent study (11) reported that Mø culture supernatants from cells exposed to cocaine, modulate mesangial cell proliferation *in vitro* altering TGFβ, as well as IL-6.

The present investigators have focused on the effects of cocaine on macrophage (Mø) functions. In previous studies, C57BL/6 mice were injected i.p. with 2.5 to 25 mg/kg cocaine. Peritoneal Mø were collected from 3 to 48 hr later and a number of alterations in function were noted. These included: an increase in the respiratory burst with a concomitant increase in phagocytosis of opsonized zymosan *in vitro* (12, 13). However, when sheep erythrocytes were injected *in vivo*, a decrease in phagocytosis was obtained. Other findings described a decrease in the production of reactive nitrogen intermediates with a concomitant decrease in the killing of P 815 target cells as measured by chromium release (14). Certain metabolites

AIDS, Drugs of Abuse, and the Neuroimmune Axis, Edited by Friedman *et al.*
Plenum Press, New York, 1996

of cocaine have also been shown to alter both reactive oxygen and reactive nitrogen intermediates (15).

The present studies can be divided into 3 distinct areas involving the effects of cocaine on Mø functions. These studies include alteration of: 1) phagocytosis and bacterial cell killing, 2) Mø cell surface receptors, and 3) viral replication in Mø. Part 1 of this study was to determine if either acute or "subchronic" exposure (14 consecutive daily injections) of cocaine affected either phagocytosis and/ or killing of bacteria by isolated peritoneal Mø. Part 2 of this study was concerned with the effects of *in vivo* exposure of cocaine on certain Mø surface markers as measured using a fluorescent activated cell sorter (FACS). Part 3 was a study of the effects of cocaine on the replication of murine hepatitis virus in thioglycollate-induced peritoneal Mø.

2. PHAGOCYTOSIS AND BACTERIAL KILLING

C57BL/6 mice were injected i.p. with either a single injection of 10 mg/kg cocaine or 1 injection per day for 14 days. At intervals of 3, 24, or 48 hr after the last injection, peritoneal Mø were collected as described previously (12). Methods employed for the culturing and opsonizing of E. coli were reported previously (13, 14), Methods used for the cultivation of Mø and subsequent staining are described briefly as follows: The number of Mø was adjusted to 1×10^6 cell/ml. One hundred µl of the cell suspension were added to each well of a 16-well tissue culture chamber slide (Nunc Inc., Naperville, IL). The cells were allowed to attach for 2 hr at 37°C under 5% CO_2. Following attachment, cultures were washed twice with 200 µl warm media to remove non-adherent cells. *E. coli*, suspended in Dulbecco's minimal essential medium (DMEM) with 10% fetal bovine serum, were added at a ratio of 10 : 1. After incubation, the cells were stained for 45 seconds with acridine orange (0.1 mg/ml). Subsequently, the slides were counter-stained for 1 min. with crystal violet (1 mg/ml) to conceal extracellular bacteria. Three 100 cell counts were done using fluorescence microscopy. Bacteria which fluoresced green were scored as live and those that fluoresced red-orange were scored as dead.

Phagocytosis was measured by counting the number of cells under the microscope which ingested *E. coli*. A minimum of 3 mice were used per group and 3, 100 cell counts were averaged per well. All experiments were repeated at least twice. A slight but significant increase in phagocytosis of *E. coli* by Mø collected from animals exposed to cocaine 3 hr previously was noted (27% Vs 32%). There was also a similar difference (P2 0.001) between cultures from control and cocaine treated animals 24 hrs after a single injection of cocaine. Following subchronic administration similar results were obtained, however, no differences were noted 48 hrs after the last exposure using either injection schedule.

Experiments were designed to determine the viability of bacteria after phagocytosis by Mø. Macrophages from mice treated using either acute or "subchronic" schedules of cocaine demonstrated a greatly increased ability to kill bacteria. After "subchronic" exposure to cocaine, the percent killing was shown to increase dramatically to 90% in the cocaine treated as compared to 1% in the controls (Fig. 1). If Mø were harvested 24 hrs after the last injection of cocaine, 61% of the bacteria were killed by Mø from cocaine treated animals compared to 3% of the bacteria killed by Mø from control animals. Results obtained with Mø from mice exposed to a single injection of cocaine were essentially the same (data not shown). When Mø were harvested 48 hr following the last injection of cocaine, using either injection schedule, there were no significant differences between PBS and cocaine treated animals.

From the above studies it should be apparent that cocaine enhances both phagocytosis and killing of bacteria. An increase in the phagocytosis of opsonized zymosan was reported

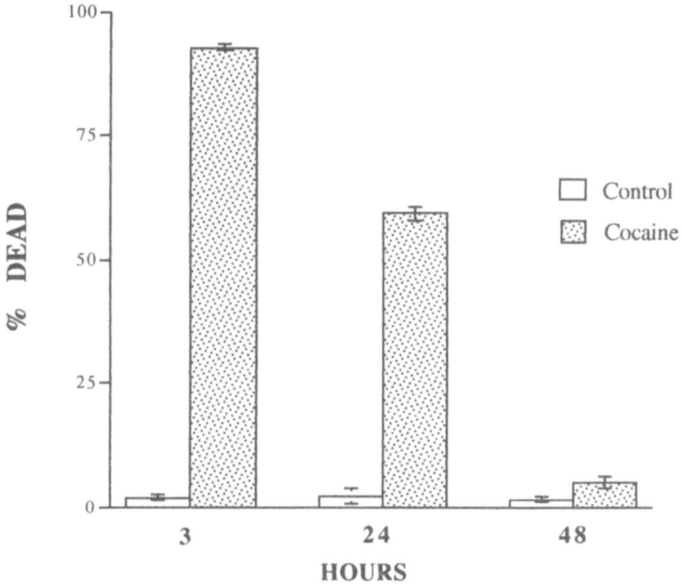

Figure 1. Effects of subchronic injections of cocaine on percent killing during *in vitro* phagocytosis of opsonized E. coli. Three mice were injected i.p. with either PBS or 10 mg/kg cocaine. Peritoneal Mø were removed at the time intervals indicated after the final injection and cultured on 16 well chamber slides. After attachment, the monolayers were washed and *E. coli* were added at a ratio of 10:1 *E. coli*/Mø. After incubation, the cells were stained with acridine orange and scored live or dead according to the color observed using fluorescence microscopy. Red-orange fluorescing bacteria were scored as dead whereas green fluorescing bacteria were scored as live. Each value represents the mean of nine 100 cell counts. P2 0.0001.

previously (12, 13), however, increased killing of bacteria represents a new finding. Because of the increase in the respiratory burst of isolated peritoneal Mø following injections of cocaine (12, 13), the induction of reactive oxygen intermediates probably represents the most likely mechanism involved in bacterial cell killing. In another study involving exposure of Mø to myeloperoxidase *in vitro*, which also caused an increase in the respiratory burst, the bactericidal role of reactive oxygen intermediates was demonstrated through the use of specific radical scavengers including superoxide dismutase, catalase, and mannitol (submitted).

Minimal differences were noted in Mø functions between a single injection or 14 injections (subchronic protocol) of cocaine. No tolerance or additive effects were noted following multiple injections. All effects of cocaine were short lived with Mø from treated animals returning to control values by 48 hrs.

3. MACROPHAGE CELL SURFACE MARKERS

Cell surface markers / receptors have been used as a measure of cellular differentiation and function providing insight into phenotypic, as well as functional capacities of cells. Engagement of various surface receptors on Mø can transduce a signal leading to cellular events that can change the phenotype, movement, gene expression, or activation of the cell. Because of studies on phagocytosis and macrophage-mediated cytotoxicity, the present studies were implemented to determine the effects of cocaine on certain surface receptors/

markers which are involved in Mø functions. Analysis using FACS was used to evaluate the effects of cocaine on the level of expression of certain Mø surface receptors and proteins, including those which could affect either phagocytosis or macrophage-mediated cytotoxicity.

Fluorescein isothiocyanate conjugated (FITC) rat monoclonal antibodies to various cell surface markers were purchased from a number of sources. Specific Mø surface markers studied included F4/80, Mac-1, Fc, MMR, and Ia. Peritoneal Mø were collected from C57BL/6 mice and suspended in PBS containing 1% bovine serum albumen (BSA) and 0.02% sodium azide. Two ml of cell suspension at a concentration of 1×10^6 cells/ml were aliquoted into polymethylpentene (PMP) jars (Nalgene, Rochester, NY). The jars were placed at 37°C under 5% CO_2 to facilitate cell adherence. After 20 minutes the cells were washed vigorously 3 to 4 times to remove contaminating non-adherent cells. The jars were then kept on ice for another 20 minutes and then vortexed to remove attached Mø. After incubation and staining with the appropriate antibody-conjugate, the cells were analyzed using a FACStar Plus flow cytometer (Becton Dickinson, Mountainview CA).

A general down regulation of peritoneal Mø receptors was noted following injections of cocaine *in vivo*. F4/80 was significantly down-regulated by an i.p. injection of cocaine 3 hrs prior to harvest. Figure 2 illustrates that F4/80 activity was still reduced at 24 hr following exposure to 10 mg/kg cocaine *in vivo*. A slight reduction in fluorescence of this marker was noted following harvest of Mø 3 hrs after the last injection using the subchronic administration protocol but considerably less than following a single injection.

The Mac-1 receptor is involved in phagocytosis of particles opsonized by complement. Figure 3 shows that control animals injected with PBS displayed three distinct cell populations with different affinities for anti-Mac-1 ligand. One population was negative, one highly positive, and one intermediate. When Mø were collected 3 hr after exposure to i.p. injections of either 5 or 10 mg/kg cocaine, a shift in the Mac-1 positive receptor populations

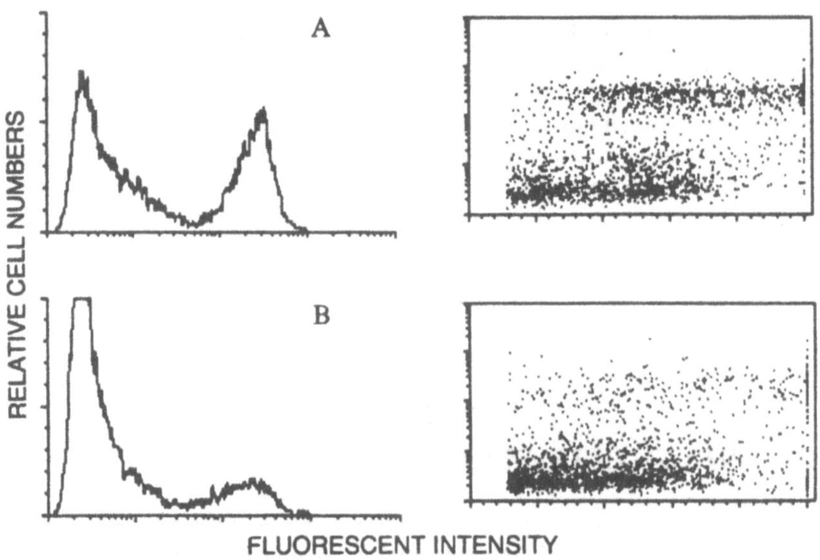

Figure 2. Macrophages were harvested from mice 3 hrs. after a single i.p. injection of either saline (A) or 10 mg/kg cocaine (B). Cells were separated by adherance, removed, and then stained with FITC conjugated anti-F4/80. Approximately 1 x 10^4 cells were counted and their relative fluorescence recorded using a fluorescent activated cell sorter.

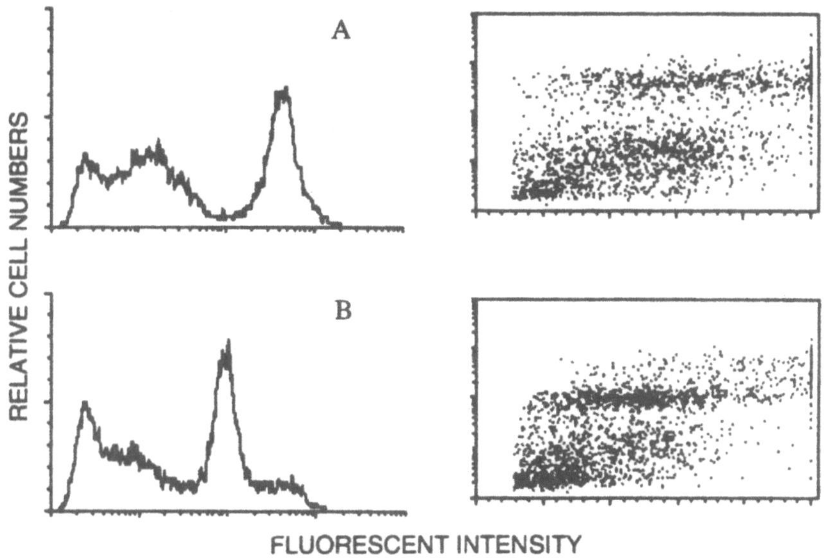

Figure 3. Macrophages were harvested from mice 3 hrs. after a single i.p. injection of either saline (A) or 10 mg/kg cocaine (B). Cells were separated by adherance, removed, and then stained with FITC conjugated anti-Mac-1. Approximately 1 x 10^4 cells were counted and their relative fluorescence recorded using a fluorescent activated cell sorter.

was observed. A fourth population appeared between population 2 and 3 of the control Mø. Part of the cells that shifted appeared to have moved to the right from population 2 representing an increase in fluorescent activity, however, a shift to the left or down-regulation was noted from the highly positive peak. When Mø were cultured 24 hrs after exposure to cocaine, only those injected with 25 mg/kg showed the above change. Subchronic exposure of cocaine on Mac-1 was less distinct with broader peaks than after a single injection (data not shown). Minimal differences were noted between control and cocaine-injected mice, suggesting a reduced effect of cocaine using this schedule Ia expression is required for the Mø to function as an antigen presenting cell to T helper cells. Mø from mice injected i.p. with either 5 or 10 mg / kg cocaine showed a major decrease in Ia expression when removed 3 hr after exposure to cocaine (Fig. 4). This reduction persisted for 24 hr. following a single 25 mg/kg injection while a single 10 mg/kg injection of cocaine produced negligible effects 24 hrs after exposure. If the subchronic protocol was employed, there was little effect on Ia expression when the Mø were harvested 3 hrs. after cocaine exposure (Fig 5).

Other receptors studied included the Fc receptors IgG_{2a} (high affinity FcR), IgG_{2b} (low affinity FcR), and the macrophage mannose receptor (MMR). Minimal changes were observed in these receptors 3 and 24 hr after exposure to cocaine (data not shown). There was, however, a slight but consistent down-regulation seen in all three receptors on Mø collected 3 hr after cocaine exposure using doses of 5-25 mg/kg. Similar results were observed with Mø harvested 24 hr following a single 25 mg/kg i.p. injection of cocaine. Macrophages collected 24 hr after a single 10 mg/kg injection of cocaine showed either very little or no effect on IgG_{2a}, IgG_{2b}, or the MMR. There were no consistent alterations of these receptors following the subchronic schedule of cocaine injection when compared to controls.

The present studies clearly show that cocaine temporarily reduces cell surface molecules which could affect both phagocytosis and macrophage-mediated cytotoxicity. This reduction appears to be more pronounced after a single injection of cocaine as compared

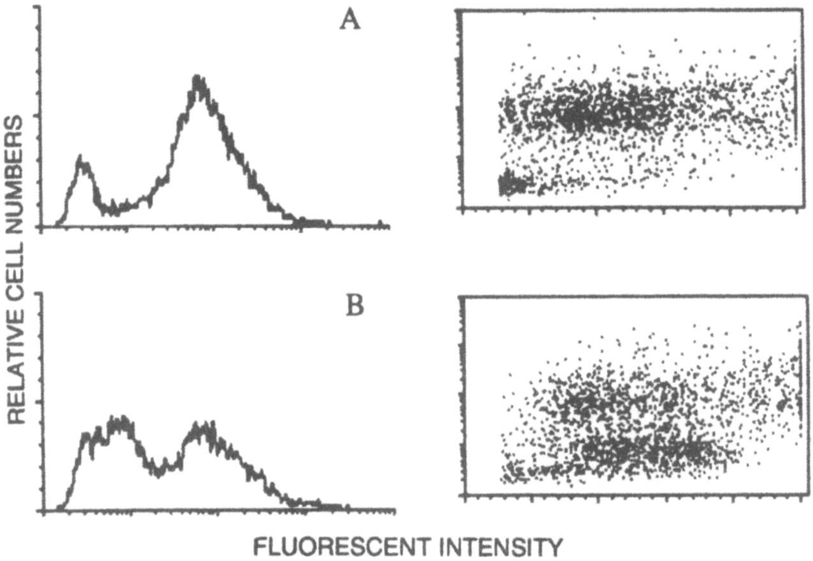

Figure 4. Macrophages were harvested from mice 3 hrs. after a single i.p. injection of either saline (A) or 10 mg/kg cocaine (B). Cells were separated by adherance, removed, and then stained with FITC conjugated anti-Ia. Approximately 1 x 10^4 cells were counted and their relative fluorescence recorded using a fluorescent activated cell sorter.

to after the subchronic exposure of consecutive injections for 14 days. This would suggest possible "tolerance" after multiple exposures and minimizes the possibility of a long term effect following continued usage of cocaine. Overall, these data may translate into a possible impairment of certain non-specific immune responses. Although levels of cocaine taken by habitual users are somewhat less than those injected into mice in these studies, frequent abuse could conceivably induce similar cellular "lesions" in man. These results taken in their

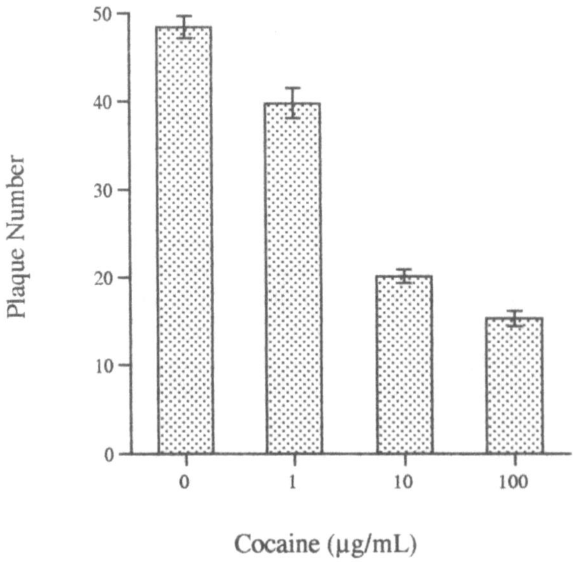

Figure 5. Monolayers of murine thioglycollate-induced macrophages were incubated 48 hr with different concentrations of cocaine dissolved in DMEM containing 2% FBS. After removal of media, these cells were infected with mouse hepatitis virus, an overlay added, and the number of viral plaques quantitated. p<0.001.

entirety suggest that the ability of cocaine to alter Mø functions could also cause a temporary alteration of responses resulting in a compromised immune system.

4. VIRAL REPLICATION IN MACROPHAGES

C57BL/6 mice, 8-16 weeks of age, were injected i.p. with 1 ml thioglycollate broth (Baltimore Biological Laboratories, Baltimore, MD). After 4 days, the animals were sacrificed by cervical dislocation. Peritoneal lavage was performed as described previously (12) and the cells resuspended at 1.5 x 10^6 cells per ml in DMEM and 100 µl of cell suspension were added to each well of a Costar (Cambridge, MA) 96 well tissue culture plate. After 2 hr incubation, cells were washed to remove non-adherent cells and 200µl of media containing 2% serum were added to each well. After overnight incubation, supernatants were removed and media containing various dilution's of cocaine from 1-100µg per ml were added to wells and incubated from 1 to 120 hours. After the allotted time, media were removed and a viral plaque assay was performed using mouse hepatitis virus (MHV) obtained from ATCC (American Type Culture Collection, Rockville, MD).

Initial studies were done in order to determine if cocaine would affect replication of murine hepatitis virus *in vitro*. Cocaine levels of 1, 3, 11, 33, and 100µg per ml were incubated with Mø for 48 hrs prior to infection with MHV. A dose-dependent inhibition of viral replication was observed in the form of a decrease in both plaque size and number (Fig. 5). After noting this anti-viral effect with as little as 1µg per ml, an experiment was done to determine the kinetics of anti-viral activity. Keeping the cocaine concentration constant at 100µg per ml, the incubation time was varied from 3 to 120 hrs. When cocaine was removed from the Mø monolayers between 3 and 6 hrs, and replaced with fresh media, no antiviral activity was found in contrast to when cocaine was left on the cells. An increase in antiviral activity was seen as early as 12 hrs (data not shown). Fig. 6 illustrates the time course between 48 to 120 hrs. Antiviral activity continued to increase for as long as 120 hrs.

In order to identify the antiviral material involved in cocaine inhibition of MHV, 4 different antisera were tested. Both anti-TGFβ and anti-TNFα had no effect on the anti-viral activity in supernatants from cocaine exposed Mø (data not shown). The addition of either anti-IFNα+β or anti-IFNβ, however, resulted in an increase in both viral plaque number and

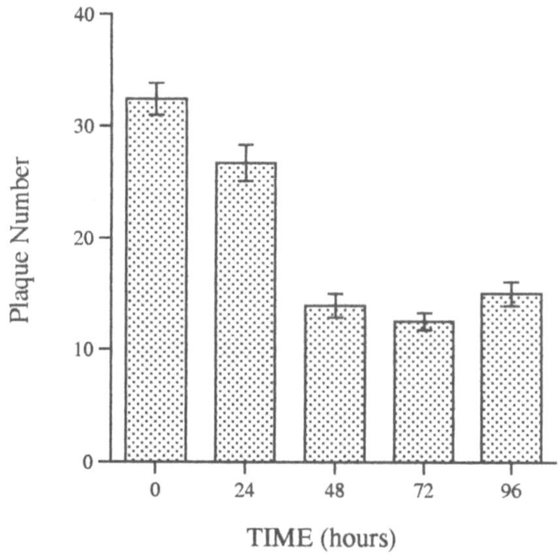

Figure 6. Monolayers of murine thioglycollate-induced macrophages were incubated for various time intervals with 100 µg/ml of cocaine dissolved in DMEM containing 2% FBS. After removal of media these cells were infected with mouse hepatitis virus, an overlay added, and the number of viral plaques quantitated. $p<0.001$.

size. This increase was greater than in the controls without serum. Anti-IFN caused a significant increase in plaque number when added to the transfer supernatants. The increase in plaque size as well as number was seen when either anti-IFNα+β or anti-IFNβ was incubated with pooled supernatants from cocaine exposed Mø.

In order to determine if the effect of cocaine on virus replication depended on intracellular calcium levels, ionomycin was added to cocaine-treated cultures. The addition of ionomycin to virus-infected cultures and subsequent removal resulted in a increase in viral plaques similar to that of the controls without cocaine (data not shown).

The present studies have reported an increase in both plaque size and plaque number after addition of anti-IFN. It is apparent that MHV caused the induction of IFN in the present system even without the addition of cocaine, since plaque size was increased in the presence of the antisera even in the controls. In order to maximize the effect of anti-IFN, a number of different designs were used including both direct exposure of cocaine-exposed cells to the antisera, as well as to the supernatants which were transferred from cocaine-exposed cells to fresh cells. In both experimental designs, both plaque size and number were increased in the presence of anti-IFN. In certain experiments, control viral plaques were slightly larger in the presence of the antisera.

Cocaine had to be continuously present in culture since removal of the cocaine within a few hrs failed to induce antiviral activity. It was noted by Watzl and Watson (1) that cocaine needed to be continuously present in order to function in certain systems. Interestingly, maximal levels of IFN were obtained after 48 hrs suggesting that this may not be a direct effect of cocaine on IFN induction, but rather an indirect effect since maximal IFN$^{\alpha+\beta}$ induction *in vitro* is usually in about 6 hrs using a classical inducer such as poly I:C.

It has been reported that cocaine interferes with calcium mobilization (15). Studies by others (16, 17) reported that both calcium inhibitors and cocaine interfere with induction of reactive oxygen intermediates and reactive nitrogen intermediates by Mø. It has been reported that calcium antagonists inhibit the replication of certain viruses including influenza virus (18) and vesicular stomatitis virus (19). The stimulation of virus replication in cocaine-exposed cultures by the calcium ionophore ionomycin suggests a similar effect in the present study. It appears that alterations of intracellular calcium levels are involved in the inhibition of viral replication. This is further supported by the observation that early removal of cocaine from Mø cultures prevents production of the antiviral effect. Preliminary studies on intracellular calcium levels support this concept. This study demonstrates that both interferon and calcium levels mediate the antiviral action of cocaine.

5. SUMMARY AND CONCLUSIONS

- Phagocytosis and Bacterial Killing
  - Peritoneal MØ obtained from C57BL/6 mice injected with 10 mg/kg cocaine demonstrated a slight increase in phagocytosis of E. coli but a highly significant increase in bacterial killing.
  - Phagocytosis and bacterial cell killing were not significantly different between Mø from mice exposed to either a single injection of cocaine or 1 each day for 14 days.
  - Increases in phagocytosis and killing were brief and persisted for 24 hrs after injection returning to control levels by 48 hrs.
- Macrophage Cell Surface Markers
  - Injection of mice with cocaine resulted in a down regulation of Mø cell surface markers as evidenced by a reduction of specific fluorescence.

- Down regulation of cell surface markers was greater following a single injection of cocaine than following the subchronic protocol.
- Density of most cell surface markers were at control levels by about 24 hrs using the lower doses of cocaine but not when exposed to 25 mg/kg.

- Viral Replication in Macrophages
  - Replication of murine hepatitis virus was inhibited in thioglycollate-induced Mø incubated with cocaine *in vitro* .
  - This inhibition of viral replication was dependent, in part, upon the alteration of intracellular calcium.

6. ACKNOWLEDGMENTS

This work was supported by NIH grant 5 R01 DA07298-02.

7. REFERENCES

1. Watzl B, and Watson RR. Immunomodulation by cocaine-A neuroendocrine mediated response. Life Sci 46: 1319-1329, 1990.
2. Pacifici R, Avico U, Belogi L, Borelli G, Croce C, Di Carlo S, Pichini S, Santiangeli C, Zuccaro P, Tubaro E. Immunological effect of cocaine and host resistance in mice. Int J Immunother Vlll 91-99, 1992.
3. Poet TS, Pillai R, Wood S, amd Watson RR. Stimulation of natural killer cell activity by murine retroviral infection and cocaine. Tox Let 59: 147-152 1991.
4. Lopez MC, Chen G-J, Huang DS, Wang Y, and Watson WW. Modification of spleen cell subsets by chronic cocaine administration and murine retrovirus infection in normal and protein-malnourished mice. Int J Immunopharm 14:1153-1163, 1992.
5. Chen GJ, Tachibana K, Huang DS, Watson RR. Cocaine modulation in vitro of tumor necrosis factor production by macrophages from retrovirally-infected mice. Life Sci 52: 1641-1647, 1993.
6. Wang Y, Huang DS, Watson RR. In vivo and in vitro cocaine modulation on production of cytokines in C57BL/6 mice. Life Sci 54: 401-411, 1994.
7. Shen HM, Kennedy JL, Ou DW. Inhibition of cytokine release by cocaine. Int J Immunopharm 16: 295-300, 1994.
8. Peterson P K, Gekker G, Chao CC, Schut R, Molitor TW, Balfour HH. Cocaine potentiates HIV-1 replication in human peripheral blood mononuclear cells: involvement of transforming growth factor-ß. J Immunol 146: 81-84, 1991.
9. Peterson P K, Gekker G, Chao CC, Schut R, Verhoef J, Edelman CK, Erice A, Balfour HH. Cocaine amplifies HIV-1 replication in cytomegalovirus-stimulated peripheral blood mononuclear cell cultures. J Immunol 149: 676-680, 1992.
10. Peterson P K, Gekker G, Chao CC, Hu S, Edelman CK, Balfour HH, Verhoef J. Human cytomegalovirus-stimulated peripheral blood mononuclear cells induce HIV-1 replication via a tumor necrosis factor-α-mediated mechanism. J Clin Invest 89: 574-580, 1992;.
11. Mattana J, Gibbons N, Singhal PC. Cocaine interacts with macrophages to modulate mesangial cell proliferation. J. Pharm Exptl Therap 271: 311-318, 1994.
12. Vaz A[a], Lefkowitz SS, Lefkowitz DL. Cocaine alters the respiratory burst and phagocytic activity of murine macrophages. Clin Immunol Immunopath 69:161-166, 1993.
13. Vaz A[b], Lefkowitz SS, Lefkowitz DL. Effects of cocaine on the respiratory burst of murine macrophages. *In:* Drugs of Abuse, Immunity and AIDS, Friedman H. et al., (Eds.), Plenum Publishers, NY 135, 1993.
14. Lefkowitz SS, Vaz A, Lefkowitz DL. Cocaine reduces macrophage killing by inhibiting reactive nitrogen intermediates. Int J Immunopharm 15:717-721, 1993.
15. Vaz A, Lefkowitz SS, Castro A, Lefkowitz DL. The effects of cocaine and its metabolites on the production of reactive oxygen and reactive nitrogen intermediates. Life Sci. 55:PL439-444, 1994.
16. Smith DL, Rommel F. A rapid micro method for the simultaneous determination of phagocytic-micro-biocidal activity of human peripheral blood leukocytes in vitro. J. Immunol. Meth.17:241-247.
17. Lian C-J, Hwang WS, Pai CH. Plasmid-mediated resistance to phagocytosis in *Yersinia enterolitica*. Infect Immun 55:1176-83 1987;.

18. Matsui K, Friedman H, Klein TW. Molecular mechanisms associated with cocaine-induced modulation of human T lymphocyte proliferation. *In:* Drugs of Abuse, Immunity and AIDS, Friedman H. et al., (Eds.). Plenum Publishers, NY 127, 1993.
19. Shen HM[a], Wiederhold MD, Ou DW. The suppression of macrophage secretion by calcium blockers and adenosine. Immunopharm and Immunotox 17:301-309, 1995.
20. Shen HM[b], Sha LX, Wiederhold MD, Ou DW. Suppression of macrophage reactive intermediates by cocaine. Int J Immunopharm 17:419-423, 1995.
21. Nugent KM, and Shanley JD. Verapamil inhibits influenza A virus replication. Archives of Virol 81:163-170, 1984.
22. Schlesinger MJ and Cahill D. Verapamil and chlorpromazine inhibit the budding of sindbis and vesicular stomatitis viruses from infected chicken embryo fibroblasts. Virology 168:187-190, 1989.

20

DIVERGENT EFFECTS OF COCAINE ON CYTOKINE PRODUCTION BY LYMPHOCYTES AND MONOCYTE/MACROPHAGES

HIV-1 Enhancement by Cocaine within the Blood-Brain Barrier

A. M. Fiala,[1] X. -H. Gan,[2] T. Newton,[3] F. Chiappelli,[4,5] P. Shapshak,[6] V. Kermani,[7] M. A. Kung,[4,5] A. Diagne,[1] O. Martinez,[8] D. Way,[9] M. Weinand,[9] M. Witte,[9] and M. Graves[10]

[1] Department of Medicine
[2] Departments of Microbiology and Immunology
[3] Department of Psychiatry
[4] Department of Neurobiology
UCLA School of Medicine, Los Angeles, California 90095
[5] Division of Diagnostic Sciences
UCLA School of Dentistry, Los Angeles, California 90095
[6] Department of Psychiatry, Neurology, and Pathology
University of Miami School of Medicine, Miami, Florida 33136
[7] Immunobiogen, Inc., Canoga Park, California 91303
[8] Departments of Obstetrics and Gynecology
UCLA School of Medicine, Los Angeles, California 90095
[9] Department of Surgery
University of Arizona School of Medicine, Tucson, Arizona 85724
[10] Department of Neurology
Department of Neurobiology
UCLA School of Medicine, Los Angeles, California 90095

ABSTRACT

Cocaine-related immunosuppression is asumed to have serious consequences, but its evaluation in drug-addicted subjects is lacking. In this study performed with materials from addicted subjects receiving intravenous cocaine and normal control subjects, acute cocaine effects on cytokine production *in vivo* and in mononuclear cells *in vitro* were determined. Acute intravenous cocaine administration resulted in (a) increased white blood cell and lymphocyte counts, (b) decreased tumor necrosis factor-α (TNF-α) and interleukin (IL)-10

AIDS, Drugs of Abuse, and the Neuroimmune Axis, Edited by Friedman *et al.*
Plenum Press, New York, 1996

serum levels; (c) depressed TNF-α, IL-10 and IL-12 production by unstimulated or LPS-stimulated mononuclear cells; (d) increased TNF-α production by PHA-stimulated mononuclear cells. These observations suggest that cocaine has stimulatory effect on TNF-α production by lymphocytes but inhibitory action on TNF-α production by monocyte/macrophages. *In vitro* cocaine treatment of monocyte-enriched preparations of mononuclear cells from normal donors resulted in suppression of cytokine production. A blood-brain barrier model was constructed using human brain microvascular endothelial cells. In this model mononuclear cell transmigration was correctly regulated by Th1 and Th2 cytokines and preferential migration of "memory" T cells was inhibited by cocaethylene. TNF-α and cocaethylene increased HIV-1 titers in the brain-side of the model.

Conclusions

Cell migration and virus transport across the blood-brain barrier are regulated by cytokines. Cocaine and cocaethylene alter cytokine production and cell migration by lymphocytes and monocytes, and virus infection of the brain compartment.

1. INTRODUCTION

Cocaine is the most commonly abused drug in the United States [Gawin, 1994] and is also instrumental in the spread of HIV-1 infection to persons utilizing non-sterile needles and in increased sexual promiscuousness. Moreover abused drugs are assumed to predispose to the acquired immunodeficiency syndrome (AIDS) by their immunosuppressive effects, which are difficult to assess in chronically-addicted, frequently non-compliant subjects. Acute effects of intravenous cocaine can be, however, evaluated by cytokine assays of blood samples from chronically-addicted subjects undergoing experimental therapy with intravenous cocaine, such as is done at the West Los Angeles VA Hospital Infusion Laboratory for the Study of Treatments of Cocaine Abuse (WLAVA laboratory).

Modulation of cytokine expression by abused drugs may play a role in the progression of AIDS and, specifically, in HIV-1 penetration across the blood-brain barrier (BBB) and infection of neural cells. We previously demonstrated that TNF-α enhances penetration of cell-free HIV-1 across a BBB model *in vitro* [Fiala et al, 1996a] and facilitates "restricted" infection of astrocytes in coculture with macrophages [Fiala et al, 1996b]. In this study cocaine was noted to increase white blood cell and lymphocyte counts *in vivo,* to modulate secretion of TNF- α, interleukin IL-10, and IL-12 *in vivo* and *in vitro*, and to alter selective migration of T cell subsets across the BBB model. Cocaethylene enhanced HIV-1 penetration or replication in the brain-side of the model.

2. MATERIALS AND METHODS

2.1 Intravenous Cocaine Administration to Subjects Undergoing Experimental Treatment of Cocaine Addiction

Chronically cocaine-addicted subjects are treated at the WLAVA Laboratory with various treatment modalities administered together with intravenous (IV) cocaine. After a 3-5 day withdrawal from cocaine abuse, the subjects in this study received 20 mg IV cocaine with selegiline or placebo. A pre-injection blood specimen was obtained 1 to 2 h before a cocaine dose and a post-injection specimen 10-30 min after the dose.

2.2 Cytokine Assays

Peripheral blood mononuclear cells (PBMC) from drug-addicted subjects or healthy control subjects were separated by Ficoll-Hypaque gradient centrifugation. Duplicate cultures of PBMC were established in a microtiter plate in RPMI1640 with 10% fetal calf serum with or without bacterial lipopolysaccharide (LPS) (Sigma) (100 ng/ml), or with phytohemagglutinin A (PHA) (Sigma) (5 μM).

Cytokines were assayed by a double-antibody sandwich ELISA technique [Gan et al, 1994] which is highly sensitive (lowest detectable level of TNF- α is about 5 -10 pg/ml, that of IL-10 is about 5 pg/ml, and that of IL-12 is about 0.1 pg/ml) and highly specific (no cross-reactivity of TNF- α with IL-1β, IL-2 or IFN-γ). Wells of 96-well ELISA plates were coated with 50 uL of monoclonal antibody to each cytokine (3-5 ug IgG/ml) for at least 1 day and then stored for up to 4 weeks at 4°C. Before the assay, coated plates were washed three times and blocked for 1 hr with ELISA phosphate-buffered saline containing 1% bovine serum albumin. The plates were washed twice and 50 μl of sample or cytokine standards were added to the wells. After overnight incubation, the plates were washed three times, and 50 μl of polyclonal antibody to each cytokine was added. Following 1 hr incubation, akaline phosphatase-conjugated goat anti-rabbit IgG (Caltag) was placed in each well and incubated for an additional one hour. Finally, the plates were washed and incubated with the substrate (Sigma 104). The plates were read 2 hr later at 405 nm using a Titertek Multiscan MCC/240 ELISA reader. The following monoclonal antibodies were used in these assays: TNF- α: monoclonal mouse from G. Trinchieri, Wistar Institute; IL-10 monoclonal (JES3-119F) from Pharmingen, San Diego; IL-12: monoclonal C8.6 from G. Trinchieri, Wistar Institute. Secondary polyclonal anticytokine antibodies were prepared in rabbits.

2.3 Blood-Brain Barrier Model

An *in vitro* BBB model (referred to as "model") consisted of a human brain microvascular endothelial cell monolayer (referred to as " brain endothelial cells") on the upper surface and an astrocytic sublayer on the lower surface of a porous membrane. The model was used in basal state and after treatment with TNF- α or abused drugs. The model was constructed by placing 0.1-0.2 ml suspension of 1 x 10^5 brain endothelial cells in E-Stim medium (Collaborative Biomedical Products, Becton Dickinson, Lincoln Park, NJ) or CS5.0 medium (Cell Systems Corp, Kirkland, WA) in the upper chamber of a 24 well tissue culture insert with a Cyclopore^R polyethylene terephthalate membrane bottom comprising 2 x 10^6 pores/cm^2 (pore diameter of 3 μ) and coated with human fibronectin (50 μg/ml) (both from Collaborative Biomedical Products). Then 0.5-0.6 ml of the same medium was placed in the lower chamber and the model was used on days 2 to 5 after seeding. Brain endothelial cell lines were obtained from two laboratories: (a) the Department of Surgery, University of Arizona (Tucson, AZ), six independent cultures were isolated from non-epileptogenic lateral temporal cortex tissues obtained during surgical removal of epileptogenic foci in the medial temporal lobe [Weinand et al, 1992]. Neural microvascular fragments obtained by microdissection were separated by unit gravity sedimentation for 2-5 min with 2-3 repetitions depending on purity. The microvascular fragments were placed in culture on a gelatin-coated tissue-culture plastic in Dulbecco's modified Eagle's medium/F-12 Ham nutrient mixture (DME/F-12) (Sigma , St. Louis, MO) with 10% fetal bovine serum and 25 mM Hepes (pH 7.2-7.4), endothelial cell growth supplement (50 μg/ml) (Collaborative Biomedical Products, Becton Dickinson, Lincoln Park, NJ) and heparin (100 μg/ml). The outgrowing cells were cultured at 37º C in a 7.5% CO_2 humidified incubator and were used with less than ten *in vitro* passages, since Sill et al [1992] showed that the permeability of bovine endothelial cells remained similar (4-11 Ohm.cm^2) up to passage 10; (b) the Applied Cell Biology

Research Institute (Kirkland, WA), brain endothelial cells were isolated from human brain tissue by microdissection, enzymatic digestion, and selection of cells reactive with monoclonal antibody against E-selectin in AIS MicroCELLector flasks (Applied Immune Science, Menlo Park, CA) as described by Dhawan et al [Dhawan et al, 1995]. Each brain endothelial cell line had cobblestone morphology and was positive for endothelial cell markers, Factor VIII related antigen and *Ulex europaeus* agglutinin, as determined by flow cytometric analysis. Glucose transporter isoform type 1 (GLUT-1) antigen was demonstrated in one line by immunocytochemical staining utilizing a rabbit polyclonal antibody to the COOH terminus of GLUT-1 [Pardridge et al, 1990]. Transmission and scanning electron microscopy revealed uniformly flat and tightly adjoining endothelial-like cells displaying areas of cell membrane fusion between adjoining cells resembling *zonula adhaerens* (desmosome) junctions [Farquahar and Palade, 1963]. Primary human fetal astrocytes were prepared as described by Tornatore et al. [1994] from discarded fetal brain tissues of gestational age 12 -20 weeks obtained during therapeutic abortions. The cultures used in these experiments were 100% positive by immunocytochemistry with polyclonal rabbit antibody to glial fibrillary acidic protein (DAKO Corp, Carpinteria, CA). The model displayed an adequate barrier function to macromolecules [Fiala et al, 1996a] and a moderate transendothelial electrical resistance (up to 58 Ohm/cm^2).

2.4 Assay of Infectious HIV-1 Penetration across the BBB Model

HIV-1 penetration was investigated in the BMVEC model in a basal state or after pretreatment with TNF-α or medium. Cell-free HIV-$1_{JR\text{-}FL}$ (0.5 ng) was placed in the upper chamber and, at indicated intervals, a 50 μl sample was removed from the lower chamber and added to a 1 ml suspension of 2 x 10^5 A3.01 cells (a human T-cell line derived from the buffy coat of a patient with lymphoblastic leukemia, which was provided by the AIDS Research and Reference Reagent Program, Division of AIDS, NIAID, NIH [Folks et al, 1985]) in RPMI medium with 10% fetal calf serum placed in a separate well. After 5 (or 10) days of incubation, the wells with A3.01 cells were harvested by centrifugation and p24 antigen concentration was measured in the supernatant by the Coulter HIV-1 p24 antigen assay (Coulter Corp, Hialeah, FL). This assay measures the presence of infectious HIV-1 in the lower chamber since undetectable amounts of the p24 antigen are replicated into pg amounts. The cell pellet was tested for HIV-1 RNA by the reverse transcriptase nested polymerase chain reaction (PCR) using the outer primers SK 149/39 and the inner primers SK 38/39 followed by the Southern blot analysis [Xin et al,1995].

HIV-1- and TNF-α-stimulated mononuclear cells were prepared by exposing $1x10^6$ peripheral blood mononuclear cells with 2 ng HIV-$1_{JR\text{-}FL}$ for 16 hr, washing the cells three times by centrifugation and resuspending them in RPMI with 10% fetal calf serum. Then $5x10^5$ of these cells were placed in the upper chamber pretreated with TNF-α (20 ng/ml) and cell migration across the model was observed by transmission electron microscopy.

2.5 Transmission Electron Microscopy

For morphological studies of transmigration, 1 x 10^6 mononuclear cells enriched in monocytes (80% monocytes) by the technique of Recaldi et al [Fogelman et al, 1988] were incubated with 1.4 ng of HIV-$1_{JR\text{-}FL}$ for 1 hr and $2x10^5$ of these cells were placed in the upper chamber of the two-layer model bathed in TNF- α (20 ng/ml). After 1 and 24 hr, the membrane filters with cells were fixed in modified Karnovsky's fixative (1.5% glutaraldehyde, 2% paraformaldehyde in 0.1M cacodylate buffer) for 2 hr at 4ºC. The filters were embedded in plastic using routine methods [Hunter, 1984]. Thick sections (1 μm) from the resultant blocks were cut at right angles to the filter so that the filter would be visualized in cross section. Selected regions were further processsed for electron microscopy examined in a Siemens electron microscope.

2.6 Mononuclear Cell Migration and Flow Cytometry

Mononuclear blood cell preparations comprising 70 - 80% lymphocytes were isolated by the Lymphoprep gradient centrifugation from peripheral venous blood of normal adult volunteers. The cells were washed, suspended at 1 x 10^6 cells/ml in AIM-V medium (Gibco BRL. Gaithersburg, MD) and stimulated with concanavalin-A (Sigma Chemical Co., St. Louis, MO) (5 μg/ml) for 2 hr [Chiappelli et al, 1993, and 1994] before use. For migration assays, the cell culture inserts were treated with: (a) (in the lower chamber) IL-1β (2 ng/ml) and TNF-α (20 ng/ml) (both from Genzyme Corp., Cambridge, MA), (b) (in the upper chamber) IL-4 (10 ng/ml) or IL-10 (10 ng/ml) (both from DNAX , Inc, Palo Alto, CA), or with IL-12 (10 ng/ml) (Genetics Institute, Cambridge, MA). After removing the medium, 0.5 ml of mononuclear cell suspension (1 x 10^6 cells/ml) was placed in the upper well and the model was incubated at 36 ºC. At intervals, the contents of the lower and upper chambers were gently resuspended three times. The cell suspension was counted using a Coulter MICRO DIFF 16 counter (Coulter Corp, Hialeah, FL). Transmigrated monocyte-derived macrophages were counted after resuspension with trypsin of adherent cells on the bottom coverslip. Lymphocyte subpopulations were identified by standard dual-color flow cytometry using fluorochrome-conjugated mouse anti-human antibodies (LeucoGATE, CD4 PE, and CD45RA FITC, Becton-Dickinson, San Jose, CA) and a FACScan instrument (Becton Dickinson, San Jose, CA) according to standard protocols.

2.7 Cultures of Monocyte-Derived Macrophages

Monocyte-derived macrophages were prepared as described elsewhere [Fiala et al, 1996b]. Briefly, monocyte-enriched preparations of mononuclear cells from healthy donors were suspended in RPMI medium with 10% autologous serum and cultivated in 6-well T.C. dishes for 5-7 days until the cells were seen to be differentiated into typical macrophages.

3. RESULTS

3.1 *In Vivo* Effects of Acute Intravenous Cocaine Administration on Blood Cell Counts

Acute intravenous administration of cocaine to three experimental cocaine-addicted subjects resulted in an elevation of total WBC, total lymphocyte, and total CD4+ counts in peripheral blood of all subjects (Table 1).

3.2 *In Vivo* Effects of Acute Intravenous Cocaine Administration on Cytokine Secretion in the Blood *in Vivo* and Cytokine Production by Mononuclear Cells *in Vitro*

In post- cocaine injection serum specimens, TNF- α and IL-10 serum levels were decreased compared to pre-injection specimens, whereas IL-12 levels were unchanged (Table 2a). Supernatant cytokine levels of mononuclear cell cultures isolated from post-cocaine injection blood specimens were depressed compared to pre-cocaine injection specimens, both in unstimulated cultures and in cultures mitogenically stimulated by LPS (a

Table 1. Effects of acute IV cocaine administration on blood counts of addicted subjects

Patient's # (treatment)[a]	Test	Cell count (per mm^3) before IV cocaine	Cell count (per mm^3) after IV cocaine
1 (placebo)	WBC count	6,200	7,500
	Lymphocyte total (%)	2,232 (36%)	3,000 (40%)
	CD4+ total (%)	982 (44%)	1,350(45%)
2 (selegiline)	WBC count	5,100	5,900
	Lymphocyte total (%)	2,244 (44%)	2,537 (43%)
	CD4+ total (%)	1,100 (49%)	1,243 (49%)
5 (selegiline)	WBC count	4,200	4,900
	Lymphocyte total (%)	2,100 (50%)	2,303 (47%)
	CD4+ total (%)	945 (45%)	967 (42%)

[a] Either selegiline or placebo were co-administered with IV cocaine to investigate the effect of selegiline on cocaine craving

macrophage stimulatory factor) [Yirmiya R et al, 1993]. In post-cocaine cultures stimulated by PHA (a T cell stimulatory factor), however, TNF- α secretion was upregulated (Table 2b). These results suggested divergent responses to cocaine stimulation by monocytes and lymphocytes. These effects were, therefore, investigated using purified cell subpopulations.

3.3 Cocaine and Cocaethylene Effects *in Vitro* on Secretion of TNF-α, IL-10, and IL-12 by Monocyte-Derived Macrophages from Normal Donors

In vitro cocaine treatment of monocyte-derived macrophages isolated from peripheral blood of normal donors suppressed cytokine production in the supernatant collected 18 hr after addition of cocaine (Table 3).

Table 2. Cytokine responses to acute intravenous cocaine administration (a) *in vivo* in the pre- and post-cocaine blood (serum) samples in three subjects. (b) *in vitro* by mononuclear blood cells isolated from pre- and post-cocaine blood samples (one subject)

Cytokine	TNF- α	TNF- α	TNF- α	IL-10	IL-10	IL-10	IL-12	IL-12	IL-12
in Vivo									
Patient #	#1	#2	#3	#1	#2	#3	#1	#2	#3
Post/Pre-cocaine serum cytokine ratio [a]	60%[*]	93%	52%	64%	102%	64%	121%	100%	91%
in Vitro									
Mitogenic stimulation	None	LPS	PHA	None	LPS	PHA	None	LPS	PHA
Post/Pre-cocaine PBMC supernatant cytokine ratio [b]	34%[*]	38%[*]	150%[*]	28%[*]	25%[*]	42%[*]	20%[*]	30%[*]	28%[*]

[a] (cytokine concentration in the serum from the post-cocaine blood specimen: cytokine concentration in the serum from the pre-cocaine blood specimen) x 100 (%).
[b] (cytokine concentration in the supernatant of mononuclear cells from the post-cocaine specimen: cytokine concentration in the supernatant of mononuclear cells from the pre-cocaine specimen) x 100 (%).
[*] indicates significant change at $P < 0.05$ in post-cocaine specimen compared to pre-cocaine specimen using paired t-test

Table 3. Secretion of TNF- α, IL-10, and IL-12 by monocyte-derived macrophages

Medium	TNF-α (pg/ml)[(a)] (mean +/- SE)
Control	380 +/-142
LPS (1 ng/ml)	2,765 +/-701
Cocaine (10^{-5} M)	255 +/-14

[(a)]In each well 800,000 monocytes were incubated in RPMI medium with 10% autologous serum for 7 days until differentiated into typical macrophages. TNF-α level in the supernatant medium was measured 18 h after addition of the indicated drug.

3.4 Effects of *in Vitro* Cocaine and Cocaethylene Treatment of Mononuclear Cells from Normal Donors on Secretion of TNF- α, IL-10, and IL-12

Two million mononuclear cells (isolated from peripheral blood of two healthy normal donors) were stimulated with PHA in the presence or absence of cocaine (10^{-5} to 10^{-4} M) or cocaethylene (10^{-5} to 10^{-4} M). PHA alone stimulated secretion of TNF- α, IL-10, and IL-12, whereas cocaine and cocaethylene with PHA suppressed cytokine secretion, significantly in the case of TNF- α and non-significantly in the case of IL-10 and IL-12 (Table 4).

3.5 Mononuclear Cell Migration in the BBB Model

The kinetics of mononuclear cell migration following cytokine treatments were investigated. At 24 hours post-migration onset, the proportion of cells in the process of adhesion or transmigration (i.e. cells not found in the upper or lower chambers) was 17 to 25% for nonactivated mononuclear cells but much higher, 73 to 74%, for Concanavalin-A activated mononuclear cells. Emigration of mononuclear cells into the lower chamber was: (a) enhanced by TNF- α and IL-1β (both at 20 ng/ml) 1.3fold (non-activated cells) to 1.8 fold (Concanavalin-A activated cells (Table 5), (b) enhanced by IL-12 (10 ng/ml) 2.125 fold (non-activated cells) , (c) depressed by IL-4 (10 ng.ml) 0.75 fold (non-activated cells). The migration data were, however, not strictly comparable since, in the experiments with TNF-

Table 4. Secretion of TNF- α, IL-10, and IL-12 by mononuclear cells of normal donors treated with abuse drugs[(a)]

Medium	TNF-α (ng/ml)	IL-10 (pg/ml)	IL-12 (pg/ml)
Control	0.2 +/-0.4	24.3 +/- 25.4	21.6 +/- 12.4
PHA	13.7 +/-0.9	236 +/-47.1	224 +/-16.1
PHA + cocaine (10^{-5} M)	10.7 +/-0.3	171 +/-10.8	221 +/-0
PHA + cocaine (10^{-4} M)	7.3 +/-0.2	174 +/-1.4	188 +/- 3.1
PHA + cocaethylene (10^{-5} M)	8.7 +/-0.04	208 +/- 15.7	232 +/- 3.8
PHA + cocaethylene (10^{-4} M)	6.4 +/- 0.4	202 +/- 1.5	237 +/- 6.1

[(a)]2 million monocyte-enriched mononuclear cells were cultivated in RPMI medium with 5% fetal bovine serum in presence of a mitogen (phytohemagglutinin A at 5 ug/ml) with or without cocaine or cocaethylene. Cytokine levels were assayed in the supernatant medium after 18 hr incubation.

Table 5. Migration of mononuclear cells across the BBB model

Prior activation of mononuclear cells	TNF-α and IL-1 β [(b)]	Mononuclear cell recovery[(a)] (mean number (x10^6) (%)) Upper chamber	Lower chamber
None	-	0.28 (56%)	0.09 (19%)
	+	0.29[(c)] (58%)	0.12 (25%)
Con-A	-	0.08 (16%)	0.05 (10%)
	+	0.04[(c)] (9%)	0.09 (18%)

[(a)]At the start of the experiment, 0.5 x 10^6 mononuclear cells were placed in the upper chamber of each of 8 replicate BBB models (2 models in each group). The data are expressed as the mean of cell counts in two BBB models and (the average percent of cells compared to the initial number of cells added to the upper chamber).
[(b)]The lower chamber was treated with TNF- α and IL-1 β at 20 ng/ml for 2 hr prior to the migration and then removed.
[(c)]Significant difference between mean cell counts in the upper chamber of normal and Concanavalin-A activated mononuclear cells (t=2.21; p=0.002).

α and IL-1β, peripheral blood mononuclear cells were used, whereas in the experiments with IL-4, IL-10 and IL-12, mononuclear cells enriched in monocytes were used.

3.6 Preferential Migration of CD4± CD45RA⁻ (Memory) Cells in the Blood-Brain Barrier Model, and Inhibition of Preferential Migration by Cocaethylene

The distribution of $CD4^+$ $CD45RA^+$ ("naive") and $CD4^+$ $CD45RA^-$ ("memory") T cells was analyzed in the upper (blood) and the lower (brain) chambers by flow cytometry. Concanavalin-A-activated mononuclear cells from two normal donors, either in the presence

Table 6. Preferential migration of CD4+ CD45RA- T cells across the BBB model and inhibition of preferential migration by cocaethylene

Mononuclear cell activation[(a)]	TNF- α + IL-1β treatment[(b)]	Chamber[(c)]	CD4+ CD45RA+ (%)[(d)]	CD4+ CD45RA- (%)[(d)]	Enrichment[(e)]
Con-A	-	upper	27	31	
	+	lower	31	48	1.55
Con-A	-	upper	40	14	
	+	lower	38	41	2.93
Con-A	-	upper	41	14	
	-	lower	43	36	2.57
-	-	upper	33	27	
	+	lower	12	36	1.33
Cocaethylene	-	upper	33	31	
	+	lower	57	17	0.55

[(a)]Normal human mononuclear cells from donors 1 and 2 were stimulated with either Concanavalin-A (5 ug/ml), con-A(5 ug/ml) and cocaethylene 10^{-6}M for 2 hours on the day of collection, or were left untreated, and 0.5 x 10^6 cells were migrated in an individual construct for each donor and treatment.
[(b)]Lower chamber was either treated with TNF-α and IL-1 α at 20 ng/ml or was left untreated.
[(c)]Chamber used for sampling the migrated cell population, i.e. upper chamber for non-migrated and lower chamber for migrated population.
[(d)]T lymphocyte data are expressed as % LeucoGATE (Becton Dickinson)- gated region in a flow cytometric analysis with anti-CD4/antiCD45RA antibodies.

or absence of TNF-α and IL-1β in the lower chamber, revealed preferential emigration of $CD4^+$ $CD45RA^-$ compared to $CD4^+$ $CD45RA^+$ T cells (Table 6). Since, as shown above, mononuclear cells responded to cocaine by modulating cytokine production, we speculated that cocaine could alter cell trafficking across the model. Mononuclear cells pretreated with cocaethylene *in vitro* showed a lower proportion of CD4+ CD45RA- and an increased proportion of CD4+ CD45RA+ in the lower chamber (Table 6). Similar results were obtained with 0.2% alcohol treatment of mononuclear cells.

3.7 Transmigration of HIV-1- and TNF-α–Stimulated Monocytes Observed by Electron Microscopy

Mononuclear cells were enriched in monocytes (80% monocytes) and preincubated with HIV-1 $_{JR\text{-}FL}$ in the presence of TNF-α (20 ng/ml). The cells were placed in the upper chamber and their migration was followed by electron microscopy. These cells were predominantly myeloid with multishaped nuclei and cytoplasmic vacuoles. One hour post-migration onset, three mononuclear cells were seen attached to an endothelial cell, but the endothelial cells remained flat and displayed scant microvilli (Fig.1A). At 24 hr post-migration onset, mononuclear cell migrated between endothelial cells (Fig.1B and C) and into pores (Fig. 1D). The endothelial cells showed increased cell thickness, cellular disorganization with gaps between cells, and displayed abundant microvilli and mitochondria (Figs. 1B, C, D). The fibronectin layer was degraded following mononuclear cell migration (Figs. 1B and D).

3.8 Cocaine Effects on HIV-1 in the Model

As will be reported elsewhere [Fiala et al, 1996a] , HIV-1 penetrates the untreated BBB model in only minute amounts (<1 pg/ml), whereas TNF-α–treated models are permeable to increasing amounts of infectious HIV-1 in time- and dose-dependent fashion. TNF-α and cocaethylene treatments of the model resulted in increased amounts of p24 antigen in the lower chamber (Table 7).

Table 7. Effects of TNF-α and cocaine on HIV-1 in the brain-side chamber the BBB model

Brain endothelial cells	TNF-α (ng/ml) or cocaine (M)	HIV-1 inoculum[(b)]	HIV-1 p24 antigen (pg/ml) in A3.01 assay a at indicated time-points post-infection (hr) 71	95	148
+	–	0.5 ng of cell-free HIV-1$_{JR\text{-}FL}$	<8, <8[c]	<8, <8	<8, <8
+	TNF- α 20 ng/ml	0.5 ng of cell-free HIV-1$_{JR\text{-}FL}$	92, 56	91,66	94,90
–	TNF- α 20 ng/ml	0.5 ng of cell-free HIV-1$_{JR\text{-}FL}$	636, 687		
+	cocaine 10^{-5}	0.5 ng of cell-free HIV-1$_{JR\text{-}FL}$	230, 196	257, 156	
	10^{-6}		178, 162	160, 281	

[(a)]A3.01 assay: A sample (50 μl) was removed from the lower chamber of each BBB model and was placed in a well with A3.01 cells (one mL of 200,000 cells). After amplification for 5 days, p24 antigen concentration was measured in the supernatant.

[(b)]HIV-1 inoculum was placed in the upper chamber.

[(c)]Results in duplicate BBB models.

4. DISCUSSION

The results of this investigation have implications for the effects of abuse drugs on (a) cytokine production *in vivo* and *in vitro*, and (b) HIV-1 replication and penetration across the BBB. With respect to the former, as observed previously in animal studies [Chen et al, 1993] [Wang et al, 1994], in human cells *in vitro* and *in vivo* abuse drugs modulated cytokine expression with complex kinetics and variable consequences, exerting depressive effects in monocyte/macrophages and enhancing effects in lymphocytes. Intravenous cocaine increased WBC counts which could be related in part to its lymphoproliferative effects [Matsui et al, 1992]. These effects were extremely rapid occurring within one hr after cocaine administration.

Regarding the consequences of cocaine abuse on HIV-1 infection in the CNS, cocaine increased p24 antigen levels in the brain compartment of the BBB model. This effect may result from enhancement of virus penetration across the BBB compounded by stimulatory effect of abuse drugs on virus replication in mononuclear cells [Peterson et al, 1991]. The transport of cell-associated virus may be enhanced *in vivo* by proinflammatory cytokines such as TNF- α, which increased cell emigration into the brain compartment in the model. The neuropathogenesis of AIDS dementia may be also augmented by the transmigration of virus-infected mononuclear cells across the BBB as migrating cells damaged the endothelial cell monolayer during emigration (Figure 1 and also [Dhawan et al, 1995]). Migration of infected monocytes, proinflammatory cytokines, and abuse drugs are the major causes of damage to the blood-brain barrier, and their aftereffects must be considered in the management of neurological dysfunction of HIV-1 infection.

ACKNOWLEDGMENTS

We thank H. Vinters and M-A. Ackers for electron microscopical observations, the UCLA Center for AIDS Research Virology Core Laboratory for p24 assays, the UCLA Clinical Immunology Laboratory for cell counting, the Flow Cytometry Laboratory of the UCLA Cancer Center for FACScan analyses, J. McMahon for fetal brain tissues, K. Conant and E. Major for fetal astrocytes, M. Navab, S. Hama, and A. Fogelman for enriched monocytes; R. Stewart for PCR determinations; and R.H. Rhodes, E.Wright, E. Pure, and M. Brightman for helpful discussions. J.E. Lindholm, P. Villanueva, P. Aslmand, P. Baharinejad, J. Ramos provided excellent technical assistance. IL-4 and IL-10 were a generous gift of R. Coffman, DNAX, IL-12 was provided by the Genetics Institute, and IL-12 monoclonal antibody by G. Trinchieri, the Wistar Institute.

Figure 1. Mononuclear cell migration across the BBB model comprising a BMVEC monolayer in a tissue culture insert on a fibronectin-coated Cyclopore membrane with 3u diameter pores. $2x10^5$ mononuclear cells (70% monocytes, 30% lymphocytes), 0.1 ml of HIV-1 (1.4 ng of p24 antigen) in E-Stim medium with TNF-α (20ng/ml) were placed in the upper chamber. Mononuclear cells were allowed to migrate for one and 24 hr (transmission electron microscopy, x 7,500). A. Adhesion phase of cell migration (1 hr post-migration onset). Two monocytoid cells are attached to each other and to an endothelial cell which remains flat and with scant microvilli except at the site of adhesion (arrowhead). B. Transmigration phase (24 hr post-migration onset). The endothelial cells display increased cell height, abundant microvilli on apical and basolateral surfaces, aggregates of mitochondria, and disorganization of the monolayer architecture with irregular spaces between the cells. One mononuclear cell is observed between the basal surface of the endothelial surface and the porous membrane. The fibronectin layer is degraded over a pore. C. Emigration phase (24 hr post-migration onset). A mononuclear cell (bearing vacuoles at the leading edge) is emigrating through a pore in the membrane. The monolayer remains disorganized with wide gaps between endothelial cells.

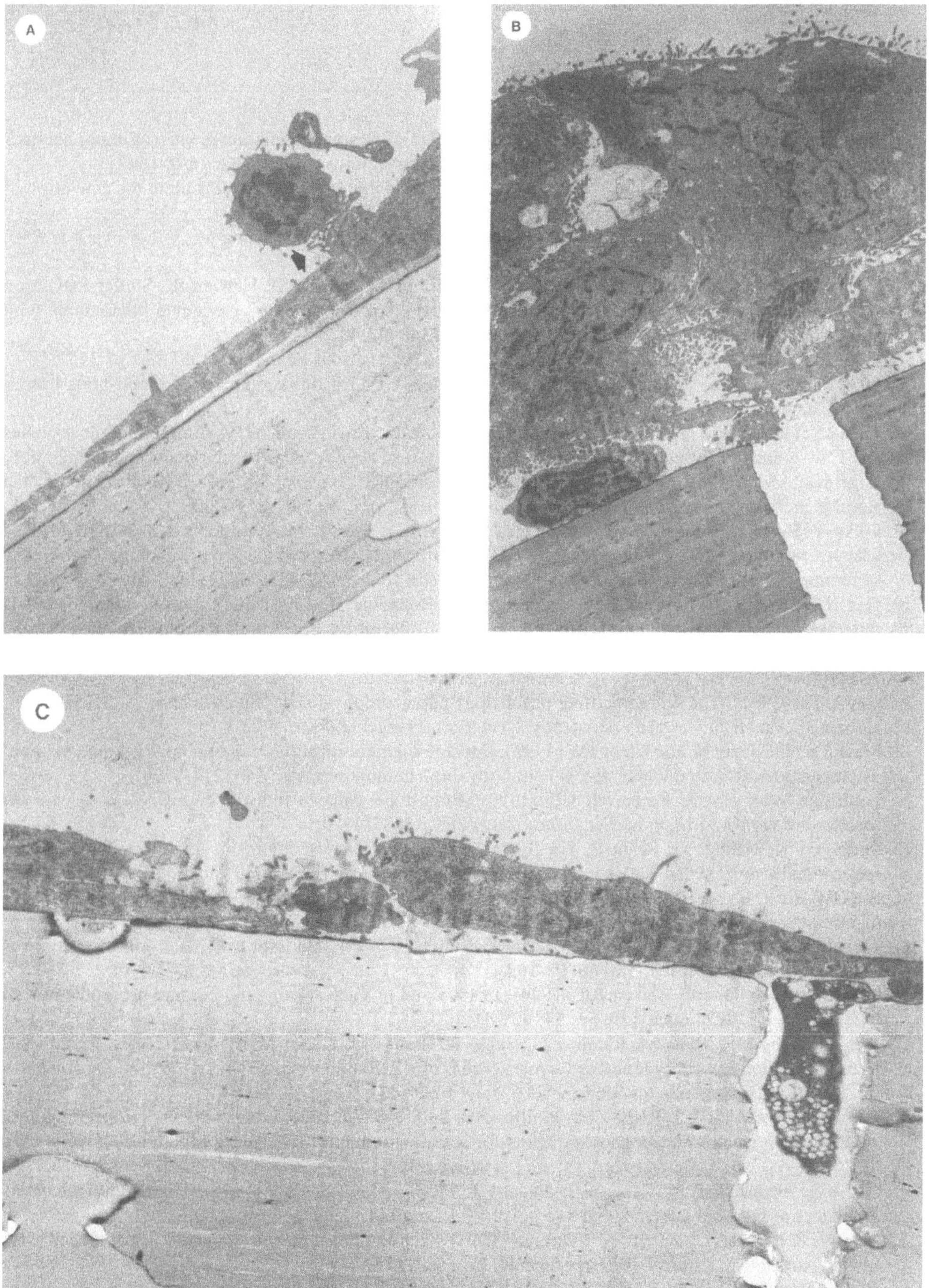
A
B
C

This work was supported by grants from the UCLA Norman Cousin's Program in Psychoneuroimmunology to M.F., NIDA DA07683 to F.C., HL48493 to M.W., and NIDA DA07909 and DA 04787 to P.S.

REFERENCES

1. Chen G, Tachibana K, Huang DS, and Watson RR (1993). Cocaine modulation in vitro of tumor necrosis factor production by macrophages from retrovirally infected mice. Life Sci 52: 1641-1647.
2. Chiappelli F, Frost P, and Wylie T. (1993). Alcohol and alcohol/cocaine mixtures blunt the activation of human CD4+T cells. *Alcologia* **5**: 221-229.
3. Chiappelli F, Frost P, Manfrini E, Lee P, Pham L, Garcia C, Daley S, Kung M. Villanueva P (1994). Cocaine blunts human CD4+ cell activation. *Immunopharmacol* **28**:233-240.
4. Dhawan S, Weeks BS, Soderland C, Schnaper HW, Toro LA, Asthana SP, Hewlett IK, Stetler-Stevenson G, Yamada SY, Yamada KM, Meltzer MS (1995). HIV-1 infection alters monocyte interactions with human microvasculare endothelial cells. *J Immunol* **154**: 422-432.
5. Farquahar MG, Palade GE (1963). Junctional complexes in various epithelia. *J Cell Biol* **17**:375-412
6. Fiala M et al (1996a) Tumor necrosis factor-α enhances HIV-1 penetration across a blood-brain barrier model. In preparation.
7. Fiala M et al (1996b) Restricted human immunodeficiency virus type 1 (HIV-1) infection of astrocytes and TNF- α and IL-6 production are enhanced in coculture of astrocytes with macrophages. In preparation.
8. Fogelman AM, Elahi F, Sykes K, Van Lenten BJ, Territo MC, Berliner JA. (1988) Modification of the Recalde method for the isolation of human monocytes. *J Lipid Res* **29**: 1243-1247.
9. Folks T, Benn S, Rabson A, Theodore T, Hoggan MD, Martin M, Lightfoote M, Sell K. (1985). Characterization of a T-cell line susceptible to the cytopathic effects of the acquired immunodeficiency syndrome (AIDS)-associated retrovirus. *Proc Natl Acad Sci USA* **82**:4539-4543.
10. Gan X-H, Robin JP, Huerta JMM, Braquet P, and Bonavida B (1994). Inhibition of tumor necrosis factor-alpha (TNF-α) and interleukin-1 beta (IL-1β) secretion but not IL-6 from activated human peripheral blood monocytes by a new synthetic demethylpodophyllotoxin derivative. J Clin Immunol 14: 280-288.
11. Gawin FH (1991). Cocaine addicition: psychology and neurophysiology. Science 251: 1580-1586.
12. Hunter EE. Practical electron microscopy. New York, Praeger, 1984.
13. Matsui K, Friedman H, and Klein TW (1992). Cocaine augments proliferation of human peripheral blood T-lymphocytes activated with anti-CD3 antibody. Int J Immunopharmac 14: 1213-1220.
14. Pardridge WM, Boado R, Farrell CR (1990). Brain-type glucose transporter mRNA is selectively localized to the blood-brain barrier. *J Biol Chem* **265**: 18035-4020.
15. Peterson PK, Gekker G, Schut R, Hu S, Balfour HH, Jr, Chao CC (1993). Enhancement of HIV-1 replication by opiates and cocaine: the cytokine connection. Adv Exper Med Biol 335: 181-188
16. Sill HW, Butler C, Hollis TM, Tarbell JM (1992). Albumin permeability and electrical resistance as means of assessing endothelial monolayer integrity in vitro. J Tiss Cult Meth 14: 253-258.
17. Tornatore, C, Meyers K, Atwood W, Conant K, Major E (1994) Temporal patterns of HIV-1 transcripts in human fetal astrocytes. *J Virol* **68**: 93-102.
18. Wang Y, Huang D, and Watson RR (1994). In vivo and in vitro cocaine modulation on production of cytokines in C57BL/6 mice. Life Sci 54: 401-411.
19. Way D, Witte MH, Fiala M, Ramirez G, Nagle R, Bernas M, Dictor M, Witte C.(1993). Endothelial transdifferentiated phenotype and cell-cycle kinetics of AIDS-associated Kaposi sarcoma cells. *Lymphology* **26**: 79-89.
20. Weinand ME, Wyler AR, Richey ET, Phillips BB, Somes GW (1992). Long-term ictal monitoring with subdural strip electrodes: prognostic factors for selecting temporal lobectomy candidates. *J Neurosurg* **77**:20-28.
21. Xin KQ, Shapshak P, Kawamoto S, Nagano I, McCoy CB, Okuda K(1995). Highly divergent *env* sequences of HIV-1 B subtype with two novel V3 loop motifs detected in an AIDS.
22. Yirmiya R, Pilati M, Chiappelli F, Taylor AN (1993). Fetal alcohol exposure attenuates LPS-induced fever in rats. Alcoholism Clinical and Experimental Research **17**:906-910.

21

EFFECTS ON MOUSE THYMOCYTE BIOLOGY

A Mini-Overview with Some New Evidence

David W. Ou,[1] Mei-ling Shen,[1] and Ken M. Anderson[2]

[1] Department of Pathology
University of Illinois at Chicago
[2] Departments of Medicine and
Biochemistry, Rush Medical College
Chicago, Illinois 60612

I. AN OVERVIEW

Cocaine

The alkaloid designated cocaine, derived from the leaves of the Anean coca bush (Erythroxylon coca) was first isolated and identified in 1860 by the German chemist, Albert Niemann. Cocaine is used medically in nasal surgery as a topical anesthesia but most of its interest is related to its potential as a powerful addicting narcotic. Its ready availability and the ease with which its use leads to psychological compulsion and physical dependency provides an important impetus for understanding its mechanisms of action, both on the nervous system and other organ systems.

Cocaine is a neuro-stimulant and initially produces an undefinable "high" associated with feelings of increased energy, work productivity and sexual prowess. But the euphoric feelings are short-lived and hours after usage are replaced by feelings of irritation, anxiety, exhaustion and depression (1). Financial hardship due to the cost of the habit, social ineptitude leading to overt paranoid psychoses are anticipated sequelae of dependent usage. Some 2 percent of young adults are estimated to use the drug with over 2 million known abusers (2). These individuals are more likely to develop endocarditis (3) and increased rates of HIV infection are associated with its use (4). Interestingly, cocaine can promote the replication of HIV-1 and CMV viruses in tissue culture (5,6). While poor nutrition and personal hygiene may contribute, the increased rate of bacterial and viral infections in chronic cocaine users or in users with an underlying disease such as diabetes (7) suggests that it exerts a deleterious effect on the immune system.

In one of the earliest studies of cocaine and the immune system, Watson (8) found that drug and related alkaloids fed to mice for 5 days inhibited immune response. Sub-

AIDS, Drugs of Abuse, and the Neuroimmune Axis, Edited by Friedman *et al.*
Plenum Press, New York, 1996

sequently there have been many reports of cocaine-related depression of the immune system in both experimental animals and cocaine abusers and of other associated disease. Cocaine has been reported to enhance (9,10) or suppress (11,12) the immune system while in a few reports no effects was seen (13,14). On balance the evidence indicates that cocaine usage produces an imbalance of the immune response.

The mechanism of the effect of cocaine on the immune system is not yet clear. Watson et al. (15) proposed that cocaine indirectly affects the immune system via neuro-endocrine factors. Metabolic products of cocaine were shown by Hosapple and coworkers (16) to be more active than the parent drug. Other reports concerning the direct addition of cocaine to immune components in vitro indicate that the drug or its metabolites can act directly on cells (17,18).

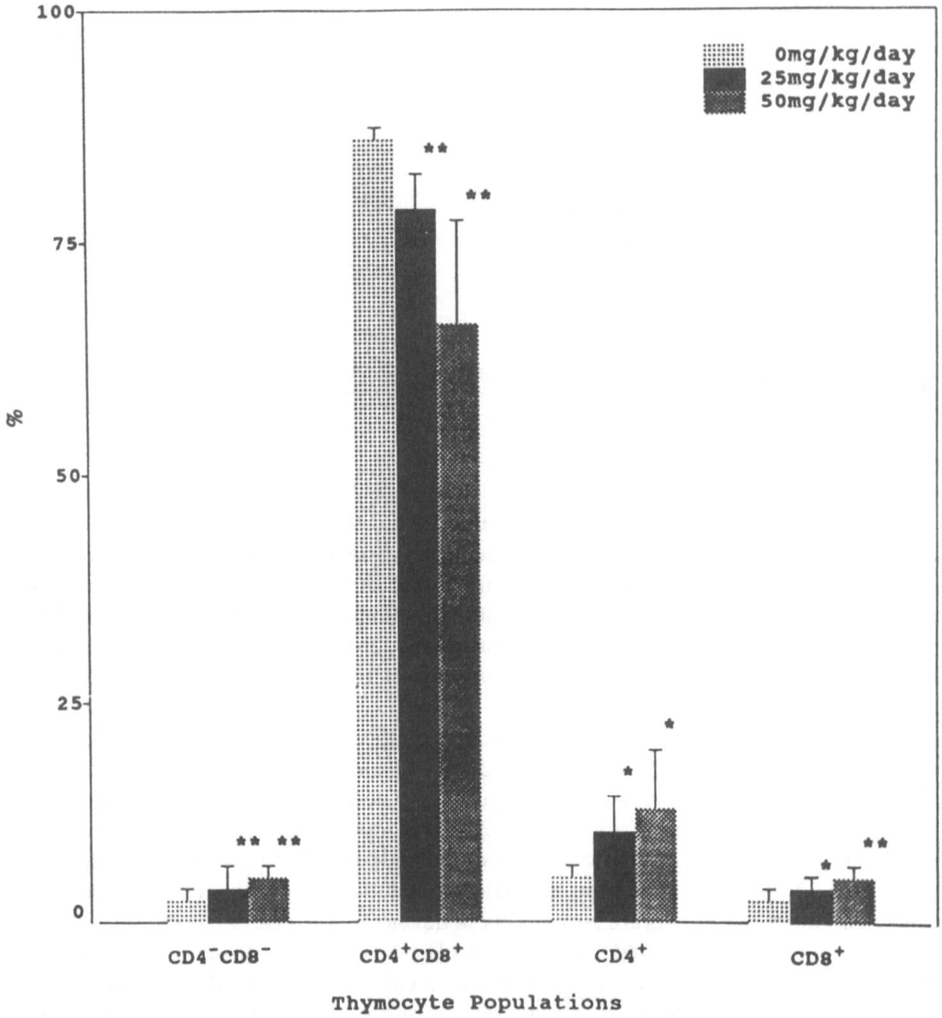

Figure 1. Mice were evenly distributed into several groups, 2 per group, and were injected i.p. with different dosages of cocaine for 5 days. Four hours after the last injection, thymus cells were stained with anti-Lyt 2, anti-L3T4, or a combination of both antibodies, and were assayed by flow cytometry. Values are means ± S.D. of 3 experiments. ** P<0.01.

The Thymus

T lymphocyte selection and maturation occurs in the thymus. $CD4^-8^-$ T cells originating from the bone marrow represent about 2% of thymocytes in adult mice. These cells mature into CD4 and CD8 double positive immature cells (85%) and with further maturation a majority of these cell dies, probably by a physiologic cell death characterized by apcptosis. The remaining cells mature into functional $CD4^+$ and $CD8^+$ cells. Mature lymphocytes exit the thymus and migrate to the secondary lymph organs including the spleen and lymph nodes, where they perform their immune functions (19). Thus, any alterations in thymocyte maturation or trafficking are expected to have direct effects on the normal immune functions.

The effect of cocaine on the thymus has not been studied extensively, despite its central role in developing immunologic defenses. Five daily cocaine injections reduces thymus weight and alters cell populations (20). However, long-term cocaine injections for 11 weeks did not cause a significant reduction in Thy 1.2 or $CD4^+$ cells but did reduce $CD8^+$ cells (21). Recently, 71+ 37 ng/mg of cocaine was detected by gas chromatograph-mass spectrometer in thymus 30 minutes after a single i.p. injection of 30 mg/kg of cocaine, but none was present at 90 minutes (22). This indicates that cocaine could transiently accumulate in the thymus.

II. COCAINE EFFECTS ON MOUSE THYMOCYTE BIOLOGY

Five daily i.p. injections of cocaine (10 mg/kg to 50 mg/kg) to C57/BL mice reduced the total thymocyte number and altered the percentage of subpopulation in a dosage-dependent manner (Fig. 1). When the percentages of each thymocyte subpopulation were multiplied by the total cell count, the number of cells in $CD4^+8^+$ and $CD8^+$ subpopulation decreased, while the $CD4^+$ subpopulation was unchanged and $CD4^-8^-$ increased. The effects were most noticeable in the $CD4^+8^+$ subpopulation (Table 1). Statistically significant changes occurred at or above 25 mg/kg and these concentrations were used in the in vivo experiments. These results suggest that the selective effects of cocaine on T cell subpopulation could results in an imbalance of the immune system.

The rapid decrease of the $CD4^+8^+$ population suggests that cocaine may decrease the number of thymocytes through apoptosis (1). Flow cytometric analysis of propidium iodide-treated cells yielded hypo and hyper diploid populations, consistent with DNA degradation in the former and DNA synthesis in the latter (Fig. 2). A dose-dependent increase

Table 1. The effects of cocaine injections on thymocyte subpopulations

Dosage Cocaine (mg/kg/day)	Cells ($x10^6$) Total	$CD4^-CD8^-$	$CD4^+CD8^+$	$CD4^+$	$CD8^+$
0.00	57.4 ± 0.8	2.2 ± 0.6	43.6 ± 1.7	7.3 ± 0.2	4.2 ± 0.3
10.00	48.6 ± 0.6	2.4 ± 0.0	35.8 ± 2.6	7.4 ± 0.4	3.0 ± 0.3
25.00	31.5 ± 0.8**	2.5 ± 0.2	18.3 ± 1.1**	6.5 ± 0.5	3.2 ± 0.5
50.00	16.7 ± 3.2**	3.0 ± 0.5**	6.5 ± 0.5**	5.4 ± 0.4	1.8 ± 0.8**

Mice were evenly distributed into several groups, 2 per group, and were injected i.p. with different dosages of cocaine for 5 days. Four hours after the last injection, thymus cells were stained with anti-Lyt 2, anti-L3T4, or a combination of both antibodies, and were assayed by flow cytometry. The number of cells was calculated by multiplying the total number of thymocytes by the percentage of the subpopulation. Values are means ± S.D. of 3 experiments. ** P<0.01

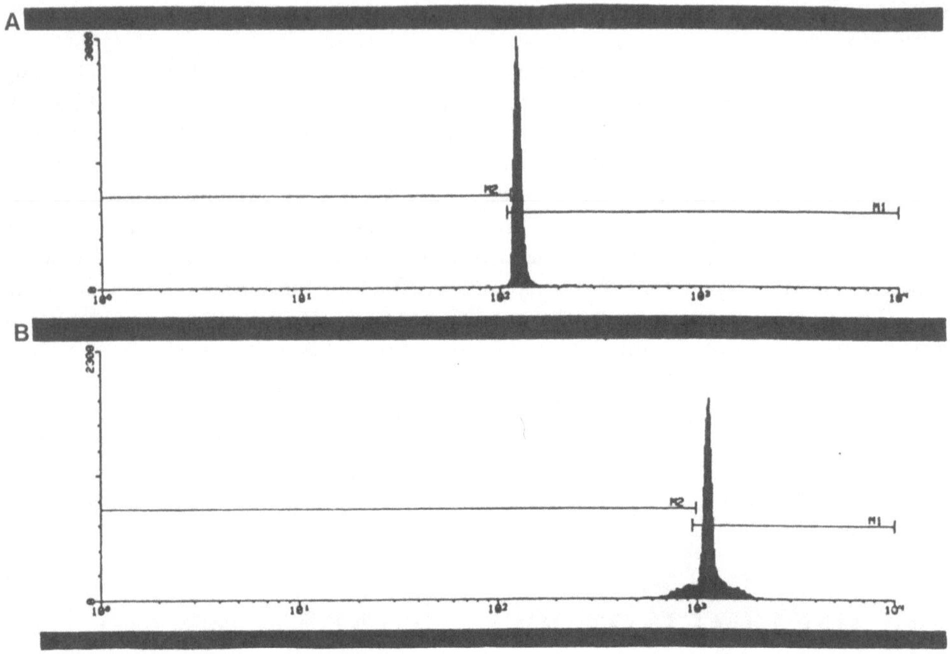

Figure 2. Mice were injected with either saline or cocaine. Four hours after the last injection, thymocytes were removed for flow cytometric analysis of apoptosis. Abscissa: relative DNA density. Ordinate: relative amount of DNA. Fig. 2A revealed a typical diploid DNA peak. Fig. 2B showed that cocaine induced a hypodiploid peak and a hyperdiploid peak, in addition to the normal diploid DNA peak. Data listed is from one representative experiment.

Table 2. Comparison of in vivo and in vitro effects of cocaine treatment on C57/BL mouse thymocytes

	In vivo			In vitro (48 hrs)		
	0 mg/kg	25 mg/kg	50 mg/kg	0 ug/ml	2.5 ug/ml	5.0 ug/ml
Cells ($x10^6$)	55.3±11.7	35.9±2.7*	27.6±2.3**	7.5[1]	6.7[1]	4.2*[1]
Apoptosis (%)	1.9±0.3	2.5±0.1*	13.4±1.7**	0.4±0.1[2]	4.6±1.1**[2]	8.0±0.6*[2]
S-Phase (%)	9.0±1.0	11.4±0.2**	19.0±0.6**	10.2±0.5	11.1±0.2**	14.1±1.3**
DNA (ug/10^6 cells)	7.8±0.2	10.8±0.6**	13.7±0.3**	8.2±0.5	10.4±0.3	11.7±0.6*
Protein (ug/10^6 cells)	2582.00±231	1672.00±109**	1246.00±113**	2338.00±71	1787.00±42	1591.00±45*

[1]Twelve million cells per 3ml were cultured.
[2]Cells were cultured for 24 hrs.
Values are means ± S.D. of 3 experiments. * P<0.05, ** P<0.01.

in the percent of apoptotic cells is shown in row 2 of Table 2. Comparable cells contained DNA which "laddered" after agarose DNA electrophoresis (not shown, manuscript submitted). Therefore, at least some of the decline in $CD4^+8^+$ cells can be accounted for by "physiologic" cell death accompanied by apoptosis as induced by cocaine.

The percent of cells in S-phase in cocaine-treated mice was dose-dependent (Table 2, row 3). DNA analysis by UV spectrometry, flowmetric analysis of Hoechst 33258-treated thymocytes and the diphenylamine method demonstrated apparently increased DNA content of cocaine-treated thymocytes (Table 2, row 4). Of course these methods do not discriminate between intact and partially degraded or laddered DNA. Protein content, on the other hand, was found to be decreased in a dose-dependent manner (Table 2, row 5).

To further elucidate the mechanism of cocaine actions, the survival of cultured thymocytes from saline or cocaine-injected mice were found to be inversely proportional to cocaine dose in culture. At 72 hr, 60% of control cells survived, while only 15% of cells from mice treated with 25 mg/kg of cocaine were viable at that time (Fig. 3). When normal

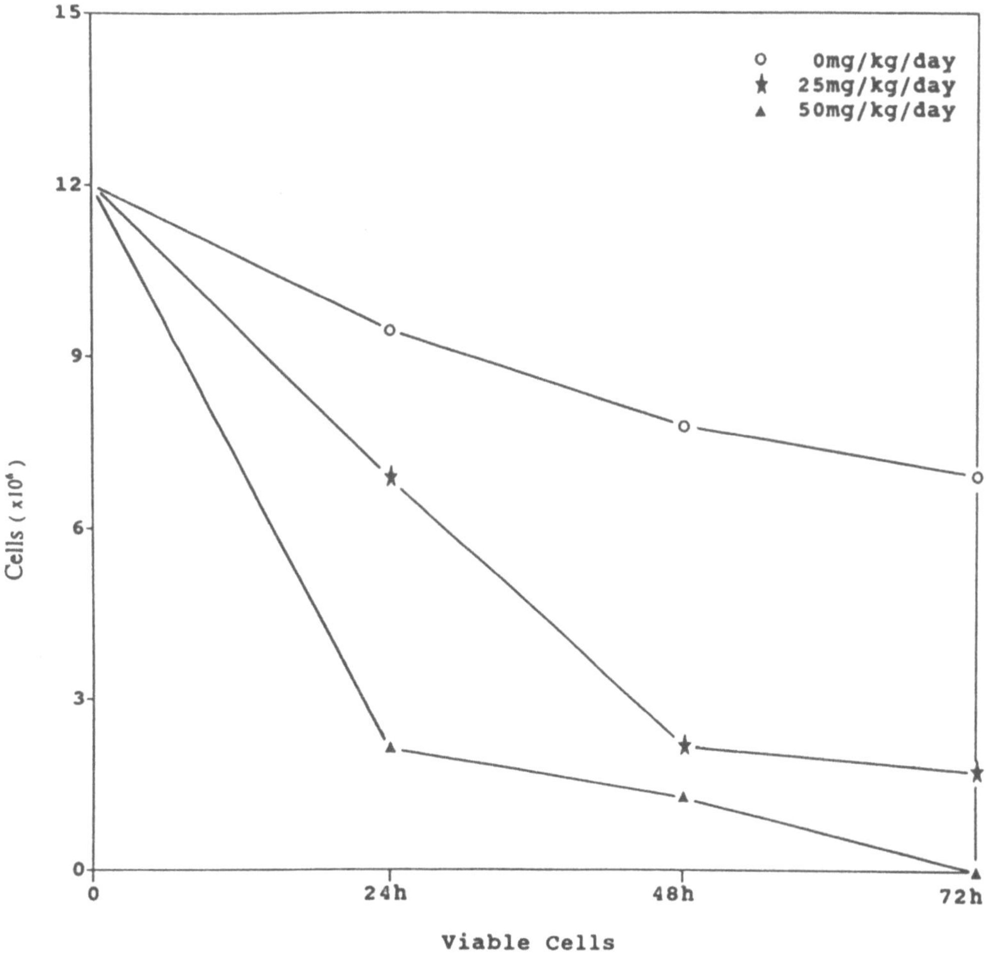

Figure 3. Four hours after the last cocaine injection, thymocytes were removed and cultured in complete medium at a concentration of 4 x 10^6/ ml in a CO_2 incubator. The number of viable cells were compared at 24, 48, and 72 hours. Data listed is from one representative experiment. Values are means ± S.D. ** P<0.01.

Table 3. The effects of cocaine on the viability of normal thymocytes in culture

Cocaine Concentration (ug/ml)	Cells (x 10^6) 0 hr	24 hr	48 hr	72 hr
0.00	12.00	9.20	7.50	8.80
5.00	12.00	7.70	4.20	4.80
10.00	12.00	2.60	0.70	0.20
20.00	12.00	2.40	0.30	0.10
50.00	12.00	0.40	0.10	0.00
100.00	12.00	0.00	0.00	0.00
200.00	12.00	0.00	0.00	0.00

Thymocytes from normal mice were cultured in vitro with different concentrations of cocaine for varying hours, and the cell number in each flask was counted. Data listed is from one representative experiment.

thymocytes were cultured with cocaine less than found after an single injection of 30 mg/kg (22), their viability decreased in a dose-dependent manner (Table 3). These findings and the evidence of apoptosis and reduction in cell number indicates that the concentrations of cocaine present in the mouse thymus after injection are sufficient to injure thymocytes, and that the effect can be direct and need not involve products of distant neuroendocrine origin.

To examine this further, normal thymocytes cultured with cocaine were examined for apoptosis, DNA and protein content, and its effect on the cell cycle (Table 2, right hand columns). After 24 hr, the percentage of apoptotic cells and of S-phase cells increased with increasing cocaine concentrations. While the number of viable cells decreased after 48 hr of culture with cocaine, significant increases in DNA and decreases in protein content were recorded at concentrations of 5 ug/ml and statistically less significant changes at 2.5 ug/ml. The in vitro results are consonant with the in vivo findings and provide additional evidence that in vivo cocaine injections could directly affect the thymus.

III. SUMMARY

We demonstrated that cocaine induces selective loss in mouse thymocyte subpopulation and increases DNA synthesis and cell proliferation. The loss of cells is in part due to apoptosis. The in vitro and in vivo responses to cocaine that were examined mirrored one another, suggesting that the in vitro system can serve as a model with which to examine at least some of the important effects of cocaine on that organ. While indirect effects of cocaine or its metabolics cannot be ruled out, even in the in vitro system, the results suggest that direct effects may be of major importance.

IV. REFERENCES

1. Farrar HC, Kearns GL, Cocaine: Clinical pharmacology and toxicology. J. Pediatr., 115,665, 1989.
2. Gawin, F, Cocaine addiction: Psychology and Neurophysiology. Science, 251, 1580 - 1586, 1991.
3. Chambers, HF, Morris DL, Tauber MG, Modin G, Cocaine use and the risk for endocarditis in intravenous drug users. Ann. Intern. Med., 106, 833 - 836, 1987.
4. Chaisson RE, Bacchetti P, Osmond MA, Brodie B, Sande MA, and Moss AR, Cocaine use and HIV infection in intravenous drug users in San Francisco. J. AM. Med. Assoc., 261, 561-565, 1989.

5. Peterson PK, Gekker G, Chao CC, Schut R, Molitor TW, and Balfour HH, Cocaine potentiates HIV-1 replication in human peripheral blood mononuclear cell cultures. J. Immunol., 146, 81 - 84, 1991.
6. Peterson PK. Gekker G, Chao CC, Schut R, Verhoef J, Edelman CK, Erice A, and Balfour HH, Cocaine amplifies HIV-1 replication in cytomegalovirus-stimulated peripheral blood mononuclear cell cocultures. J. Immunol., 140, 676-680, 1992
7. D'Elia JA., Weinrauch LA, Paine DF, Domey PE, and Kaldany A, Increased infection rate in diabetic dialysis patients exposed to cocaine . Am. J. Kidney Dis., 18, 349-352, 1991.
8. Watson ES, Murphy JC, Elsohly MA, Elsohly HN, and Turner CE, Effects of the administration of coca alkaloids on the primary immune responses of mice: interaction with delta-9-tetrahydrocannabinol and ethanol, Toxicol. Appl. Pharmacol., 71, 1. 1983.
9. Matsui K, Freidman, H, and Klein TW, Cocaine augments proliferation of human peripheral blood T-lymphocytes activated with anti-CD3 antibody. Int. J. Immunopharmac., 14, 7, 1213-1220, 1992
10. Van Dyke C, Stesin A, Jones R, Chuntharapal A, Seaman W, Cocaine increases natural killer cell activity, J. Clin. Invest., 77, 1387, 1986.
11. Ou DW, Shen ML, and Luo YD, Effects of cocaine on the imnmune system in Balb/C mice. Clin. Immuno. Immunopathol., 52, 305-312, 1989.
12. Klein TW, Matsui K, Newton CA, Young J, Widen RE, and Friedman H, Cocaine suppresses proliferation of phytohemagglutinin-activated human peripheral blood T-cells. Int. J. Immunopharmac., 15, 1, 77-86, 1993
13. Lu F, and Ou DW, Cocaine or delta 9-tetrahydrocannabinol does not affect cellular cytotoxicity in vitro. Int. J. Immunopharmac. 11,849, 1989.
14. Havas HF, Dellaria M, Schiffiman G, Geller EB, Adler MW, Effect of cocaine on the immune response and host resistance in Balb/C mice. Int. Archs. Allergy Appl. Immun., 83, 377-383, 1987.
15. Waltz B., and Watson RR., Immunodulation by cocaine - A neuroendocrine mediated response. Life Sci., 46, 1319-1329, 1990.
16. Jeong TC, Matulka RA., Jordan SD, Yang KH, Holsapple MP, Role of metabolism in cocaine-induced immunoisuppression in splenocyte cultures from B6C3F1 female mice. Immunopharmac., 29, 37-46, 1995.
17. Klein TW, Newton C., and Friedman H, Cocaine effects on cultured lymphocytes. Drugs of Abuse, Immunity, and Immunodeficiency, 151-158, 1991.
18. Delafuente JC, and DeVane L, Immunologic effects of cocaine and related alkaloids. Immunopharmac. Immunotoxicol., 13 (1&2), 11-23, 1991.
19. Abbas AK, Lichtman AH, and Pober JS, Cellular & Molecular Immunology, 179-182, 1991.
20. Hagen KL, Shen ML, and Ou DW, The effects of cocaine on cellularity, subclass composition, and apoptosis of the mouse thymus. J. Immunol., 152,6, 113 (3328), 1994
21. Lopez MC, Colombo LL, Huang DS, Wang YJ, and Watson RR, Modification of thymic cell subsets induced by long-term cocaine administration during a murine retroviral infection producing AIDS. Clin. Immunol. Immunopathol., 65, 1, 45-52, 1992.
22. Kump DF, Matulka RA, Edinboro LE, Poklis A, and Holsapple MP, Disposition of cocaine and norcocaine in blood and tissues of B6C3F1 mice. J. Anal. Toxicol., 18, 342-345, 1994.

22

IMMUNOPATHOGENESIS OF HIV INFECTION

Role of Alcohol and HIV Peptides

Madhavan P. N. Nair* and Stanley A. Schwartz

Departments of Medicine and Microbiology
State University of New York at Buffalo

ABSTRACT

We examined the in vitro effects of ethyl alcohol and a recombinant HIV-1, fusion peptide, env-gag, corresponding to portions of the gp-41 envelope (env) and internal core (gag) proteins on the natural killer (NK) cell activities of lymphocytes from healthy donors. Preculture of large granular lymphocytes (LGL) from normal donors with 0.3% alcohol for 72 hr significantly inhibited NK activity compared to untreated controls. Direct addition, without preculture, of alcohol (0.1%, 0.2% and 0.3%) and env-gag peptide (10 ng/ml) at concentrations which did not affect NK activity when either was added alone, produced a significant, synergistic, inhibitory effect on NK activity when added together. This synergistic effect of alcohol and HIV-derived soluble products is consistent with a model proposing that alcohol abuse may be a co-factor involved in the progression of HIV infections.

INTRODUCTION

Previous studies have shown that chronic alcohol consumption is associated with abnormalities of humoral and cellular immunity, including dysfunction of suppressor, helper and cytotoxic functions of lymphocytes and the production of soluble immune mediators (Jerrels et al 1989, Watson et al 1988). Infection by the human immunodeficiency virus (HIV) causes profound abnormalities of cellular and humoral immune response (Rosenberg and Fauci, 1989) including significant inhibition of NK cell activities, especially during the later stage of disease (CDC 1986). NK cell dysfunction has been noted despite normal numbers of NK cells as identified by several monoclonal antibodies (Voth et al 1988). These observations suggest that either the virus or soluble products derived therefrom may be

* Send all correspondence to: Madhavan P. N. Nair, Ph.D., Division of Allergy and Immunology, Buffalo General Hospital, 100 High Street, Buffalo, New York 14203.

AIDS, Drugs of Abuse, and the Neuroimmune Axis, Edited by Friedman *et al.*
Plenum Press, New York, 1996

responsible for the inhibition of NK cell function noted in HIV infected patients. It has been reported that many people who are exposed to or infected with HIV do not necessarily manifest rapid progression of disease to frank AIDS. Consequently cofactors may exist which may hasten the course of HIV infections ultimately leading to AIDS. It has been hypothesized that repeated exposure to HIV, malnutrition, coincident infections, and use of recreational drugs such as heroin, marijuana, cocaine, alcohol, etc. may further suppress an already compromised immune system. This investigation examines the synergistic effect of the direct addition of alcohol and an HIV-derived peptide on the NK activity of lymphocytes from healthy donors.

MATERIALS AND METHODS

Normal Subjects and Preparation of Effector Cells for NK Assay

Normal donors were apprised of this study and consents were obtained consistent with the policies of the State University of New York at Buffalo, the Buffalo General Hospital, and the National Institutes of Health. Peripheral blood from healthy (HIV^-), nonalcoholic individuals was drawn into a syringe containing heparin (20 units/ml). Peripheral blood mononuclear cells (PBMC) were isolated from heparinized (20 U/ml) venous blood using a modified method of Boyum (1968). PBMC in RPMI 1640 medium containing 10% fetal calf serum were depleted of adherent cells by passage through a 7 ml column of Sephadex G-10 beads (Pharmacia Fine Chemicals, Piscataway, NJ). After 45 min of incubation at 37°C, nonadherent peripheral blood lymphocytes (PBL) were washed through the column with medium at 37°C. Cell recovery was >70% of the total input and monocyte contamination as indicated by nonspecific esterase staining was <2%. LGL enriched for NK activity were prepared on a discontinuous density gradient of Percoll as described (Nair et al., 1990).

Tumor Target Cells and Assay for NK Activity

The human erythroleukemia cell line, K562, was used as targets for NK cells. NK activity was determined in a direct ^{51}Cr-release assay as described (Nair et al., 1990). Briefly, varying concentrations of viable effector cells in complete medium were added to triplicate cultures of ^{51}Cr-labeled target cells in 0.2 ml volumes in V-bottomed microtitration plates (Dynatech Labs, Alexandria, VA). After centrifugation at 40 x g for 2 min, the cells were incubated at 37° C in a humidified atmosphere of 5% CO_2 in air for 4 hr. Percent cytotoxicity was calculated as follows:

$$\%\ \text{Cytotoxicity} = \frac{\text{experimental release} - \text{spontaneous release}}{\text{total release} - \text{spontaneous release}} \text{ X } 100$$

where total release represents counts obtained in an aliquot of 1×10^4 target cells, and spontaneous release represents counts released into the medium in control wells containing only 1×10^4 target cells. Spontaneous release of ^{51}Cr was always in the range of 2-5% of total labeling. Because the maximum releasable counts (total labeling) determined by counting an aliquot of unlysed labeled target cells (always comparable to lysed cells). Alcohol at a final concentration of 0.1%, 0.2%, or 0.3% and HIV env-gag peptide at 10 ng/ml were added directly to the mixture of effector and target cells, incubated for 4 hr and the NK activity was measured. Control cultures containing media alone instead of alcohol/HIV peptide were examined concomitantly.

Env-Gag Fusion Protein

Env-gag is a recombinant fusion product containing conserved and antigenic epitopes from the env and gag regions of the HIV genome. The sequence of expressed env-gag fusion protein used in the present experiments includes the following amino acid sequences, env 560-639 and gag 87-276, totalling 270 amino acids. The env-gag protein is expressed in *Escherichia coli* as a single polypeptide without any evidence of premature termination or internal initiation. Twenty-one extra amino acids are encoded by the expression vector genome. Env-gag is purified on 10-20% SDS-PAGE gradient gels under reducing conditions and migrates at ~33kDa. The protein was further analysed by HPLC on a TSK 4000 column in Na phosphate buffer, pH 6.8, in the presence of 10mM dithiothreitol and produced single peak. The protein concentration of our preparation was ~0.27 mg/ml based on OD 280 nm with E/mg =0.487. Our rationale for selecting the env-gag peptide in this investigation is based on the observation that virtually 100% of all serum samples from HIV positive donors contain antibodies that react with it. Further, env-gag showed significant immunomodulatory activities on both T and B cell functions in vitro (Nair et al., 1988).

RESULTS

Effect of Alcohol on the NK Activity of Lymphocytes

In view of the findings that alcoholics are more susceptible to various infections and malignancies than nonalcoholics (Pollack et al 1984), we examined the direct effect of alcohol on the NK activity of lymphocytes from normal donors. Data presented in Table 1 show the effect of preculture with alcohol on the cytotoxic activities of purified NK cells against K562 target cells. Alcohol at a 0.1% initial concentration had no effect at a 2.5:1 effector to target cell ratio against K 562 target cells compared with control cultures (27% versus 28% cytotoxicity, respectively). Alcohol at a 0.2% initial concentration produced a slight decrease in NK activity (20% cytotoxicity) compared to control cultures. Lymphocytes precultured with alcohol at the highest concentration, 0.3%, produced significantly lower levels of NK activity (16.4% cytotoxicity, $p < 0.05$). It should be noted that evaporation of alcohol from our cell cultures reduced its concentration by 38% after 24 hr, 47% after 48 hr, and 59% after 72 hr as quantitated by gas chromatography. Therefore the actual concentration

Table 1. Effect of alcohol on NK activity of large granular lymphocytes

% Ethanol Added at Initiation of Culture	% Ethanol Present at 72 hr Culture	% Cytotoxicity
0	0	27.7 + 4.0
0.1%	0.059%	28.7 + 5.7 (P-NS)
0.2%	0.118%	20.3 + 3.4 (P-NS)
0.3%	0.177%	16.4 + 3.3 (P<.05)

Lymphocytes precultured with different initial concentrations of alcohol for 72 hr were washed and tested for NK activity against K562 target cells at a 2.5:1 E:T cell ratio. LGL were prepared on a discontinuous density gradient of Percoll. The least dense fraction of lymphocytes banding at the 37% Percoll interface consistently showed the highest NK activity and was used as LGL. Recovery of the cell was ~85% of the input with a yield of 7 to 10% at the 37.5% Percoll interface. Using staining with the HNK1 monoclonal antibody, 7—80% of the LGL were positive. Values are the mean ±SD of three experiments performed in triplicate.

Table 2. Synergistie effect of direct addition of alcohol and HIV-1 ENV-gag peptide on NK activity of normal lymphocytes[a]

Lymphocytes Treated With	Percent Cytotoxicity
Medium	26.7 ± 2.5
Ethanol 0.1%	24.5 ± 2.2 (NS)
Ethanol 0.2%	23.8 ± 1.8 (NS)
Ethanol 0.3%	21.4 ± 2.5 (NS)
Env-gag 10 ng/ml	26.6 ± 2.4 (NS)
Ethanol 0.1% + Env-gag	22.1 ± 1.8 (NS)
Ethanol 0.2% + Env-gag	18.3 ± 1.5 (P<.025)
Ethanol 0.3% + Env-gag	15.2 ± 1.0 (P<.01)

[a]Final concentrations of 0.1, 0.2, 0.3% ethanol or Env-gag (10ng/ml) alone or env-gag plus ethanol were added directly to a mixture of normal effector cells plus targets and incubated for 4 hr, and the NK activity was measured against K562 target cells. Values represent mean % cytotoxicity ± SD of triplicate determinations from 4 experiments at 25:1 E:T cell ratio. Statistical significance of differences in the mean values was determined by a single tailed student's 't' test.

of alcohol which produced significant suppression of NK activity at the end of the incubation period may be considerably less than the starting concentration. For example, alcohol at an initial concentrations of 0.3%, 0.2%, and 0.1% will become 0.17%, 0.11% and 0.05% respectively at the end of the 72 hr incubation period.

Synergistic Effects of Alcohol and HIV Protein on NK Cell Activty

Because of the potential association between alcohol abuse and AIDS (McGregor, 1987), we examined the effect of alcohol and HIV env-gag protein separately and in combination on the NK activity of lymphocytes. Data presented in Table 2 demonstrate the synergistic effect of alcohol and env-gag on NK activity when both are added directly to the mixture of effector and the target cells without preincubation. Ethanol at concentrations of 0.1, 0.2, and 0.3% did not produce any modulatory effects on the NK activity of normal lymphocytes with cytotoxicities of 24, 23 and 21% respectively compared to 26% cytotoxicity produced by control cultures. Direct addition of env-gag at 10 ng/ml concentration also did not affect NK activity, the cytotoxicity being 26%, identical to control cultures (26% cytotoxicity). However in combination experiments, env-gag (10 ng/ml) plus ethanol at concentrations of 0.2% and 0.3% which did not affect NK activity when either was added alone, produced a significant synergistic inhibitory effect. The cytotoxic activities were 18% (p<.025) and 15% (p<0.01) respectively for 0.2% and 0.3% alcohol concentrations.

DISCUSSION

Previously we reported that patients with a history of intravenous drug abuse, often associated with excessive alcohol consumption, demonstrated decreased levels of NK and antibody-dependent and lectin-dependent cellular cytotoxic activities (Nair et al 1990). These effects appeared to be due, in part to decreased production of interferon and interleukin 2. We also reported that alcohol selectively suppressed the NK activity of lymphocytes from AIDS patients in contrast to cells from normal donors which were not affected by similar concentrations of alcohol (REF).The reduced NK activity observed in AIDS patients despite normal numbers of NK cells suggests that exogenous factors such as soluble HIV-specific products may play a significant role in the immunopathogenesis of AIDS. Release of HIV proteins into circulation during HIV infection may thus cause, in part, the suppression of NK activity seen with active disease. Our current study demonstrates that direct addition of an HIV protein to the mixture of effector and target cells did not affect NK activity; neither did direct addition of alcohol produce any significant effects. However, direct addition of env-gag together with alcohol to the mixture of effector and target cells resulted in significant inhibition of NK activity. The suppression of NK activity caused by alcohol and env-gag was not due to selective effects on target cells because in control experiments, target cells preincubated with alcohol or HIV peptide separately or in combination for 4 hr were as sensitive to NK lysis as untreated target cells. The decrease in cytotoxicity observed also was not due merely to toxic effects of alcohol or env-gag on effector cells, as treated cells showed levels of viability comparable to untreated control cultures.

Several investigators have proposed a potential relationship between AIDS and alcohol abuse (MacGregor 1987). Recently it was demonstrated that moderate alcohol ingestion increased the in vitro susceptibility of normal peripheral blood mononuclear cells to infection with HIV (Bagasara et al., 1989). Thus alcohol may compromise residual, protective lymphocyte responses to HIV infection such as NK activities. Earlier we showed that HIV peptides also selectively suppressed the NK activities of lymphocytes from AIDS patients in comparison to normal controls (Nair et al., 1989). The current study demonstrates that alcohol in synergy with the HIV peptide, env-gag, significanatly downregulates the NK activty of normal lymphocytes. This observation may have implications in vivo and may in part, explain the role of alcohol as a cofactor in susceptibility to HIV infection and clinical progression to AIDS.

ACKNOWLEDGMENTS

This work was supported in part by NIH grants 1P50AA07378, 1RO1MH47225 and the following grants: The Buffalo General Foundation # G23, The Margaret Duffy and Robert Cameron Troup Memorial Funds for Cancer Research, The Buffalo General Hospital # 229893 and the State University of New York at Buffalo Multidisciplinary grant # 150-8288P.

We wish to express our appreciation to Carol Sperry and Gerry Sobkowiak for their excellent secretarial assistance.

REFERENCES

1. Bagasra O, Balla AK, Lischner HW. Effects of alcohol ingestion on in vitro susceptibility of peripheral blood mononuclear cells to infection with HIV and of selected T cell functions. Alcoholism: Clinical and Experimental Research. 1989; 13:636-643.
2. Boyum A. Isolation of mononuclear cells and granulocytes from human blood. Isolation of mononuclear cells by one centrifugation and of granulcoytes by combining centrifugation and sedimentation. Clin. lab. Invest. 1968; 21(suppl) 97:77.
3. Centers for Disease Control, MS Department of Health and Human Services. Morb. Mort. Wkly. Report. 1986; 35:76-78.
4. Jerrells TR, Peritt D, Marietta C and Eckardt MJ. Mechanisms of suppression of cellular immunity induced by ethanol. Alcoholism Clin. Exp. Res. 1989; 13:490-493.
5. MacGregor RR. Alcohol and drugs as cofactors for AIDS. Advan. Alcohol. Sub. Abuse. 1987; 7(2):47-71.
6. Nair MPN, Pottathil R, Heimer EP, Schwartz SA. Immunoregulatory activities of human immunodeficiency virus (HIV) proteins: Effect of HIV recombinant and synthetic peptides on immunoglobulin synthesis and proliferative responses by normal lymphocytes. Proc. Natl. Acad. Sci. USA 1988; 85:6498-6502.

7. Nair MPN, Schwartz SA, Kronfol ZA, Heimer EP, Pottahil R. Immunoregulatory activities of human immunodeficiency virus (HIV) proteins. Inhibitory effect on natural killer (NK) cell functions (Abstract). 7th Intnatl Cong of Immunology, Berlin, Germany, 1989.
8. Nair MPN, Kronfol ZA, Schwartz SA. Effect of alcohol and nicotine on cytotoxic responses of human lymphocytes. Clin. Immunol. Immunopathol. 1990; 54:395-409.
9. Pollack ES, Nomura AM, Heilburn LK, Stemmermann GN, Green SB. Prospective study of alcohol consumption and cancer. N. Engl. J. Med. 1984; 310:617-621.
10. Rosenberg ZF, Fauci AS. Immunopathogenic mechanisms of HIV infection. Clin. Immunol. Immunopathol. 1989; 50:5149-5156.
11. Voth R, Rossol S, Graff E, Laubenstein RHP, Schroder HC, Muller WE, Meyer zum Buschenfelde KH, Hess G. Natural killer cell activity as a prognostic parameter in the progression to AIDS. J. Infect. Dis. 1988; 157:851.
12. Watson RR, Prabhala RH, Darban HR, Tahya MD, Smith TL. Changes in lymphocyte and monophages subset due to morphin and ethanol treatment during retrovirus infection causing murine AIDS. Life Sciences. 1988; 43:5-11.

23

HIV-1 NEUROPATHOGENESIS AND ABUSED DRUGS

Current Views, Problems, and Solutions

P. Shapshak,[1-3,6*] K. A. Crandall,[7] K. Q. Xin,[8] K. Goodkin,[1,5] R. K. Fujimura,[1] W. Bradley,[2] C. B. McCoy,[4,5] I. Nagano,[9,11] M. Yoshioka,[9] C. Petito,[3] N. C. J. Sun,[10] A. K. Srivastava,[12] N. Weatherby,[4,6] R. Stewart,[1] S. Delgado,[1] A. Matthews,[1] R. Douyon,[1] K. Okuda,[8] J. Yang,[1] B. T. Zhangl,[8] X. R. Cao,[8] S. Shatkovsky,[1] J. B. Fernandez,[1] S. M. Shah,[6] and J. Perper[13]

1 Departments of Psychiatry and Behavioral Sciences
2 Department of Neurology
3 Department of Pathology
4 Department of Epidemiology
5 Department of Psychology
6 Comprehensive Drug Research Center
University of Miami Medical School, Miami, Florida
7 Department of Zoology
University of Texas, Austin, Texas
8 Department of Bacteriology
Yokohama City Medical School, Yokohama, Japan
9 Department of Neurology
Johns Hopkins Medical School, Baltimore, Maryland
10 Department of Pathology
Harbor-UCLA Medical Center, Los Angeles, California
11 Department of Neurology
Tohoku University Medical School, Sendai, Japan
12 Department of Viral Diseases
Walter Reed Army Institute of Research, Washington, DC
13 Broward County Medical Examiner's Office
Ft. Lauderdale, Florida

* Corresponding author: Dr. Paul Shapshak, Professor and Director of the HIV Laboratory, Elliot Bldg., RM 2026, University of Miami School of Medicine, 1800 NW 10th Avenue, Miami, Florida 33136. Tel. 305-243-3352; Fax. 305-243-4772; e-mail. pshapsha2@mednetnewssun.med.miami.edu.

AIDS, Drugs of Abuse, and the Neuroimmune Axis, Edited by Friedman *et al.*
Plenum Press, New York, 1996

1. ABSTRACT

HIV Associated Dementia (HAD) and peripheral neuropathy result from HIV-1 infection and several parameters impact on their initiation and course. These parameters include properties of the virus such as sequence heterogeneity of the envelope protein and virus and host gene expression in infected and uninfected macrophages in HIV infected individuals. The infection of brain cells such as macrophage/microglia may influence the course and duration of HAD through the elaboration of toxic molecules and viral host by-products of infection. Drugs of abuse complicate our interpretation of the resulting pathologies and affect the molecular and biochemical processes involved in HIV-1 infection and its life cycle. Furthermore, abused drugs may modulate the biology and function of macrophage/microglia as well as other cells in brain. Total HIV-1 virus load in the brain may also impact the clinical consequences of infection. Although specific strains of HIV-1 may inflict HAD by interactions at the molecular level, other mechanisms may operate in the initiation and development of peripheral neuropathy. An important aspect of these studies is the determination of their accuracy, specificity, sensitivity, and reproducibility. We describe important caveats involved in the performance, analysis, and interpretation of the results.

2. INTRODUCTION

HIV associated Dementia (HAD) in HIV-1 infected patients may result from HIV-1 infection (11, 28, 29); neuropathology in both HAD and peripheral neuropathy in these patients may result from toxic molecules produced in situ in these tissues. HIV-1 probably enters the brain early after infection (73, 88, 95) and we are analyzing the association of brain sequence heterogeneity and brain virus load of HIV-1 and the incidence and course of HIV-1 related neuropsychiatric diseases. The heterogeneity of human immunodeficiency virus type 1 (HIV-1) may be a primary cause of its resilience and resistance to suppression (27, 34, 54, 77). There appears to be discontinuity in the arrays or clusters of sequences which are detected for HIV-1, both spatially (in different tissues in infected individuals and in different geographical locations) (22, 24, 46, 47, 57, 58, 81, 85, 97, 109) and temporally (during the course of infection in each individual and world-wide during the course of the epidemic) (27, 54, 58, 109). In addition, the virus may contribute to host destruction (pathology) by autostimulatory mechanisms in which the virus appears to promote cytokine production and other host-derived gene products. These viral and host products derange the host's immune defenses. When this occurs in the nervous system the result is nervous system damage (105, 106, 108, 117, 119) as well as direct damage by HIV and virus by-products. We discuss several factors, including drug abuse, possibly involved in the pathogenesis of HIV-related neurological diseases (82). We also discuss important caveats for the interpretation of DNA sequence analysis and reduction of the dangers of contamination.

3. MATERIALS AND METHODS

3.1 Specimens and Cell/Viral Culture

We used the definition of AIDS disease as previously defined (18CDC). Clinical histories were summarized previously (60, 61, 85, 115, 118, 119). Methods to obtain brain tissue from several regions including frontal, temporal (hippocampal and amygdala regions), parietal, and occipital lobes and midbrain (peri-aqueductal grey areas) for in situ hybridization (ISH) and immunohistochemistry (IHC) have been previously described (87, 90). Formalin fixed paraffin embedded and cryopreserved tissue were used in our studies. Cell and virus culture methods have also been previously described (87, 90). Normal peripheral blood mononuclear cells and macrophages were purified according to standard procedures (87, 90) and purification of macrophages from brain are also described (98).

3.2 In Situ Hybridization (ISH), Immunohistochemistry (IHC), and Combined ISH and IHC

ISH, IHC, and the combined procedures used to detect HIV-1 (pol gene) and host cell gene products have been described in detail previously (60, 61, 85 86, 87, 89, 90, 98, 118, 119). Apoptotic cells were detected using an immune labeling kit (Apoptag kit, Oncor, Gaithersburg, MD).

3.3 Polymerase Chain Reaction

Our DNA and RNA extraction and PCR procedures have been previously described (85, 119). Controls included DNA extracted and purified from cultured cells and also provided in the PCR kits. Sentinel tubes are used as an additional means to monitor potential contamination (80). We have not as yet detected any contamination in our negative controls. During the studies described here and previously published (84, 85, 115), the laboratory clone, HXB2 (72), was never used. However, contamination from this clone is still a danger due to its widespread use as discussed below.

3.4 DNA Sequencing and Phylogenetic Analysis

The PCR primers specific for the HIV-1 env V1-V5 variable region, nucleotide numbers, 6,564-7,660, and amino acid numbers 2,188-2,553 and the PCR-cloning and DNA sequencing procedures were described previously (85, 115). Sequences were aligned using Clustal 5 (36). Neighbor-joining trees (79) were estimated using PAUP* (100) incorporating the HKY85 model of nucleotide evolution (35). Confidence in resulting relationships is assessed using 500 replications of the bootstrap procedure (25).

3.5 Comparative Quantitative PCR HIV-1 PCR in Brain

Methods that depend on PCR amplification of DNA are extremely sensitive and are used to establish correlation between HIV load and pathology (20). A linear response PCR technique was developed for the comparative quantitative analysis of HIV DNA in tissue specimens (26). The ratio of the amount of HIV DNA amplified to that of endogenous cellular genomic DNA (e.g. β-actin DNA) is determined for each tissue DNA, and the ratio is converted to the ratio of the number of HIV DNA copies per cellular genome for comparison among tissue specimens. A standard curve is made for each set of experiments using the standard DNA amplified with each set. Each specimen is amplified at three concentrations. PCR amplification with β-actin primers is carried out first. This will determine the DNA concentration dependent range of amplification, and the value obtained will be used for the denominator of the ratio of amplified products. Then PCR amplification for an HIV-1 DNA with SK 38/39 primers is carried out at three DNA concentrations; optimum amounts determined from respective β-actin data. Amplified products are labeled with 5' 32P labeled primers for the last cycle of amplification and the amount of product is determined using a phosphorimager.

3.6 Methods to Prevent Background Reaction and Contamination

The following are methods that we practice to maintain Biosafety and to prevent potential contamination from occurring at all stages of our work.

3.6.1 Autopsy. 1. Double gloves, gown and masks must be worn. 2. No cerebrospinal fluid (CSF) taps with blood are utilized; we label such tubes as "bloody tap" and do not use this fluid in any sequencing experiments. 3. We change scalpels between each new area or section at autopsy. 4. All tissues and cutting boards are rinsed with sterile phosphate buffered saline (PBS) at the Medical Examiner. 4. We change the outermost set of gloves when handling a new brain region or tissue. 5. All tubes wiped with gauze saturated with 70% ethanol before and after use. 6. We use clean knives to cut the brain and rinse them with 100% bleach, 70% ethanol, and wipe clean and dry before use. Also, we clean and disinfect spatulas to transport tissue from the cutting board to conical tubes. We do not do this by hand. All personnel involved in utilization of tissue are vaccinated against Hepatitis B and monitored with the tuberculin test annually.

3.6.2 Virology/Tissue Culture. 1. We use only sterile conical tubes, Eppendorf tubes and petri dishes and do not use glass. 2. Scalpels are changed with each new region of tissue to be cut and discarded immediately in puncture resistant containers. 3. All tissue must be rinsed with sterile PBS. 4. We cut only one tissue at a time in the tissue culture hood. 5. Any tissue to be discarded should be sprayed with 100% bleach before it is discarded. It is placed in freshly made 1% osyl and autoclaved the same day. 6. We wipe all tubes with gauze saturated with 100% bleach and then 70% ethanol before and after using them. 7. We are careful to label tubes correctly and to have a carefully written inventory. 8. All the equipment used in processing should be autoclaved immediately after each use. 9. 100% undiluted bleach and 70% ethanol bottles must be installed at each work station. 10. Should any contamination occur in cultures we adhere to the following procedure. We clean contaminated wells with undiluted bleach followed by 70% ethanol. We use care when doing this so as not to generate splash droplets. 11. Cryopreserved tissue is stored at -85 °C. 12. Tissues and fluids are aliquoted and stored in cryovials in 10-20 aliquots per tissue or fluid from each case. Tissues and fluids from not more than one case are stored per box. 13. Subsequent analyses are done on one tissue or fluid specimen at a time.

3.6.3 Molecular Biology. 1. To prevent contamination, we utilize modified published recommendations (16, 43, 71, 116, 121). Each operation is carried out in a space specifically designated for that purpose: PCR reaction tubes are set up in a hood in a room specifically reserved for PCR. 2. Target DNA's are added in a hood in a separate room, the PCR amplification unit is placed in another room, radioactive reaction tubes are set up in another hood, and the products are used for analysis at a bench near an electrophoresis unit. 3. We keep all glassware carefully cleaned and baked. 3. When retrieving tissue for sequencing, we do not remove more than 1 tube of tissue or fluid specimen at a time and we note date, time, and location. 4. Cross contamination is avoided by using aerosol free tips for each addition into each tube for all the ingredients. These tubes are wiped with 70% ethanol solution after each ingredient is added, and gloves are changed after each set of operations. 5. Cross contamination during the entire procedure is monitored by including a tissue DNA sample from an HIV-negative patient extracted at the same time as the HIV positive tissue specimens as well as sentinel tubes (80, 84, 85). 6. In addition, the laboratory is exposed to UV light when not in use. 7. We process one specimen at a time and process purified DNA and RNA, separately, as well.

3.6.4 In Situ Hybridization and Immunohistochemistry. Comparisons of hybridization (signal) and background (noise) are utilized in both these procedures. Various artifacts may contribute to background including chemical and procedural artifacts. During in situ hybridization, stray light can induce artifacts during autoradiography. The selection of controls is a very important step: in a specimen, a region of staining or grains of hybridization may be compared with surrounding areas without stain or grains (86, 89, 90, 101, 102, 104, 119). In the case of staining for a particular antigen, positive and negative cells are counted and the numbers compared (119). In addition, sections from non-disease controls may be compared with the specimens. Furthermore, non-immune antibody and control probes may be used for their respective procedures. For example, anti-sense riboprobes or DNA probes (for example, generated by asymmetric PCR) may be compared to corresponding sense riboprobes or DNA probes so that the sense and anti-sense sequences are complementary with each other. The advantage of manual autoradiographic techniques is that grains may be counted over specific histologically defined objects such as cells or nuclei and signal to noise ratios calculated. Generally, background grains occur below 2 grains per cell and positive cells contain more than 10 grains per cell. The student t-test is applied to confirm the significance of the results. These are standard methods that are utilized extensively in this field and have been developed in detail during the last 10-15 years (86, 89, 90, 102). In addition, artifacts can be reduced by optimizing experimental conditions by performing melting curve in situ hybridization (varying the stringency of the hybridizations and washes), as is done for Southern blot hybridizations. These procedures are time-consuming but confirm the specificity of the methods, as has been shown for several viruses, including HIV-1, by this laboratory (86, 89, 90, 102, 119). The combined immunohistochemical and in situ hybridization techniques are similarly optimized with the same criteria as for each procedure alone (86, 89, 90, 119, 120).

3.7 Methods to Deal with Potential Problems in DNA Sequencing

Several problems can occur during DNA sequencing and multiple appropriate strategies, in response, are required (32). DNA sequence primers are used in opposing (3' and 5') directions to deal with the potential problem of unknown and potentially unidentified errors that may occur during sequencing due to the problem of the lack of fidelity of the taq-polymerase and related enzymes. In addition, the patience and skill of the sequencer to specifically review every base from the computer file output from automated DNA sequencers is necessary to confirm all sequences and also to adjudicate lack of assignments when they occur. In addition, it is useful for the sequencing and alignment procedures to be repeated as one does for any other scientific discipline. Timing of processing samples and order of analysis are also important in attempting to determine if contamination has occurred in DNA sequencing studies.

Other problems that occur can be of a less obvious nature and require additional comparisons of sequences with each other. Comparisons of DNA and amino acid sequences with similar categories of sequences in data bases should be done as well. These problems are a specific aspect of HIV sequence analysis because of the heterogeneity of HIV-1. An additional concern is that these potential problems are supernumerary to the fundamental problem of contamination that can occur during DNA and RNA purification and during the original PCR steps (discussed above).

In this regard, two specific problems have been addressed in the literature recently (41, 44, 58, 109 and personal communication from Drs. B. Korber, B. Foley [Los Alamos, NM], G. Learn, and J. Mullins [Seattle, WA]): a. when sequences are extremely similar—possibly, due to contamination or b. When similarities occur for non-epidemiologically linked specimens—possibly, due to generation of artefactual recombinants and sample mix-up (discussed below).

4. RESULTS

In this article we deal with two aspects of this laboratory's research on neuropathogenesis in AIDS: results suggesting molecular mechanisms of neuropathogenesis and an analysis of the reproducibility and validity of some of these analyses.

4.1 Cocaine/Cocaethylene and Macrophage Surface Marker Expression, in Vitro, and Neuroimmunology

We found that macrophages purified from brain and treated with cocaethylene (a by product of co-ingestion of cocaine and alcohol) result in down-regulation (reduced expression) of macrophage surface markers, CD11c, CD14, CD 68, and HLA-DR, compared to untreated controls (at 7 days post-treatment). On the other hand, cocaine treatments stimulated expression of these surface markers compared to controls at early times (3 days post treatment, data not shown). These results are obtained in the context of our studies on Neuroimmunology in the HIV-1-infected nervous system (post-mortem). We find increased numbers of nodules of Nageotte in dorsal root ganglia from AIDS patients and increased IL-6 (endothelial cells), IL-1, TNF-α, γ-interferon (macrophages), and reduced parvalbumin expression (neurons) (60, 61, 85, 117, 118, 119).

4.2 Determination of the Quantitative Distribution of HIV DNA in Brains from HIV-1 Infected Patients (Quantitative PCR)

The method described in section 3.5 was evaluated using mixtures of DNA purified from HIV-1 infected cells (TH4-7-5) that are known to harbor one copy of HIV-1 DNA per genome (10) and DNA from uninfected human cells (H9) (26). Mixtures were made to simulate conditions in the brain where only a small fraction of cells may be infected (63). On the basis of this study, the list of crucial conditions that have to be met for the quantitative PCR amplification is compiled (26). These conditions are: 1) the copy number of proviral HIV DNA in the standard must be known accurately; 2) when test specimens are chromosomal DNA, then the standard DNA should be chromosomal DNA; 3) The efficiency of amplification should be uniform among the experiments being compared; 4) Specimens are compared within the DNA concentration range where the degree of amplification is dependent on the amount of target DNA; and 5) Variations in the amount of amplified products due to variations in experimental conditions are corrected by the standard curve constructed for each experiment from the standard DNA's included in each set of samples amplified. We observed that when the standard curves for different conditions are parallel, then this indicates that their amplification efficiencies are the same and the results can be compared. See Table 1.

4.3 DNA Sequencing of HIV DNA and RNA Derived from Brain, CSF, and Blood from HIV-1 Infected Patients

We are characterizing the HIV-1 DNA and RNA sequences present in post-mortem brain, CSF, and blood from HIV-1 infected patients who were drug abusers or not and died with and without HIV associated dementia. Using techniques mentioned above, DNA and

Table 1. HIV DNA load in 5 neuroanatomical locations in a case with early HAD. Relative quantitative PCR was done in DNA purified from cryopreserved brain tissue

Specimen	Cellular DNA (ng)	SK 38/39 Net PIU	ß 1/2 Net PIU	SK/ß	HIV DNA copies/10^3 host genomes
Hippocampus	10	300,000	19,000	15.8	580
Frontal Lobe	10	94,000	22,000	4.3	40
Parietal Lobe	10	48,000	31,000	1.5	11
Basal Ganglia	10	30,000	53,000	0.57	1.5
Cerebellum	10	55,000	100,000	0.55	1.4

Methods are described in the text
PIU = phophorimager unit
ß 1/2 = primers in actin gene
HAD = HIV Associated Dementia
SK 38/39 = HIV primers in gag gene

RNA are purified from brain, CSF, and blood, subjected to PCR across the V1-V5 regions of the HIV envelope gene (reverse transcription is performed prior to the PCR step for RNA). Cloning of individual sequences is done and DNA sequencing is performed. Phylogenetic analyses are then carried out (85). We find that sequences tend to cluster according to tissue or fluid of origin and that there are increased similarities for RNA-derived sequences compared to DNA-derived sequences (data not shown). We find that there may be similarities between HIV-1 sequences in the brain of HIV-1 infected patients and the complexities of this analysis are discussed below.

5. DISCUSSION

5.1 Viral and Host Neuroimmunology

HIV-1 infection of the brain occurs early after HIV-1 infection of the patient (62, 73, 88, 95, 103) and may result in toxicity due to virus proteins, including gp120, or subsequent host gene expression. HIV-1 invasion may result in local autoimmune and hyperimmune reactions in AIDS. Our studies include analyzing the involvement of the following in neuropathogenesis (data not shown). We quantitate nodules of Nageotte in the PNS because they are indicative of neuronal death in dorsal root ganglia (DRG) and their numbers are increased in HIV infected individuals compared to age-matched individuals who are HIV-seronegative (60, 61, 120). In the central nervous system (CNS) we characterize microglial nodules and multi-nucleate giant cells. In HIV infected patients, these are increased in the brain and spinal cord and are often infected with HIV-1 (23, 66, 67, 85, 111, 120 Eilbot, Petito, Shapshak, Wieser, Yoshioka). Cytokine expression (e.g. TNF-α, IL-1, IL-6, and γ-interferon) occurs in several cell types including macrophages, astrocytes, and endothelial cells (60, 61, 96, 105, 106, 108, 110, 117). Cytokines may be expressed in early stages and may induce successive reactions in pathogenesis such as nitric oxide synthase and apoptosis (60, 61, 110). In addition, end-stage damage (apoptosis) may also be due to convergent mechanisms such as gp120 effects on neurons via the NMDA receptor (as reviewed 45, 117).

Parvalbumin and calbindin are calcium binding proteins, and parvalbumin shows reduced expression in AIDS whereas calbindin is unchanged (60, 61). Possibly, this shows that specific neuronal sub-type damage can occur due to either specific susceptibility or specific results of the effectors of damage. An example of specific neuronal susceptibility may be dopaminergic neurons in the substantia nigra. Early cognitive-motor symptoms associated with HIV-1 infection include Parkinsonian symptoms of bradyphrenia and bradykinesia as well as postural instability, gait abnormalities, masked fascies, and slowed saccadic eye movements. In addition, lowered dopamine level has been demonstrated in the CSF of those with HIV-related neurological disease (7, 29). Chronic ICV administration of α-interferon has been associated with Parkinsonian symptomatology in rats (83), and this has been related to changes in neuronal structure. Endogenous α-interferon has also been related to increased likelihood of HIV disease progression (56Mildvan et al.,1992). Recent work suggests that glial derived neurotrophic factor (GDNF) — a cytokine that is a member of the TGF-β super-family — is protective against MPTP-induced substantia nigra toxicity (an animal model for Parkinson's disease) (5). Hence, there may be a dynamic equilibrium between two cytokines — α-interferon and GDNF — at the dopaminergic neuronal level in the substantia nigra that determines the structural response to challenge by whole virions and/or virus products such as gp120 (29). This equilibrium may be further influenced by use of abused substances such as cocaine, which is known to cause inhibition of dopaminergic reuptake, resulting in a euphoric experience associated with dopaminergic stimulation of the ventral tegmental area of the midbrain as well as the nucleus accumbens and frontal cortex (39, 74). Cocaine withdrawal may result in the opposite manifestation — anhedonia — upon withdrawal, related to decreased dopamine availability and possible increased likelihood of an equilibrium shift toward dopaminergic neuronal damage in response to HIV-1.

A complex set of interactions in the nervous system subsequent to HIV infection apparently result in pathogenesis of central and peripheral nervous system neurological disease as well as neuropsychiatric disease (117). A unifying feature of pathogenesis in both the CNS and PNS appears to involve cytokines and toxic molecules such as nitric oxide, possibly resulting in apoptosis. The macrophage is the focus of intense studies in pathogenesis and is responsible for the elaboration of much of the detected toxicity (60, 61, 105, 106, 117). Our studies include peripheral nerves, dorsal root ganglia, spinal cord, and the brain. (Morphometry is currently being performed for the peripheral nerves in our studies on peripheral neuropathy). There appear to be common pathways of pathogenesis in both central and peripheral nervous systems in spite of more frequent detection of HIV-1 RNA in the CNS than in the PNS (60, 61, 85, 105, 106). Subsequent to HIV-1 infection, the elaboration of cytokines, increased nitric oxide synthase (NOS) expression, reduction of parvalbumin expression, and increased apoptosis may be associated with pathogenesis such as Nodules of Nageotte in the peripheral nervous system (in dorsal root ganglia, DRG) and possibly with microglial nodules and multinucleate giant cells in the CNS. Other effectors of tissue destruction include quinolinic acid (a product of tryptophan metabolism) and increased intra-neuronal free calcium cation (as reviewed 28, 117). The effects of abused drugs including cocaine (and its by-product of co-ingestion with ethanol, cocaethylene) are complicating factors in unraveling the complex patterns associated with neuropathogenesis. Intravenous use of cocaine increases the risk for HIV-1 infection (2, 15, 17, 49) and may be associated with neurological abnormalities (29, 51, 82, 92); however, there is disagreement with the possible relationship of chronic drug use and neurological disease (19Concha). We find that cocaine and cocaethylene may effect brain macrophages and result in perturbed surface marker expression. These studies may provide additional basis for developing models for macrophage function and neuropathogenesis in drug abusers.

5.2 PCR to Quantitate HIV DNA Distribution in the Brain

Virus load may be another parameter of virus infection that is associated with onset or progression of HAD. Our recent analysis of virus load in the AIDS brain using quantitative

PCR shows that the hippocampus may have an elevated virus load compared to other regions. Most prior studies of HIV-1 DNA load in the brain analyzed only the frontal lobe (6, 9, 63, 91, 94, 107, 113), and the HIV-1 DNA distribution has not been done on large enough samples to make definitive statements. However, other studies have shown that HIV-1 associated abnormalities (predominantly HIV encephalitis and atrophy) are most severe in the basal ganglia (4, 11, 14, 21, 66). On the basis of immunohistochemical analysis, it was hypothesized by Masliah, Wiley and their associates that HIV associated neuropathology results from local abundance of HIV-1 and is associated with severity of motor-cognitive disorders (48, 112, 113). In one study by PCR (1), HIV-1 DNA load was shown to be greater in basal ganglia than in cortical white matter or cerebral gray matter. To our knowledge, the report by Bockstahler and his associates (8) was the first that analyzed by PCR, HIV-1 proviral DNA distribution in several regions of the brain by a qualitative PCR. They determined the frequency of occurrence of the amplified product at each neuroanatomical location in only three brains. This was extended to quantitative comparison as discussed in the previous section. The method was used to analyze specimens from two brains — one with and one without neuropathological symptoms (26). In both cases, the frontal lobe white matter had approximately 50 proviral DNA copies per 103 cellular genomes, which is at the higher end of the values reported by Pang and his associates (63). However, the hippocampus had about 250 proviral DNA per 103 cellular genomes, the highest amount of HIV DNA in both brains (26). It remains to be determined if this may be correlated with detection of CD4 receptor density in the hippocampus (65). These HIV-1 quantitation results suggest that more extensive quantitative comparisons of HIV-1 DNA with respect to neuroanatomical regions in the brains of AIDS patients are needed to increase the sample size and to further explore neuropathogenesis and its possible relationship with cognitive-motor disorders at the molecular level.

5.3. Sequence Heterogeneity and Tropism of HIV-1

Sequence heterogeneity of HIV-1 may be crucial and facilitate its escape from the humoral neutralization of the HIV-1 gp120 and cell mediated immune response against HIV-1 infected cells. Specific HIV-1 strains that evolve during the immune response may be involved in neuropathogenesis and the variable regions of gp120 may reflect this. We performed DNA sequencing across the V1-V5 region of the envelope gene of HIV-1 from post-mortem brain, CSF, blood, spinal cord, and sensory dorsal root ganglia (DRGs) from injecting DUs (IDUs) from the Medical Examiner. We published phylogenetic analyses of 86 sequences of the V4 variable region of the env gene of HIV from brain, CSF, and blood (see Figure 3 in 85). At the time of publication, our preliminary analyses indicated that one patient, XSH149 may have a separate subtype. However, we subsequently determined that sequences from this case were an extreme variant of the B subtype (115). The significance of this finding is under investigation.

Some additional analyses have been performed with these sequences. There are several potential problems that can occur during the management of DNA sequencing projects (41, 44) and we apply these insights to our DNA sequence analyses. These studies are ongoing and current conclusions and future studies are pointed out here. In our phylogenetic study of the HIV-1 env V4 region, 86 sequences derived from the brain, CSF, and blood from three drug users were shown (see Figure 3 in 85 Shapshak 1994). Additional analyses have shown that 11 of these sequences have a higher similarity (more than 97%) to HIV-1B (HXB2, 72) than to the other sequences derived from the three individuals in the study (44; Crandall, Shapshak, and Xin, unpublished observations). The clones with this property are: XSH141 R2D, R4D, R5D, R6D, R7D, XSH144 C3R, C6R, C9R, C12R, C13R, and L1D. A possible mechanism for these findings is direct contamination during the procedures due to HXB2-like sequences; however, several of the sequences exhibit a higher similarity at the 5' end than elsewhere in the clone and so the possibility of PCR-related recombination has been proposed (44). This process depends on specific conditions of primer concentrations and elongation reaction times during PCR and could result in recombination between any of the patient HIV sequences as well as between the patient HIV sequences and the potential external HIV contaminant (55). We are performing additional experiments to test the conditions and underlying mechanisms for these types of putative contaminating events. Another explanation for these findings is that there may be an HXB2-like wild-type strain present contemporaneously, a wild-type strain which had remained relatively unchanged during the last 10-12 years. Individuals with these sequences would thus have super-infections of more than 1 strain of HIV-1. Though infrequent, superinfection in a few patients by two strains of HIV-1 has been detected (68, 114, 122) and recombination, in vivo, has been documented in several studies (33, 37, 52, 75, 76, 78). The possibility of infection of patients during the last few years by HIV-1B-like strains has been published (3). Additional work is required to assess the extent to which such vestigial strains of HIV-1 may exist in the HIV-1 infected population at large vs. the omnipresent danger of contamination by HXB2 due to its widespread use. Similarly, HIV-1 infected cell cultures and DNA clones derived from these cultures, can possibly become contaminated with HTLV-III, LAV, LAI, or laboratory strains derived from isolates such as these. Direct cloning and sequencing from tissue obviates the problem of cell culture contaminants.

We found that 13 out of 31 (42%) of the brain-derived V4 env sequences from patients 141 and 144 were more similar to each other than to their own blood and CSF sequences (see Figure 3 in 85). From this it was inferred that there is tissue specificity of HIV-1 infection and that neurotropic HIV-1 strains or sequences may exist (85). These possibilities are supported in the literature (22, 24, 30, 40, 42, 59, 64, 69, 70, 81, 97). However, the question was raised as to whether these results may be due to a sample mix-up (44). The clones in question are XSH141 R1R, R3R, R7R, R8R, and R9R (see Figure 3 in 85). Similar questions have been raised about five CSF clones: XSH144 C3D, C4D, C7D, C8D, and C10D (see Figure 3 in 85). We are investigating this further by doing additional sequencing and by performing synonymous-non-synonymous codon profile searches of the sequences in our studies (58). Percent similarity data base searches and synonymous-non-synonymous profile calculations will become routine in order to establish base-lines for comparisons in these studies. Potential contamination and sample mix-up have also been proposed as problems (12, 41) in studies on maternal-perinatal transmission of HIV-1 (13). Several studies, however, support the occurrence of similarities of HIV sequences from different individuals who are not linked by transmission, i.e. convergent evolution or tissue-specific evolution of HIV-1 sequences in different individuals (12, 31, 38, 50, 93, 99) and at times extremely close similarities for those who are linked epidemiologically (demographically) (53) as well as similarities to the HXB2 type sequences (3).

6. CONCLUSIONS

There is evidence that HIV-1 invasion of the brain occurs early in HIV-1 infection and that host and viral factors are involved in neuropathogenesis in AIDS. Drug abuse is an additional complicating factor in these studies and we present evidence that cocaine and cocaine-by-products alter macrophage marker expression. In order to provide a firm work foundation we discuss the requirements for accuracy, specificity, and reproducibility in DNA sequencing analysis, comparative quantitative PCR, as well as for in situ hybridization, immunohistochemistry, and other aspects of laboratory procedures.

7. ACKNOWLEDGMENTS

We thank Drs. B. Korber and B. Foley (Los Alamos, NM), and Drs. J. Mullins and G. Learn (Seattle, WA) for critical discussions. Ms. X.R. Cao (Yokohama, Japan), Ms. M. Perez, Mr. M. Epler, Mr. C. Carpentieri, Ms. V. Laird, Mr. B. Henry, Mr. Y. Jeanty and Mr. C. Bess (Miami, FL) are thanked for technical assistance. The NIAID Resource is thanked for research reagents. We thank Dr. R.A. Bitonte (Los Angeles, CA) for fetal brain tissue. Our research is supported by Research Grants DA04787, DA07909, DA09229, NS26584, NS35331, MH48628, and NIMH OD920004.

8. REFERENCES

1. Achim, C. L., Wang, R., Miners, D. K., and Wiley, C. A. Brain Viral Burden in HIV Infection. J. Neuropathol. Exp. Neurol. 53, 284-294, 1994
2. Anthony JC, Vlahov D, Nelson KE, Cohn S, Astemborski J, and Solomon L, New evidence on intravenous cocaine use and the risk of infection with HIV-1, Am J of Epidemiol, 134, 1175-1189, 1991
3. Antonioli IM, Baumberger C, Yerly S, and Perrin L, V3 sequences in primary HIV-1 infection, AIDS, 9, 11-17, 1995
4. Aylward, E.H., Henderer, J.D., McArthur, J.C., et al. Reduced basal ganglia volume in HIV-1 associated dementia complex: results for quantitative neuroimaging. Neurology, 43, 2099-2104, 1993
5. Beck KD, Valverde J, Alexi T, Poulsen K, Moffat B, Vandlen RA, Rosenthal A, Hefti F: Mesencephalic dopaminergic neurons protected by GDNF from axotomy-induced degeneration in the adult brain. Nature 1995; 373: 339-341
6. Bell, J. E., Busuttil, A., Ironside, J. W., Rebus, s., Donaldson, Y. K., Simmonds, P., and Peutherer, J. F. Human Immunodeficiency Virus and the Brain: Investigation of Virus Load, and Neuropathologic Changes in Pre-AIDS Subjects. J. Inf. Diseases, 168, 818-824, 1993
7. Berger JR, Kumar M, Kumar A, Fernandez JB, and Levin B: Cerebrospinal fluid dopamine in HIV infection, AIDS, 8, 67 -71, 1994
8. Bockstahler, L. E., Werner, T., Festl, H., Weis, S., Einhaeupl, K. M., Erfle, V., and Brack-Werner, R. Distribution of HIV genomic DNA in brains of AIDS patients. Clin Diagn Virol, 3, 61-72, 1995
9. Boni, J., Emmerich, B. S., Leib, S. L., Wiestler, O. D., Schupbach, J., and Kleihues, P. PCR identification of HIV-1 DNA sequences in brain tissue of patients with AIDS encephalopathy. Neurology, 43, 1813-1817, 1993
10. Brack-Werner, R., Kleinschmidt, A., Ludvigsen, A., Mellert, W., Neumann, M., Herrmann, R., Khim, M. C. L., Burny, A., Muller-Lantzsch, N., Stavrou, D., and Volker, E. Infection of human brain cells by HIV-1: restricted virus production in chronically infected human glial cell lines. AIDS, 6, 273-285, 1992
11. Brew, B. J., Rosenblum, M., Cronin, K, and Price, R. W. AIDS Dementia Complex and HIV-1 Brain Infection: Clinical-Virological Correlations, Ann Neurol, 38, 563-570, 1995
12. Briant L, Puel J, Wade CM, Leigh Brown AJ, and Guyader M, Protecting HIV databases- Reply, Nature, 378, 243-244, 1995
13. Briant L, Wade CM, Puel J, Leigh Brown AJ, and Guyader M, Analysis of envelop sequence variants suggests multiple mechanisms of mother-to-child transmission of HIV-1, J Virol, 69, 3778-3788, 1995
14. Budka, H. et al. (33 authors). HIV-Associated disease of the nervous system: Review of nomenclature and proposal for neuropathology-based terminology. Brain Pathology, 1, 143-152, 1991
15. Chaisson RE, Bachchetti P, Osmond D, et al, Cocaine use and HIV infection in intravenous drug users in San Francisco, JAMA, 261, 561-565, 1989
16. Chelley J and Kahn A, RT-PCR and mRNA quantitation, in the polymerase chain reaction, eds. KB Mullis, F Ferré, and RA Gibbs, Birkhauser Press, Boston, 1994, pp. 97-109
17. Chitwood DD, McCoy CB, Inciardi J, et al, HIV seropositivity of needles from shooting galleries in South Florida, Am J Public Health, 80, 150-152, 1990
18. Centers for Disease Control and Prevention. Revision of the CDC surveillance case definition of AIDS. JAMA, 258, 1143-1154, 1987
19. Concha M, Graham NMH, Muñoz A, Vlahov D, Royall III, W, Updike M, Nance-Sproson T, Selnes OA, and McArthur JC, Effect of chronic substance abuse on the neuropsychological performance of intravenous drug users with high prevalence of HIV-1 seropositivity, Am J of Epidemiol, 136, 1338-1348, 1992
20. Cotter, F. E. The role of polymerase chain reaction in pathology. J. Histotechnology, 17, 253-259, 1994

21. Dal Pan, G.J., McArthur, J.H., Aylward, E., Selnes, O.A., Nance-Sproson, T.E., Kumar, A.J., Mellits, E.D., and McArthur, J.C. Patterns of cerebral atrophy in HIV-1-infected individuals: Results of a quantitative MRI analysis. Neurology, 42, 2125-2130, 1992
22. Delassus S, Cheynier R, and Wain-Hobson S, Non-homogeneous distribution of HIV-1 proviruses in the spleen, J of Virol, 66, 5642-5645, 1992
23. Eilbot DJ, Peress N, Burger H, et al, HIV-1 in spinal cords of AIDS patients with myelopathy: expression and replication in macrophages, PNAS, 86, 3337-3341, 1989
24. Epstein LG, Kuiken C, Blumberg BM, Hartman S, Sharer LR, Clement M, and Goudsmit J, HIV-1 V3 domain variation in brain and spleen of children with AIDS: tissue-specific evolution within host-determined quasispecies, Virol, 180, 583-590, 1991
25. Felsenstein J, Confidence limits on phylogenies: an approach using bootstrap, Evolution, 39, 783-791, 1985
26. Fujimura, R. K. and Bockstahler L. E. PCR Method for determining ratios of HIV proviral DNA to cellular genomic DNA in brain tissue of HIV-infected patients. J Vir Method, 55, 309-325, 1995
27. Goodenow M, Huert T, Saurin W, Kwok S, Sninsky J, and Wain-Hobson S, HIV-1 isolates are rapidly evolving quasispecies: evidence for viral mixtures and preferred nucleotide substitutions, J of AIDS, 2, 344-352, 1989
28. Goodkin K, Shapshak P, Bradley WG, Yoshioka M, Nagano I, Kumar M, Fletcher MA, and Fujimura RK, Immune function, brain, and HIV-1 infection, in Goodkin K, and A Visser (eds): Psychoneuroimmunology: Stress, Mental Disorders and Health, Washington, DC: American Psychiatric Association Press, Inc., in press, 1996
29. Goodkin K: HIV-related complications of the central nervous system. In: Beckett A, Fernandez F, Goodkin K and McDaniel JS. HIV-related neuropsychiatric complications and treatments. An AIDS Training Curriculum for Psychiatrists. Commission on AIDS, M. Forstein (Chair), American Psychiatric Association, Washington, DC, 1995, pp. 1-64
30. Goswami KK, Miller RF, Harrison MJ, Hamel DJ, Daniels RS, and Tedder RS, Expression of HIV-1 in the CSF detected by the PCR and its correlation with CNS disease, AIDS, 5, 797-803, 1991
31. Grez M, Dietrich U, Balfe P, von Briesen H, Maniar JK, Mahambre G, Delwart EL, Mullins JI, and Waigmann HR, Genetic analysis of HIV-1 and -2 mixed infections in India reveals a recent spread of HIV-1 and HIV-2 from single ancestor for each of these viruses, J Virol, 68, 2161-2168, 1994
32. Gribskov M and Devereux J, Sequence Analysis Primer, WH Freeman and Co, New York, 1992
33. Groenink M, Andeweg AC, Fouchier RAM, Broersen S, Van der Jagt RCM, Schuitemaker H, De Goede REY, Bosch ML, Huiseman HG, and Tersmette M, Phenotype associated env gene variation among eight related HIV-1 clones: evidence for in vivo recombination and determinants of cytotropism outside the V3 domain, J Virol, 66, 6175-6180, 1992
34. Hahn BH, Shaw GM, Taylor ME, Redfield RR, Markham PD, Salahuddin SZ, Wong-Staal F, Gallo RC, Parks ES, and Parks WP, Genetic variation in HTLV-III/LAV over time in patients with AIDS or at risk for AIDS, Science, 232, 1548-1553, 1986
35. Hasegawa M, Kishino H, and Yano T, Dating the human ape splitting by a molecular clock of mitochondrial DNA, J Molec Evol, 22, 160-174, 1985
36. Higgins DG, Bleasby AJ, and Fuchs R, Clustal V: improved software for multiple sequence alignment, Comput Appl Biosci, 8, 189-191, 1992
37. Howell RM, Fitzgibbon JE, Noe M, Ren Z, Gocke DJ, Schartzer TA, and Dubin DT, In vivo sequence variation of the HIV-1 env gene: evidence for recombination among variants found in a single individual, AIDS Res and Hum Retrov, 7, 869-876, 1991
38. Kalisch ML, Baldwin A, Raktham S, Wasi C, Luo C, Schochetman G, Mastro TD, Young N, Vanichseni S, Rübsamen-Waigmann H, von Briesen H, Mullins J, Delwart E, Herring B, Esparza J, Heyward WL, and Osmmanov S, The evolving molecular epidemiology of HIV-1 envelope subtypes in injecting drug users in Bangkok, Thailand: implications for HIV vaccine trials, AIDS 9, 851-857, 1995
39. Koob GF, Bloom FE: Cellular and molecular mechanisms of drug dependence. Science 1988; 242:715-723
40. Korber BTM, Kunstman KJ, Patterson BK, et al, Genetic differences between blood- and brain-derived viral sequences from HIV-1-infected patients: evidence for conserved elements in the V3 region of the envelope protein of brain-derived sequences, J of Virol 68, 7467-7481, 1994
41. Korber BTM, Learn G, Mullins JI Hahn BH, and Wolinsky SM, Protecting HIV databases, Nature, 378, 242-243, 1995.
42. Kuiken CL, Goudsmit J, Weiller GF, Armstrong, Hartman S, Portegies P, Dekker J, and Cornelissen M, Differences in HIV-1 V3 sequences from patients with and without AIDS dementia complex, J of Gen Virol, 76, 175-180, 1995

43. Kwok S, Procedures to minimize PCR-product carry-over, in PCR-protocols and applications- A Laboratory Manual, 1990
44. Learn G, Korber BTM, Foley B, Hahn BH, Wolinsky SM, and Mullins JI, Maintaining the integrity of human immunodeficiency virus sequence databases, J of Virol, submitted, 1995
45. Lipton SA, Memantine prevents HIV coat protein-induced neuronal injury in vitro, Neurology, 42, 1403-1405, 1992
46. Louwagie J, McCutchan F, van der Groen G. et al. Genetic comparison of HIV-1 isolates from Africa, Europe, and North America. AIDS Res Hum Retroviruses, 8, 147-9, 1992
47. Louwagie J, McCutchan FE, Peeters M. et al. Phylogenetic analysis of gag genes from 70 international HIV-1 isolates provides evidence for multiple genotypes, AIDS, 7, 769-80, 1993
48. Masliah, E. Achim, C. L., Ge, N., De Teresa, R., Terry, R. D., and Wiley, C. A. Spectrum of Human Immunodeficiency Virus-associated Neocortical Damage. Ann Neurol, 32, 321-329, 1992
49. McCoy CB, Shapshak P, Rivers JE, McCoy HV, Weatherby NL, Chitwood DD, Shah SM, Inciardi JA, McBride DC, and Watters JK, The risks of injection practices and compliance to risk reduction protocols in the prevention of HIV-1 among injecting drug users, J of AIDS, 7, 773-776, 1994
50. McCutchen FE, Hegerich PA, Brennan TP, Phanuphak P, Singharaj P, Jugsudee A, Berman PW, Gray AM, Fowler AK, and Burke DS, Genetic variants of HIV-1 in Thailand, AIDS Res and Hu Retr, 8, 1887-1895 1992
51. KcKegney FP, O'Dowd MA, Feiner C, et al, A prospective comparison of neuropsychologic function in HIV-seropositive and seronegative methadone-maintained patients, AIDS, 4, 565-569, 1990
52. Leitner T, Escanilla D, Marquina S, Wahlberg J, Bronstrom C, Hansson HB, Uhlen M, and Albert J, Biological and molecular characterization of subtype D, G, and A/D recombinant HIV transmission in Sweden, Virology, 209, 136-146, 1995
53. McNearney T, Westervelt P, Thielan BJ, Trowbridge DB, Garcia J, Whittier R, and Ratner L, Limited sequence heterogeneity among biologically distinct HIV-1 isolates from individuals involved in a clustered infectious outbreak, PNAS, 87, 1917-1921, 1990
54. Meyerhans A, Cheynier R, Albert J, Seth M, Kwok S, Sninsky J, Morfeldt-Månson L, Asjö, and Wain-Hobson S, Temporal fluctuations in HIV quasispecies in vivo are not reflected by sequential HIV isolations, Cell, 58, 901-910, 1989
55. Meyerhans A, Vartanian JP, and Wain-Hobson S, DNA recombination during PCR, Nucleic Acids Res, 18, 1687-1691, 1990.
56. Mildvan D, Machado SG, Wilets, I, Grossberg SE: Endogenous interferon and triglyceride concentrations to assess response to zidovudine in AIDS and advanced AIDS-related complex. Lancet 1992; 339:453-456.
57. Myers G, Berzofsky JA, Korber B, Smith RF, Pavlakis GN. Human retroviruses and AIDS. Los Alamos, NM: Dept. of Theoretical Biology and Biophysics, Los Alamos National Laboratory, 1993
58. Myers G and Korber B, The Future of HIV, in The Evolutionary Biology of Viruses, ed. S.S. Morse, Raven Press, Ltd., New York, 1994, Chapter 10, pp. 211-232.
59. Monken CE, Wu B, and Srinivasan A, High resolution analysis of HIV-1 quasispecies in the brain, AIDS, 9, 345-349, 1995
60. Nagano I, Shapshak P, Yoshioka M, Xin Kq, Nakamura S, and Bradley WG, Parvalbumin and calbindin D-28k immunoreactivity in dorsal root ganglia in AIDS, J Neuroimmunol, in press, 1996
61. Nagano I, Shapshak P, Yoshioka M, Xin KQ, Nakamura S, and Bradley WG, Increased NADPH-diaphorase reactivity and cytokine expression in dorsal root ganglia in AIDS, J Neuro Sci Res, in press, 1996
62. Palmer DL, Hjelle BL, Wiley CA, Allen S, Wachsman W, Mills RG, Davis LE, and Merlin TL, HIV-1 infection despite immediate combination antiviral therapy after infusion of contaminated white cells, Am J of Med, 97, 289-295, 1994
63. Pang, S., Koyanagi, Y., Miles, S., Wiley, C., Vinters, H. V., and Chen I. S. Y. High levels of unintegrated HIV-1 DNA in brain tissue of AIDs dementia patients, Nature, 343, 85- 89, 1990
64. Pang S, Vinters HV, Akashi T, O'Brien WA, and Chen ISY, HIV-1 Env sequence variation in brain tissue of patients with AIDS-related neurologic disease, J of AIDS, 4, 1082-1092, 1991
65. Pert, C. B., Ruff, M. R., Ruscetti, F., Farrar, W. L., and Hill, J. M. HIV Receptor in Brain and Deduced Peptides That Block Viral Infectivity. in Psychological, Neuropsychiatric, and Substance Abuse Aspects of AIDS. Bridge, T. P. et al. (eds) Raven Press, New York, 1988; pp73-83
66. Petito, C. K., Cho, E-S., Lemann, W., Navia, B.A., and Price, R. W. Neuropathology of Acquired Immunodeficiency Syndrome (AIDS): Autopsy Review. J Neuropathol Exp Neurol, 45, 635-646, 1986
67. Petito CK and Roberts B, Evidence of apoptotic cell death in HIV encephalitis, Am J of Pathol, 146, 1121-1130, 1995

68. Pieniazek D, Janini LM, Ramos A, Tanuri A, Schechter M, Peralta JM, Vicente ACP, Pieniazek NJ, Schochetman G, and Rayfield MA, HIV-1 patients may harbor viruses of different phylogenetic subtypes: implications for the evolution of the HIV/AIDS pandemic, Emerging Infect Dis, 1, 86-88, 1995
69. Power C, McArthur JC, Johnson RT, Griffin DE, Glass JD, Dewey R, and Chesebro B, Distinct HIV-1 env sequences are associated with neurotropism and neurovirulence, in HIV and Dementia, eds. MBA Oldstone and L Vitkovic (1995) Cur Topics in Microb and Immunol, 202, pp. 89-104
70. Power C, McArthur JC, Johnson RT, Griffin DE, Glass JD, Perryman S, and Chesebro B, Demented and nondemented patients with /AIDS differ in brain-derived HIV-1, envelope sequences, J of Virology, 68, 4643-4649, 1994
71. Presley LA and Budowle B, The Application of PCR-based technologies to forensic analysis, in PCR Technology Current Innovations, ed. HG Griffin and AM Griffin, CRC Press, Boca Raton, 1994, pp. 259-276
72. Ratner L, Haseltine W, Petarca R, Livak KJ, Starcich B, Josephs SF, Doran ER, Rafalski JA, Whitwhoen EA, Baumeister K, Ivanoff L, Petteway SR, Pearson ML, Lautenberger JA, Papas TS, Ghrayeb J, Chang NT, Gallo RC, and Wong-Staal F, Complete nucleotide sequence of the AIDS virus HTLV-III, Nature, 313, 277-285, 1985
73. Resnick L, Berger JR, Shapshak P, Tourtellotte WW: Early penetration of the blood-brain-barrier by HTLV-III/LAV, Neurology, 38, 9-15, 1988
74. Ritz MC, Lamb RJ, Goldberg SR, Kuhar MJ: Cocaine receptors on dopamine transporters are related to self administration of cocaine. Science 1987; 237:1219-1223.
75. Robertson DL, Hahn BH, and Sharp PM, Recombination in AIDS viruses, J of Molec Evol, 40, 249-259, 1995
76. Robertson DL, Sharp PM, McCutchan FE, and Hahn BH, Recombination in HIV-1, Nature, 3374, 124-126, 1995
77. Saag MS, Hahn BH, Gibbons J, Li Y, Parks E, Parks WP, and Shaw GM, Extensive variation of HIV-1 in vivo, Science, 334, 440-444, 1989
78. Sabino EC, Shpaer EG, Morgado MG, Mullins JI, and Mayer A, The identification of HIV-1 envelope genes recombinant between subtypes B and F, in two epidemiologically linked individuals from Brazil, J of Virology, 68, 6340-6346, 1995
79. Saitou N and Nei M, The neighbor-joining method: a new method for reconstructing phylogenetic trees, Mol Biol Evol, 4, 406-425, 1987
80. Saksena NK, Dwyer D, and Barré-Sinoussi F, A "sentinel" technique for monitoring viral aerosol contamination, J of Infect Dis, 164, 1021-1022, 1991
81. Sala M, Zambruno G, Vartanian JP, Marconi A, Bertazzoni U, and Wain—Hobson S, Spatial discontinuities in HIV-1 quasispecies derived from epidermal Langerhans cells of a patient with AIDS and evidence for double infection, J of Virol, 68, 5280-5283, 1994
82. Sanchez-Ramos JR, Neurological Emergencies related to drugs of dependence, in Urgent and Emergent Neurology, ed. WJ Wiener, Futura Press, NY, 1995, pp. 487-507
83. Saphier D: Central nervous system effects of interferon-α in man and animals. Presented at the Psychoneuroimmunology Research Society Meeting. 11/16/94-11/20/94, Key Biscayne, FL
84. Shah SM, Shapshak P, Rivers JE, Weatherby NL, Xin KQ, Stewart RV, Chitwood DD, Page JB, Mash DC, Vlahov D, and McCoy CB, Detection of HIV-1 DNA in needle/syringes, paraphernalia, and washes from shooting galleries in Miami: preliminary laboratory results, J of AIDS, in press, 1996
85. Shapshak P, Nagano I, Xin KQ, Bradley W, McCoy CB, Sun NCJ, Stewart NCJ, Yoshioka M, Petito C, Goodkin K, Douyon R, Srivastava AK, Crandall KA, HIV-1 heterogeneity and cytokines: neuropathogenesis, in The Brain Immune Axis and Substance Abuse, B. Sharp, T. Eisenstein, J. Madden, and H. Friedman, eds. Adv. in Exp. Med. And Biol., vol. 373, Chapter 31, pp 225-236, 1995
86. Shapshak P, Sun N, Resnick L, Hsu M, Tourtellotte WW, Schmid P, Conrad A, M. Fiala, and D. T. Imagawa, The detection of HIV by in situ hybridization. Modern Pathology, 3, 146-153, 1990
87. Shapshak P, Sun NCJ, Yoshioka M, Shah SM, Schiller PC, Resnick L, and Imagawa DT, Detection of HIV-1 in the CNS: explant culture, immunocytochemical, and in situ hybridization techniques, AIDS, 6, 915-923, 1992
88. Shapshak P, Tourtellotte WW, Resnick L, Osborne MA, Schmid P, Lee M, Rubinshtein G, Imagawa DT, Mitsuyasu R, Gottlieb M, Gallo RC: HTLV-III can cross the blood brain barrier. The Fourth Colloquium in Biological Sciences, Blood Brain Transfer. Annals of the NY Academy of Sci, 529, 291-294, 1988
89. Shapshak P, Tourtellotte WW, Wolman M, Verity N, Verity MA, Schmid P, Syndulko K, Bedows E, Boostanfar R, Darvish M, Nakamura S, Tomiyasu U: Search for virus nucleic acid sequences in post-mortem human brain tissue using in situ hybridization technology with cloned probes: Some solutions and results on PML and SSPE tissue. J of Neurosci Res 16: 281-301, 1986

90. Shapshak P, Yoshioka M, Sun NCJ, and Schiller P, The use of combined immunocytochemistry and in situ hybridization to detect HIV-1 in formalin fixed paraffin embedded brain tissue, Modern Pathology, 5, 649-654, 1992
91. Shaw, G. M.. et al. (14 authors) HTLV-III Infection in Brains of Children and Adults with AIDS Encephalopathy, Science, 227, 177-182, 1985
92. Silberstein CH, McKegney FP, O'Dowd MA, et al, A prospective longitudinal study of neuropshychological and psychosocial factors in individuals at risk for HTLV-III/LAV infection in a methadone program: preliminary findings, Int J of Neurosci, 32, 669-676, 1987
93. Simmonds P Balfe P, Ludlam CA, Bishop JO, and Brown AJL, Analysis of sequence diversity in hypervariable regions of the external glycoprotein of HIV-1, J of Virol, 64, 5840-5850, 1990
94. Sinclair, E., Gray, F., Ciardi, A., and Scaravilli, F. Immunohistochemical changes and PCR detection of HIV provirus DNA in brains of asymptomatic HIV-positive patients. J. Neuropathol. Exp. Neurol. 1994; 53: 43-50
95. Singer EJ, Syndulko K, Fahy-Chandon BN, Shapshak P, Resnick L, Schmid P, Conrad AJ, and Tourtellotte WW, Cerebrospinal fluid p24 antigen levels and intrathecal immunoglobulin G synthesis are associated with cognitive disease severity in HIV-1, AIDS, 8, 197-204, 1994.
96. Sippy BD, Hofman FM, Wallach D, and Hinton DR, Increased expression of TNF-α receptors in the brains of patients with AIDS, J of AIDS, 10, 511-521, 1995
97. Steuler H, Storch-Hagenlocher B, and Wildemann B, Distinct populations of HIV-1 in blood and CSF, AIDS Res and Hum Retrovir, 8, 53-59, 1992
98. Stewart RV, Shapshak P, Matthews A, Bradley W, Sun NCJ, Mash DC, Perez M, Shah SM, Yoshioka M, Nagano I, Bitonte RA, Sundar KS, Fiala M, and Arguello JC, Effects of cocaethylene and HIV-1 infection on surface marker expression of macrophages isolated from human brain using antibody coated magnetic beads: a preliminary study, submitted, 1996
99. Strunnikova N, Ray SC, Lisingston RA, Rubalcaba E, and RP Viscidi, Convergent evolution within the V3 loop domain of HIV type 1 in association with disease progression, J of Virol, 69, 7548-7558, 1995
100. Swofford DS, PAUP* 4.0 d21, Sinauer Assoc, Sunderland, MA, 1995
101. Sun NCJ, Shapshak P, Lachant NA, Hsu MY, Sieger L, Schmid P, Beall G, and Imagawa DT: Bone marrow examination in patients with AIDS and AIDS related complex (ARC): morphologic and in situ hybridization studies: Am J of Clin Pathol, 92, 589-594, 1989
102. Tourtellotte WW, Schmid P, Pick P, Verity N. Martinez S, Shapshak P: Quest for a reliable, valid, and sensitive in situ hybridization procedure to detect viral nucleic acids in the central nervous system. Neurochem Res 12/6: 565-571, 1987
103. Tourtellotte WW, Singer E, Syndulko K, Shapshak P, and Resnick L, Intra-blood-brain-barrier IgG synthesis in HIV, in Enzymes as Targets for Drug Design, MG Palfreyman, PP McCann, W Lovenberg, JG Temple, A Sjoerdsma, Merrell Dow Research Institute, Academic Press, San Diego, pp. 211-217, 1990
104. Tourtellotte WW, Verity N, Schmid P, Martinez S, Shapshak P: Covalent binding of formalin fixed paraffin embedded brain tissue sections to glass slides suitable for in situ hybridization. J Virol Methods 15: 87-99, 1987
105. Tyor WR, Glass JD, Griffin JW, et al, Cytokine expression in the brain during AIDS, Ann Neurol, 31, 349-360, 1992
106. Tyor WR, Wesselingh SL, Griffin JW, McArthur JC, and Griffin DE, Unifying hypothesis for the pathogenesis of HIV-associated Dementia Complex, Vacuolar myelopathy, and sensory neuropathy, J of AIDS and Human Retrovirology, 9, 379-388, 1995
107. Vazeux, R., Lacroix-Ciaudo, C., Blanche, S., Cumont, M-C., Henin, D., Gray, F., Boccon-Gibod, L. and Tardieu, M. Low levels of human immunodeficiency virus replication in the brain tissue of children with severe acquired immunodeficiency syndrome encephalopathy. Am. J. Pathol. 1992; 140: 137-144
108. Vitkovic L, da Cunha A, and Tyor WR, Cytokine expression and pathogenesis in AIDS brain, in "HIV, AIDS and the Brain", eds. RW Price and SW Perry, Raven Press Ltd, New York, 1994
109. Wain-Hobson S, Is antigenic variation of HIV important for AIDS and what might be expected in the future? in The Evolutionary Biology of Viruses, ed. S.S. Morse, Raven Press, Ltd., New York, 1994, Chapter 9, pp. 185-209
110. Wesselingh SL, Power C, Glass JD, Tyor WR, McArthur JC, Farber JM, Griffin JW, and Griffin DE, Intracerebral cytokine messenger RNA expression in AIDS dementia, Ann Neurol, 33, 576-582, 1993
111. Wieser B, Peress N, La Neve D, Eilbott DJ, Seidman R, and Burger H, HIV-1 expression in the CNS correlates directly with extent of disease, PNAS, 87, 3997-4001, 1990
112. Wiley, C. A., Masliah, E., and Achim, C. L. Measurement of CNS HIV burden and its association with neurologic damage. Adv Neuroimmunol 1994; 4:319-325

113. Wiley, C. A., Schrier, R. D., Nelson, J. A., Lampert, P. W., and Oldstone, M. B. A. Cellular localization of human immunodeficiency virus infection within the brains of acquired immune deficiency syndrome patients. Proc. Natl. Acad. Sci. USA 1986; 83: 7089-7093
114. Xin KQ, Ma XH, Crandall KA, Bukawa KH, Ishikasubo Y, Kawamoto S, and Okuda K, Dual infection with HIV-1 Thai subtype B and E, The Lancet, 346, 1372-1995, 1995
115. Xin KQ, Shapshak P, Kawamoto S, Nagano I, McCoy CB, and Okuda K, Highly divergent env sequences of HIV-1 B subtype with two novel V3 loop motifs detected in an AIDS patient in Miami, AIDS Res and Hu Retrov, Sequ Note, 11, 1139-1141, 1995
116. Yap EPH, Lo YMO, Fleming KA, and McGee JO'D, False-positives and contamination in PCR, in PCR Technology Current Innovations, ed. HG Griffin and AM Griffin, CRC Press, Boca Raton, 1994, pp. 249-258
117. Yoshioka M, Bradley WG, Shapshak P, Nagano I, Stewart RV, Xin KQ, Srivastava AK, and Nakamura S, Role of immune activation and cytokine expression in HIV-1-associated neurologic diseases, Adv. in Neuroimm, 5, 335-358, 1995
118. Yoshioka M, Shapshak P, Nakamura S, Nagano I, Nelson SJ, and Kogure K, TNF producing cells in AIDS brain, Neurology, 42 (suppl. 3), 236, 1992
119. Yoshioka M, Shapshak P, Srivastava AK, Nelson SJ, Bradley WG, Berger JR, Rhodes RH, Sun NCJ, Stewart RV, and Nakamura, Role of immune activation, interleukin-6 expression and HIV-1 in the pathology of dorsal root ganglia of patients with AIDS, Neurology, 44, 1120-1130, 1994
120. Yoshioka M, Shapshak P, Sun NCJ, Svenningsson A, Nelson S, Resnick L, Tate L, Ferritin immunoreactivity in microglial nodules in AIDS brain, Acta Neuropathologica, 84, 297-306, 1992
121. Young LS, The polymerase chain reaction: a new tool for the histopathologist, in Molecular Biology in Histopathology, ed J Crocker, J Wiley Publ, New York, 1994, pp. 39-55
122. Zhu T, Wang N, Carr A, Wolinsky S, and Ho DD, Evidence for coinfection by multiple strains of HIV-1 subtype B in an acute seroconverter, J of Virol, 69, 1324-1327, 1995

24

INHALED ISOBUTYL NITRITE PRODUCED LUNG INFLAMMATION WITH INCREASED MACROPHAGE TNF-α AND NITRIC OXIDE PRODUCTION

L. S. F. Soderberg, L. W. Chang, and J. B. Barnett

[1] Departments of Microbiology and Immunology and Pathology
University of Arkansas for Medical Sciences
Little Rock, Arkansas
[2] Department of Microbiology and Immunology
West Virginia University School of Medicine
Morgantown, West Virginia

1. INTRODUCTION

Isobutyl nitrite is representative of a group of nitrite inhalants, commonly called "poppers." When inhaled, these chemicals cause vasodilation and relaxation of smooth muscles. The principal abusers are male homosexuals and adolescents. Abuse of nitrite inhalants has been correlated with seropositivity to human immunodeficiency virus (HIV)[1] and to Kaposi's sarcoma among AIDS patients.[2] It is possible that abuse of these drugs might increase susceptibility to infectious agents.

Abusers expose themselves to very high levels, about 7,000 ± 260 ppm,[3] of the inhalants intermittently over several hours, sometimes daily. To reflect abuser exposures, we have developed a mouse inhalation model in which groups of mice are exposed to a constant 900 ppm isobutyl nitrite in an inhalation chamber for 45 minutes per day. Following 14 days of such exposures, mice had severely depressed immunity, including a 60% reduction in T-dependent antibody induction,[4] a 40% decrease in T cell-mediated cytotoxicity,[5] and a 60% decrease in peritoneal exudate macrophage tumoricidal activity (-60%).[6] This was accompanied by a decrease in nitric oxide (NO) induction and an increase in tumor necrosis factor-α (TNF-α) production. In the present study, we examined the effects of inhalation exposure to isobutyl nitrite on the activity of alveolar macrophages.

2. MATERIALS AND METHODS

2.1. Isobutyl Nitrite Treatment

Female 6-8 week old C57BL/6 mice (Charles River) were exposed to isobutyl nitrite (Aldrich) at 900 ppm in an inhalation chamber for 45 min per day for 14 days. Groups of 5 or 6 mice were assayed for immune activity 1 day after the last exposure to isobutyl nitrite.

2.2. Macrophage Tumoricidal Assay

Alveolar macrophages were harvested by lung lavage. Three consecutive lavages were pooled and the cells were washed and counted. Cells were maintained in 96 well plates at 7 x 10^4 cells/well in RPMI 1640 with 10% fetal calf serum, 50 nM 2-mercaptoethanol, 100 U/ml penicillin, and 100 μg/ml streptomycin. After 1 hr incubation, nonadherent cells were removed by washing. Cells were then incubated for 24 hr in medium containing 100 U/ml interferon-γ (IFN-γ) (Genzyme) and 1 μg/ml lipopolysaccharide (LPS, *E. coli* 055:B5, Sigma Chem. Co.). Target P815 cells were used in a standard 18 hr ^{51}Cr-release assay, as previously described.[6] Alveolar macrophage supernatants were collected after 24 hr and assayed for inducible nitric oxide (NO) production using the Greiss assay.[7] Significance was determined by t-test.

3. RESULTS AND DISCUSSION

The number of alveolar macrophages recoverable from the lungs of mice exposed to isobutyl nitrite was twice that of control mice (Table 1). Hematoxylin and eosin stained lung sections from mice exposed to the inhalant showed a distinct increase in cellularity with thickened alveolar walls. The increase in lung cellularity was unexpected, since we previously found that such treatment decreased the numbers of spleen cells by 23%,[4] of peritoneal exudate macrophages by 27%,[6] and of peripheral blood cells by 21%.[3] However, the increase in lung cellularity was not sufficient to account for the much larger losses of cells from other organs.

Table 1 shows that the tumoricidal activity of alveolar macrophages from treated mice was increased by 60%. Consistent with the cytotoxic activity of alveolar macrophages, inducible NO was increased by 2.5-fold following 14 daily exposures to the inhalant. We previously reported[6] that the inducible nitric oxide synthase inhibitor, nitro^{G}-methyl-arginine, blocked both NO production and tumoricidal in peritoneal exudate cells, suggesting

Table 1. Alveolar macrophage activity following subchronic exposure to isobutyl nitrite

	Control	Nitrite[a]	Change	Significance[b]
Cells x 10^5/lung	0.90 ± 0.05	2.09 ± 0.29	+ 100%	$p<0.005$
Cytotoxicity (%)[c]	12.6 ± 0.4	20.5 ± 0.7	+ 60%	$p<0.005$
NO (nM)[d]	2,717 ± 374	6,733 ± 338	+ 150%	$p<0.0001$
TNF-α (pg/ml)[e]	3,934 ± 532	6,395 ± 121	+ 60%	$p<0.005$

[a]Mice were exposed to 900 ppm isobutyl nitrite for 45 min/day for 14 days.
[b]t-test.
[c]An 18 hr ^{51}Cr-release assay using P815 target cells.
[d]Nitric oxide (NO) was measured by the Greiss assay.
[e]Tumor necrosis factor-α (TNF-α) was measured by an ELISA assay.

that NO was largely responsible for the cytotoxic activity of these cells for P815 target cells. Thus, the increase in inducible NO in alveolar cells was consistent with their increased tumoricidal activity. The heightened activity and increased numbers of alveolar cells suggests that there was an influx of inflammatory cells into the lungs, probably in response to the inhalant.

In addition, alveolar macrophage production of TNF-α was increased by 65% following exposure to the inhalant (Table 1). We previously reported[6] that peritoneal exudate macrophages similarly produced increased levels of TNF-α, following the inhalant exposure. Even low levels of TNF-α have been shown to increase the replication of HIV[8] and also to increase the proliferation of Kaposi's sarcoma cells in culture.[9] Thus, a combination of persistent increases in TNF-α production and immunosuppression[4-6] resulting from chronic inhalant abuse could promote HIV replication and the proliferation of KS cells, while impairing immune resistance.

4. ACKNOWLEDGMENTS

Supported by USPHS grant DA06662.

5. REFERENCES

1. Seage, G.R., III, Mayer, K.H., Horsburgh, C.R., Jr., Holmberg, S.D., Moon, M.W., Lamb, G.A. (1992) The relation between nitrite inhalants, unprotected receptive anal intercourse, and the risk of human immunodeficiency virus infection. *Amer. J. Epidem.* **135,** 1-11.
2. Haverkos, H.W., Pinsky, P.F., Drotman, D.P., Bregman, D.J. (1985) Disease manifestation among homosexual men with acquired immunodeficiency syndrome: A possible role of nitrites in Kaposi's sarcoma. *Sex. Trans. Dis.* **12,** 203-208.
3. Soderberg, L.S.F., J.T. Flick, and J.B. Barnett (1996) Leukopenia and altered hematopoietic activity in mice exposed to the abused inhalant, isobutyl nitrite. *Exp. Hematol.* In press.
4. Soderberg, L.S.F. and J.B. Barnett (1993) Inhaled isobutyl nitrite compromises T-dependent. but not T-independent antibody induction. *Int. J. Immunopharmacol.* **15,**821-827.
5. Soderberg, L.S.F. (1994) T cell functions are impaired by inhaled isobutyl nitrite through a T-independent mechanism. *Toxicol. Lett.* **70,** 319-329.
6. Soderberg, L.S.F. and J.B. Barnett (1995) Inhalation exposure to isobutyl nitrite inhibits macrophage tumoricidal activity and modulates inducible nitric oxide. *J. Leukocyte Biol.* **57,**135-140.
7. Ding, A.H., Nathan, C.F., Struehr, D.J. (1988) Release of reactive nitrogen intermediates and reactive oxygen intermediates from mouse peritoneal macrophages. *J. Immunol.* **141,** 2407-2412.
8. Folks, T.M., Clouse, K.A., Justement, J., Rabson, A., Duh, E., Kehrl, J.H., and Fauci, A.S. (1989) Tumor necrosis factor induces expression of human immunodeficiency virus in a chronically infected T cell clone. *Proc. Nat. Acad. Sci. USA* **86,** 2365-2368.
9. Roth, W.K., Brandstetter, H., Stürzl, M. (1992) Cellular and molecular features of HIV-associated Kaposi's sarcoma. *AIDS.* **6, 895-913.**

25

CYTOKINE ACTION IN THE NERVOUS SYSTEM AT PATHOPHYSIOLOGICAL VERSUS PHARMACOLOGICAL CONCENTRATIONS

Carlos R. Plata-Salamán*

School of Life and Health Sciences
University of Delaware
Newark, Delaware 19716-2590

Cytokines induce a variety of neurological actions.[15] Cytokine action in the nervous system may present different profiles depending on the cytokine concentration or dosage. Pathophysiological and pharmacological analyses of cytokine neuroactivity have been assessed with an integrative approach organized through neurological → behavioral → cellular → molecular → genetical levels. Cytokine-induced anorexia represents an example of this integrative approach.

1. ANOREXIA DURING DISEASE

Anorexia is a neurological manifestation that frequently accompanies acute (inflammatory, infectious) and chronic (neoplastic, necrotic, infectious) pathophysiological processes in human and other species.[13] Anorexia is a nonspecific (occurs in multiple diseases), but significant clinical manifestation. Anorexia also occurs during immunotherapy with cytokines (for viral diseases or cancer) in humans, or during exogenous cytokine administration (acute or chronic) in experimental paradigms.[13] Therefore, cytokine-induced anorexia is an appropriate model to study aspects of the pathophysiological and pharmacological profile associated with cytokine action.

2. ANOREXIA INDUCED BY CYTOKINES

Acute and chronic disease stimulate the synthesis and release of cytokines.[15] Pathophysiological processes and immunotherapy with cytokines are associated with anorexia.[13]

* Phone: 302-831-2647; FAX: 302-831-2647; E. Mail: 04189@brahms.udel.edu.

Therefore, anorexigenic cytokines including interleukin-1 (IL-1),[17] IL-6,[13] IL-8[19] and other chemokines/intercrines,[20] tumor necrosis factor-α (TNF-α),[13] and interferon (IFN)[16] could participate in the anorexia observed during pathophysiological processes and immunotherapy.

3. ANOREXIA INDUCED BY CYTOKINES: NEUROLOGICAL LEVEL

Anorexia is one of the most common clinical manifestations. Pathophysiological levels of cytokines have been reported in the cerebrospinal fluid (CSF) of several species during disease.[1,8,12,29,30] The presence of cytokines in the brain-CSF can result from local synthesis by microglia,[9] astrocytes,[9] intrinsic and blood-derived macrophages,[28] activated T-lymphocytes and polymorphonuclear leukocytes that cross the blood-brain barrier during inflammatory processes,[6] endothelial cells of the cerebrovasculature,[15] and possible neuronal components.[11] The transport of IL-1β[3] and TNF-α[4] from the peripheral circulation to the CNS through the blood-brain barrier has also been proposed. Cytokines may also gain access to the brain by passing through the circumventricular organs that lack blood-brain barrier. The CNS synthesis and release of cytokines in various pathophysiological processes is suggested by their increased levels in the CSF accompanied by lower levels in the peripheral circulation in samples from the same individuals.[5,29,30] Cytokines may also signal the brain via afferent signalling through the peripheral and autonomic nervous systems as has been demonstrated for other peptides.

4. ANOREXIA INDUCED BY CYTOKINES: BEHAVIORAL LEVEL

Pivotal immunomodulatory cytokines (IL-1β, IL-8, TNF-α, IFN) induce anorexia when administered peripherally (intravenous, intraperitoneal, or subcutaneous; microgram range)[10,13] or centrally (into the CSF or hypothalamic parenchyma; picogram-nanogram range).[13] Administration of microbial products (bacterial endotoxin or lipopolysaccharide from gram-negative, and muramyl dipeptide from gram-positive bacteria) that induce anorexigenic cytokine release also results in anorexia.[18] Intracerebroventricular (ICV, into the third ventricle, i.e, close to the critical hypothalamic regions that participate in the regulation of feeding) microinfusion of cytokines induce anorexia at estimated pathophysiological concentrations (picogram-low nanogram range: fentomolar-picomolar range) reported in the CSF.[13,16,17,19] Because the peripheral administration of cytokines consistently requires doses in the microgram range to induce anorexia, the data suggest that low doses of cytokines administered into the brain induce anorexia by direct action in the CNS.

4.1. Mechanisms Involved in Cytokine-Induced Anorexia

Feeding behavior involves a variety of psychological factors, neuronal and humoral mechanisms, and gastrointestinal, metabolic and nutrient factors.[14] During pathophysiological conditions, modifications in one or various components participating in the regulation of feeding will result in anorexia. Cytokine-induced anorexia has been proposed to involve: action in peripheral and CNS sites; modulation of hypothalamic-feeding associated sites; prostaglandin-dependent mechanisms; modifications of neurotransmitter systems (catecholamines, serotonin); and gastrointestinal and endocrine factors.[13,15]

4.2. Pathophysiological Versus Pharmacological Profile of Cytokine-Induced Anorexia

Different alterations in the microstructure of feeding (assessed by computerized behavioral-monitoring systems) are observed when cytokines are administered into the brain at estimated pathophysiological versus pharmacological concentrations.

4.2.1. Interleukin-1. The ICV microinfusion of estimated pathophysiological concentrations—based on mathematical models—of IL-1β (e.g., 1.0 ng has been estimated to yield concentrations within the pathophysiological range in the CSF when administered acutely) decrease feeding in the rat by reducing meal size (MS) and meal duration (MD) dose-dependently;[17] eating rate (MS/MD) decreases and this indicates a greater effect on meal size than on meal duration.[17] Pharmacological concentrations of IL-1β ($\geq$ 4.0 ng ICV, acutely) also decrease meal frequency (MF), prolong postprandial intermeal intervals and induce a generalized behavioral depression.[17] These effects of IL-1β are blocked by the IL-1β receptor antagonist,[17,21] a compound that binds to the cell surface IL-1 receptors and blocks the binding of IL-1β without inducing cellular responses.[2] Therefore, the anorexigenic effect induced by the ICV administration of IL-1β is a receptor-mediated phenomenon. This also indicates specificity of IL-1β action.

4.2.2. Interleukin-8. IL-8, on the other hand, induces a different profile: estimated pathophysiological concentrations (20 ng ICV, acutely) decreases feeding by reducing MS exclusively, while higher concentrations produce less anorexic effect with a consequent inverted bell-shaped dose-response curve.[19] This profile induced by ICV IL-8 and other chemokines/intercrines[20] suggests the production of inhibitory molecules for autoregulatory control, the involvement of negative cooperativity to maintain chemokine/intercrine sensitivity at low concentrations but attenuation of cellular responses to higher concentrations, differential activation of high and low affinity receptors, or the down-regulation process accompanied by a decreased number of membrane-bound chemokine/intercrine receptors. The anorexic effect induced by ICV IL-8 is blocked by anti-IL-8 monoclonal antibodies suggesting specificity of action in the CNS.

4.2.3. Interferon. IFN induces anorexia by reducing MS and MD without affecting MF, and these effects are observed only during the first two hours after administration.[16] The anorexigenic effect by IFN is observed at estimated pathophysiological concentration in the CSF, and this effect plateaus at pharmacological concentrations.[16] Furthermore, species specificity to the type of IFN preparation used is observed in immunological and behavioral experimental models including IFN-induced anorexia.[16] This IFN-associated species specificity is dependent on receptor mechanisms.[16]

Interleukin-1, IL-8 and IFN represent three different cytokine categories whose receptors are coupled to distinct signal transduction systems. The data show that IL-1, IL-8, and IFN are capable of inducing anorexia; however, they induce specific alterations in the microstructure of feeding with different potencies. The specific modifications of feeding parameters (meal size, meal frequency, meal duration, postprandial intermeal intervals) suggest that IL-1, IL-8 and IFN induce anorexia through different modes of action.

4.2.4. Cytokine Interactions. Administration of a particular cytokine induces the secondary release of other cytokines.[15] In fact, concomitant cytokine administration—at estimated pathophysiological concentrations—induces anorexia with additive or synergistic activities (*Am. J. Physiol.*, submitted). Cytokine interactions may participate in disease- and immunotherapy-associated anorexia.[25] This interactive model of cytokine-induced anorexia is consistent with the multicytokine interaction that occurs during activation of the immune system.[15]

4.2.5. Significance of Cytokine-Induced Anorexia and Relationship to Cytokine-Induced Fever. IL-1β is significantly more potent ($p< 0.01$) than IL-8, IFN and other cytokines (IL-6, TNF-α, and the chemokine/intercrine subfamily α and β) to induce anorexia.[13,16,20] Cytokine-induced and microbial products-induced anorexia can be dissociated from their fever-inducing effect. This has been verified in models were cytokine-induced anorexia and cytokine-induced changes in body and CSF-brain temperatures have been studied simultaneously in the same animal.[16,19,25] In addition, sodium salicylate and other antipyretics block fever induced by bacterial endotoxin but does not restore appetite. This is consistent with the clinical observation that patients receiving antipyretic therapy exhibit anorexia. Evidence also show that the threshold of cytokine concentrations required to induce anorexia is lower relative to the threshold needed to induce fever.

Anorexia and pyrogenesis, however, are interactive (and probably essential) contributors to the host recovery from disease. Temporary anorexia during acute disease may be beneficial to an organism since a restriction in the intake of micro- and macro-nutrients will inhibit bacterial growth. Long-term anorexia during chronic disease, however, is deleterious to an organism and may be associated with cachexia, a life threatening condition observed in chronic pathological processes including cancer, human immunodeficiency virus (HIV) infection, and other chronic diseases. Cytokines (including IL-1β, IL-6, IFN, and TNF-α) have been proposed to participate in the development and/or progression of cachexia. On the other hand, fever can suppress the growth of microorganisms and enhance immunological responses.

5. ANOREXIA INDUCED BY CYTOKINES: CELLULAR LEVEL

Cellular approaches indicate that modulation of hypothalamic activity is involved in cytokine-induced anorexia. Cytokine action involves the modulation of specific neurons that are proposed to participate in the control of feeding, i.e., glucose-sensitive neurons in the lateral hypothalamic area (LHA) and hypothalamic ventromedial nucleus (VMN).[14,15] This model predicts that inhibition of LHA and activation of VMN will result in anorexia. Direct application of IL-1β or TNF-α specifically and reversibly suppresses the neuronal activity of the glucose-sensitive neurons in the LHA,[13,15] while IL-1β- or IFN-α excites the glucose-sensitive neurons in the VMN.[7] IL-1β, TNF-α and IFN-α have little effect on the glucose-insensitive neurons in the LHA and VMN indicating specificity of action.[7,13,15] These findings support a direct and specific effect of cytokines on a subpopulation of LHA and VMN neurons. In fact, the feeding patterns induced by IL-1β are consistent with an action on LHA and VMN. An action in the LHA (a site associated with the integrative regulation of meal initiation) may be expressed by the suppression of meal frequency and prolongation of postprandial intermeal intervals, while an action in the VMN (a site associated with the integrative regulation of meal termination) may be expressed by the suppression of meal size. Furthermore, the long latency and duration of action of IL-1β on LHA and VMN neurons may be associated with the activation of intracellular mediators.[23]

6. ANOREXIA INDUCED BY CYTOKINES: MOLECULAR LEVEL

At the molecular level, IL-1β[23] and IL-2[22] inhibit the neuronal inward calcium channel currents at pathophysiological concentrations in the CSF. The IL-1β-induced inhibition of calcium channel currents reaches a plateau between 11 and 31.2 pg IL-1β/10 μl (i.e., within the pathophysiological range) in VMN and hippocampal[23] neurons. (Clinical studies have shown, for example, that 55% of patients with pyogenic meningitis present >5 pg IL-1β/10 μl in the CSF and 40% of patients >10 pg IL-1β/10 μl CSF.)[8] Pharmacological concentrations (up to 2000 pg IL-1β/10 μl) do not induce a further depression of the calcium channel current.[23] However, at concentrations ≥7.9 pg IL-1β/10 μl, there is essentially no reversibility of the IL-1β-induced depression of the calcium channel current.[23]

The number of IL-1 receptors in any cell type is low and maximal biological activity by IL-1 appears to involve only 1-10% of the receptors. The maximal depressive action of IL-1β on VMN or hippocampal neuronal calcium channel currents that plateaus between 11 and 31.2 pg IL-1β/10 μl, with no further depression observed at pharmacological concentrations, may be related to the number of receptors activated, down-regulation process with decreased number of membrane bound receptors without change in their affinity, or levels of intracellular mediators. These data suggest that various experimental models are associated with distinct pathophysiological/pharmacological profiles of IL-1β action in the CNS.

The modulation of the inward calcium channel currents by IL-1β is mediated by G-proteins and by activation of protein kinase C and is blocked by the IL-1 receptor antagonist.[23] Modulation of calcium permeability by IL-1β may play a role in regulating neuronal excitability and neurotransmitter release-associated mechanisms. This is supported by the characteristics of the IL-1β-induced long-lasting LHA and VMN neuronal activity modulation that may be associated with the long-term anorexia induced by the cytokine. A decrease in calcium influx in LHA glucose-sensitive neurons may result in inhibition, while a decrease in calcium influx in VMN glucose-sensitive neurons may inhibit the defined calcium-dependent potassium conductance in these neurons leading to maintenance of intracellular potassium, then depolarization and increase in neuronal activity.

IL-2 also depresses a fraction of the neuronal calcium channel current.[22] This IL-2-induced depression is dose-dependent, reversible and blocked by the application of anti-rhIL-2 monoclonal antibodies.[22] Thus, the depression of voltage-gated calcium channel currents by IL-1β and IL-2 in neurons present different characteristics including the concentration-effect curve and the reversibility of the response.[22,23] Consequently, different cytokines may have selective actions on the neuronal ionic channel currents.

7. ANOREXIA INDUCED BY CYTOKINES: GENETICAL LEVEL

The VMN is an important feeding regulatory site.[14] VMN neurons exhibit an array of G-protein α-subunit subclasses during in vitro and in vivo studies.[27] Chronic ICV microinfusion of IL-1β (at estimated pathophysiological concentrations adjusted for chronic administration) induces a dose-dependent long-term anorexia (without decreasing drinking), and modifies the profile of G-protein α-subunit subclasses in the VMN depending on the concentrations used.[26] Estimated pathophysiological concentrations (lower range, chronically administered ICV) of IL-1β increase the Gαi1+2 protein content; however, estimated pathophysiological concentrations (higher range) may also decrease both, the Gαi1+2 and GαO common protein contents.[26] This suggests that even within the estimated pathophysiological range (low versus high), a different cytokine action profile may be obtained. IL-1 receptor antagonist blocks the IL-1β-induced long-term anorexia and the effects of IL-1β on the G-protein α-subunit VMN profile. These data indicate specificity of action and receptor mediated phenomena.

8. CONCLUSIONS

Cytokine action in the CNS present different profiles depending on the cytokine used, its concentration or dosage, duration and timing of administration, and experimental model. The distinct pathophysiological and pharmacological profiles induced by IL-1 in behavioral, cellular, and molecular approaches is an example of diverse cytokine action in the CNS depending on the concentration or dosage. In fact, profiles obtained within the pathophysiological range also may be different when comparing the low versus high range. Therefore, caution is essential in interpreting the significance (physiological, pathophysiological, pharmacological, toxicological) of results obtained with cytokines. This applies not only to anorexia and other neurological manifestations induced by cytokines, but also to other models; for example, evidence suggest that low concentrations of IL-1β may be neuroprotective in vitro (by depressing inward calcium channel currents)[23] and in vivo (by enhancing CNS blood flow),[24] while high concentrations may be associated with neurodegeneration.[23]

REFERENCES

1. Akalin, H., A. C. Akdis, R. Mistik, S. Helvaci and K. Kilicturgay. Cerebrospinal fluid interleukin-1β/interleukin-1 receptor antagonist balance and tumor necrosis factor-α concentrations in tuberculous, viral and acute bacterial meningitis. *Scand. J. Infect. Dis.* 26: 667-674, 1994.
2. Arend, W.P. Interleukin 1 receptor antagonist. A new member of the interleukin 1 family. *J. Clin. Invest.* 88:1445-1451, 1991.
3. Banks, W.A., L. Ortiz, S.R. Plotkin and A.J. Kastin. Human interleukin (IL) 1α, murine IL-1α and murine IL-1β are transported from blood to brain in the mouse by a shared saturable mechanism. *J. Pharmacol. Exp. Ther.* 259:988-996, 1991.
4. Gutierrez, E.G., W.A. Banks and A.J. Kastin. Murine tumor necrosis factor alpha is transported from blood to brain in the mouse. *J. Neuroimmunol.* 47:169-176, 1993.
5. Halstensen, A., M. Ceska, P. Brandtzaeg, H. Redl, A. Naess and A. Waage. Interleukin-8 in serum and cerebrospinal fluid from patients with meningococcal disease. *J. Infect. Dis.* 167:471-475, 1993.
6. Hickey, W. F., B. L. Hsu and H. Kimura. T-lymphocyte entry into the central nervous system. *J. Neurosci. Res.* 28:254-260, 1991.
7. Kuriyama, K., T. Hori, T. Mori and T. Nakashima. Actions of interferon-α and interleukin-1β on the glucose-responsive neurons in the ventromedial hypothalamus. *Brain Res. Bull.* 24:803-810, 1990.
8. López-Cortés, L. F., M. Cruz-Ruiz, J. Gómez-Mateos, D. Jiménez-Hernández, J. Palomino and E. Jiménez. Measurement of levels of tumor necrosis factor-α and interleukin-1β in the CSF of patients with meningitis of different etiologies: Utility in the differential diagnosis. *Clin. Infect. Dis.* 16:534-539, 1993.
9. Merrill, J.E., Y. Koyanagi, J. Zack, L. Thomas, F. Martin and I. S. Y. Chen. Induction of interleukin-1 and tumor necrosis factor alpha in brain cultures by human immunodeficiency virus type 1. *J. Virol.* 66:2217-2225, 1992.
10. Moldawer, L.L., C. Andersson, J. Gelin and K.G. Lundholm. Regulation of food intake and hepatic protein synthesis by recombinant-derived cytokines. *Am. J. Physiol.* 254:G450-G456, 1988.
11. Molenaar, G. J., F. Berkenbosch, A.-M. van Dam and C. M. J. E. Lugard. Distribution of interleukin 1β immunoreactivity within the porcine hypothalamus. *Brain Res.* 608:169-174, 1993.
12. Ohga, S., T. Aoki, K. Okada, H. Akeda, K. Fujioka, A. Ohshima, T. Mori, I. Minamishima and K. Ueda. Cerebrospinal fluid concentrations of interleukin-1β, tumour necrosis factor-α, and interferon gamma in bacterial meningitis. *Arch. Dis. Childhood* 70:123-125, 1994.
13. Plata-Salamán, C.R. Immunomodulators and feeding regulation: A humoral link between the immune and nervous systems. *Brain, Behav. Immunity* 3:193-213, 1989.
14. Plata-Salamán, C.R. Regulation of hunger and satiety in man. *Digest. Dis.* 9:253-268, 1991.
15. Plata-Salamán, C.R. Immunoregulators in the nervous system. *Neurosci. Biobehav. Rev.* 15:185-215, 1991.
16. Plata-Salamán, C.R. Interferons and central regulation of feeding. *Am. J. Physiol.* 263:R1222-R1227, 1992.
17. Plata-Salamán, C.R. Meal patterns in response to the intracerebroventricular administration of interleukin-1β in rats. *Physiol. Behav.* 55:727-733, 1994.

18. Plata-Salamán, C.R., and J.P. Borkoski. Centrally administered bacterial lipopolysaccharide depresses feeding in rats. *Pharmacol. Biochem. Behav.* 46:787-791, 1993.
19. Plata-Salamán, C.R., and J.P. Borkoski. Interleukin-8 modulates feeding by direct action in the central nervous system. *Am. J. Physiol.* 265:R877-R882, 1993.
20. Plata-Salamán, C.R., and J.P. Borkoski. Chemokines/intercrines and central regulation of feeding. *Am. J. Physiol.* 266:R1711-R1715, 1994.
21. Plata-Salamán, C.R., and J.M.H. ffrench-Mullen. Intracerebroventricular administration of a specific IL-1 receptor antagonist blocks food and water intake suppression induced by interleukin-1β. *Physiol. Behav.* 51:1277-1279, 1992.
22. Plata-Salamán, C.R., and J.M.H. ffrench-Mullen. Interleukin-2 modulates calcium currents in dissociated hippocampal CA1 neurons. *NeuroReport* 4:579-581, 1993.
23. Plata-Salamán, C.R., and J.M.H. ffrench-Mullen. Interleukin-1β inhibits calcium channel currents in isolated hippocampal CA1 neurons through protein kinase C. *Eur. J. Pharmacol.* 266:1-10, 1994.
24. Plata-Salamán, C.R., G. Kelly, C. Agresta, K. Taylor and S.K. Salzman. Interleukin-1β enhances spinal cord blood flow after intrathecal administration in the normal rat. *Am. J. Physiol.* 269 (38), in press, 1995.
25. Plata-Salamán, C.R., G. Sonti and J.P. Borkoski. Modulation of feeding by β2-microglobulin, a marker of immune activation. *Am. J. Physiol.* 268:R1513-R1519, 1995.
26. Plata-Salamán, C.R., G. Sonti, C.D. Wilson and J.M.H ffrench-Mullen. Chronic intracerebroventricular (ICV) microinfusion of cytokines: i) differential effects on feeding; ii) profile of Gα-protein subunit subclasses in the ventromedial hypothalamic nucleus (VMN). *Soc. Neurosci. Abst.* U.S.A. 21:966, 1995.
27. Plata-Salamán, C.R., C.D. Wilson, G. Sonti, J.P. Borkoski and J.M.H. ffrench-Mullen. Antisense oligodeoxynucleotides to G-protein α-subunit subclasses identify a transductional requirement for the modulation of normal feeding dependent on $G\alpha_{OA}$ subunit. *Mol. Brain Res.* 33:72-78, 1995.
28. Thomas, W. E. Brain macrophages: Evaluation of microglia and their functions. *Brain Res. Rev.* 17:61-74, 1992.
29. Van Deuren, M., J. van der Ven-Jongekrijg, A.K.M. Bartelink, R. van Dalen, R.W. Sauerwein and J. W. M. van der Meer. Correlation between proinflammatory cytokines and antiinflammatory mediators and the severity of disease in meningococcal infections. *J. Infect. Dis.* 172:433-439, 1995.
30. Waage, A., A. Halstensen, T. Espevik and P. Brandtzaeg. Compartmentalization of TNF and IL-6 in meningitis and septic shock. *Mediat. Inflamm.* 2:23-25, 1993.

BEHAVIORAL AND NEUROPHYSIOLOGICAL EFFECTS OF CNS EXPRESSION OF CYTOKINES IN TRANSGENIC MICE

Lisa H. Gold,[1] Charles J. Heyser,[1] Amanda J. Roberts,[1] Steven J. Henriksen,[1] Scott C. Steffensen,[1] George R. Siggins,[1] Frederick P. Bellinger,[1] Chi-Shiun Chiang,[1] Henry C. Powell,[2] Eliezer Masliah,[2] and Iain L. Campbell[1]

[1] Department of Neuropharmacology
The Scripps Research Institute
La Jolla, California 92037
[2] Department of Pathology
The University of California San Diego
La Jolla, California 92093

1. CYTOKINES AND THE CENTRAL NERVOUS SYSTEM

Numerous studies have documented the altered expression of various cytokines or their genes in the brain in a variety of central nervous system (CNS) pathologic states such as multiple sclerosis (MS), acquired immunodeficiency syndrome (AIDS) encephalopathy, stroke, Alzheimer's disease, scrapie (spongiform encephalopathy), other infectious diseases and trauma. Whether the presence of cytokines in these neuropathologic states represents a primary or secondary event and the extent to which these factors may contribute to the development and progression of clinicopathologic alterations in these disorders remains largely unknown. We have focused on these issues by utilizing a transgenic approach to direct the constitutive expression of a variety of cytokines to astrocytes in the intact CNS of mice.[1-4] Transgenic expression of cytokines in the CNS of mice allows not only the investigation of complex cellular responses at a localized level in the intact brain, but also more closely recapitulates the expression of these mediators as found in pathogenetic states.

2. TRANSGENIC MODELS OF CYTOKINE EXPRESSION

To develop transgenic mice, expression of the murine cytokines IL-6 or IL-3 was targeted to astrocytes using glial fibrillary acidic protein (GFAP) fusion gene constructs (Fig. 1). The coding region of each cytokine cDNA was inserted in the first exon of a murine GFAP genomic DNA construct, downstream from the GFAP promoter and other 5' regulatory

AIDS, Drugs of Abuse, and the Neuroimmune Axis, Edited by Friedman *et al.*
Plenum Press, New York, 1996

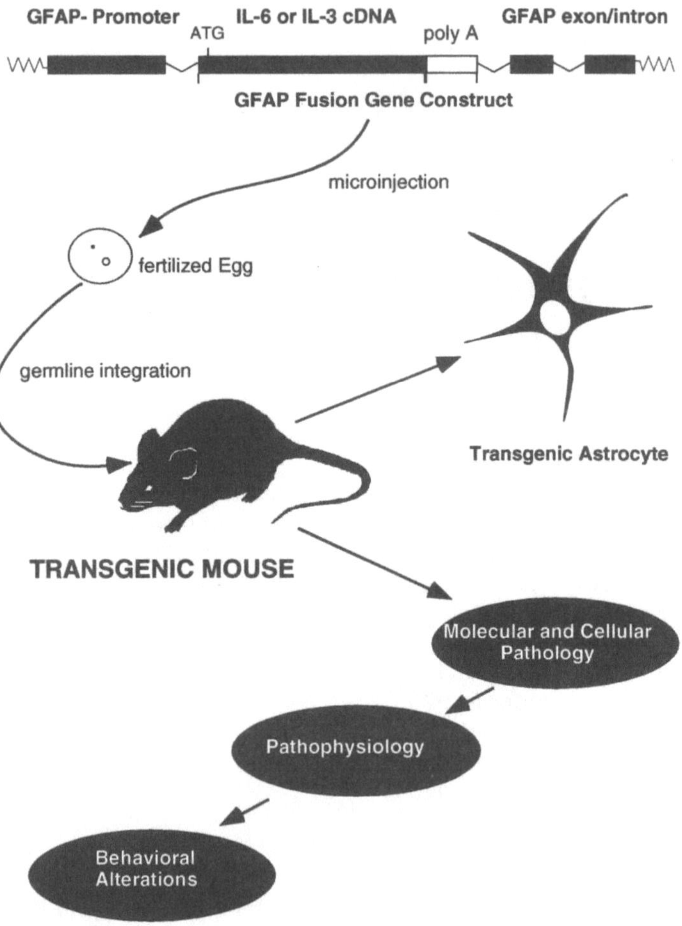

Figure 1. General scheme for the expression of cytokines in the CNS and subsequent evaluation of transgenic mice. The cDNA's encoding murine IL-6 or IL-3 were inserted downstream of the GFAP- promotor and other 5' regulatory elements in the first exon of a modified murine GFAP genomic DNA [1]. These DNA constructs (transgenes) were then used to generate mutant mice with stable integration of the transgene. Mice found to express the transgene at the RNA and protein levels were evaluated further at multiple levels for structural and functional alterations.

regions. The hybrid (transgene) DNA was subsequently microinjected into the germline of mice to generate transgenic offspring. Expression of the transgene derived cytokines in astrocytes was confirmed at both the RNA and protein levels.

2.1. GFAP-IL6 Transgenic Mice

2.1.1. Molecular and Cellular Pathology. Interleukin-6 (IL6) is a pro-inflammatory cytokine and a primary mediator of the acute-phase response. Transgenic mice with low levels of IL-6 expression developed progressive neuropathy with end stage motor impairment, tremor and seizure, progressive neuronal injury and degeneration [1-3]. Hippocampal dendritic vacuolization, reduced branching of dendritic spines in CA1 neurons, and loss of parvalbumin reactive interneurons, and cerebellar atrophy and loss of molecular and granular layer neurons were prominent. Ultrastructural studies revealed demyelination as well as oligodendrocyte injury, spongiosis and axonal dystrophy prevalent throughout the cerebellum. In association with these degenerative changes, GFAP-IL6 mice had pronounced diffuse gliosis with activation of astrocytes and microglia. Besides glial cell hypertrophy, both GFAP (astrocyte) and Mac-1 (microglia) mRNA and protein levels were significantly increased. In spite of its proimmunoinflammatory actions, expression of IL-6 in the CNS of the GFAP-IL6 mice was not associated with prominent infiltration of the brain with inflammatory cells, although, discrete perivascular accumulation of mononuclear cells was seen in vessels in the cerebellar sulci and brainstem. Additional changes to the cerebrovascular endothelium included persistent angiogenesis, increased expression of von Willebrand factor and disruption of the blood-brain barrier. Consistent with its actions in the periphery, expression of IL-6 in the CNS of the GFAP-IL6 mice resulted in activation of the acute-phase response genes α1-antichymotrypsin and complement C3. Besides the transgene derived IL-6, expression of other cytokine genes including IL-1α, IL-1β and TNF-α genes was also increased in the brain. Thus, transgenic expression of IL-6 in the CNS of mice provokes a largely localized inflammatory response with features that closely resemble those found in human chronic neuroinflammatory disorders e.g. AIDS dementia.

2.1.2. Functional Analysis in GFAP-IL6 Transgenic Mice

2.1.2.1. Neurobehavioral Alterations. The relationship between the neurological disease exhibited by GFAP-IL6 transgenic mice and functional neurobehavioral outcomes is under analysis. Transgenic mice were tested for their ability to learn to avoid the onset of a mild footshock in a Y-maze nonconditional spatial discrimination task[5]. The discriminated avoidance task was chosen as a representative short-term memory task involving trial independent memory processes (reference memory) and has previously been shown to be sensitive to learning impairments produced by persistent viral infection [6]. Mice were tested for 5 trials per day for 6 days and the number of correct avoidance responses, as well as the number of errors made during training, was taken as a measure of acquisition. Mice heterozygous or homozygous for IL6 transgene expression and normal age- sex-matched littermates were tested at 3, 6 and 12 months of age. GFAP-IL6 transgenic animals showed a significant age- and transgene dose-related decline in their ability to perform this task. Homozygous mice showed a significant impairment at the earliest age tested (3 mo.) and further declined with age. Heterozygous animals which were indistinguishable from controls at 3 months of age regressed to similar levels of impairment as their homozygous littermates by 12 months of age. No correlation was observed between the impaired learning ability of the transgenic groups and motor function, measured as escape (correct responses that occur after the onset of footshock) latencies. These data suggest that progressive cognitive decline follows closely the course of molecular and cellular neuropathology observed in GFAP-IL6 mice.

2.1.2.2. Neurophysiological Alterations. GFAP-IL6 transgenic mice exhibit hippocampal neuropathology and pathophysiology which may mediate the observed learning deficits. GFAP-IL6 homozygous mice exhibit anomalous paroxysmal discharges and suppressed theta rhythm compared to controls [7]. Analysis of hippocampal field responses revealed site-specific increases in recurrent inhibition in the dentate gyrus, and an absence of the cholinergic component of septohippocampal conditioning of dentate-evoked activity. These results suggest a functional pathophysiology of hippocampal cholinoceptive target neurons in GFAP-IL6 transgenic mice.

In contrast to the *in vivo* studies, *in vitro* studies did not reveal significant differences in paired-pulse potentiation and inhibition in the dentate gyrus of hippocampal slices from

GFAP-IL6 homozygous mice compared with nontransgenic controls [8]. However, long-term potentiation in the dentate was significantly reduced in slices from GFAP-IL6 transgenic mice when compared with wild-type control mice. Such disruption of long-term potentiation could contribute to the altered cognitive function observed in the transgenic mice.

2.2. GFAP-IL3 Transgenic Mice

2.2.1. Molecular and Cellular Pathology. Transgenic mice expressing the macrophage/microglia activation factor IL-3 develop a motor disorder (gait abnormality, tremor, ataxia then quadriplegia) in adulthood which progresses to severe incapacitation and death[3,4]. Neurohistologic and electron microscopic analysis in symptomatic transgenic mice revealed multi-focal hypercellular, plaque-like, white matter lesions in cerebellum and brainstem. Lesions showed extensive primary demyelination and remyelination in association with the accumulation of large numbers of macrophage/microglia , many of which contained numerous lipid rich vacuoles and/or crystalline 'pole-shaped' inclusions. In addition to recruitment from the periphery and possibly other brain areas, significant proliferation of the macrophage/microglia cells in white matter was also observed. Lesion-associated macrophage/microglia cells were shown to be activated with markedly increased expression of the complement C3 receptor and MHC class II (Ia) molecules. Mast cells were also identified in the white matter lesions while lymphocytes were rarely, if at all present. Thus, transgenic mice with low levels of cerebral IL-3 expression develop, in later life, a progressive motor disorder as a result of a vigorous T-cell independent macrophage/microglia -mediated demyelination process. Many of the pathologic manifestations of this disorder resemble those observed in acute MS, indicating the GFAP-IL3 transgenic mouse represents a significant new model to study the role of macrophage/microglia in the pathogenesis of inflammatory demyelinating disease.

2.2.2. Functional Analysis in Gfap-Il3 Transgenic Mice. Motor performance was tested using a rotorod apparatus that has been used successfully to characterize drug-induced changes in motor coordination as well as developmental behavioral abnormalities [9,10]. Rotorod balancing requires a variety of proprioceptive, vestibular, and fine-tuned motor abilities.

GFAP-IL3 transgenic mice and wild-type controls were tested on the rod rotating at a fixed speed of 5 revolutions per minute (rpm). Performance for mice at 4 and 6 months of age and normals is shown in Figure 2. The 4 month old transgenics performed as well as nontransgenic mice (Fig. 2A), however, a marked deficit in rotorod performance was observed in the 6 month old GFAP-IL3 transgenic mice for all 3 trials (Fig. 2B).

In order to better characterize the onset of the rotorod deficit, an additional study was performed in naive mice starting at 5 months of age. In this case, mice were placed on a stationary rod which began to rotate at an acceleration of 20 rpm. The amount of time each mouse remained on the rod was recorded and rpm calculated. Overt signs of motor disease, such as head leaning and tremor, and body weights were recorded prior to each rotorod test. Transgenic mice showed impaired rotorod performance relative to controls starting at approximately 5.25 months of age (Fig. 2C). This difference was significant even when only approximately 20% of the transgenic mice showed any overt motor deficits and before significant differences in body weights had developed (Fig. 2D). These results suggest that rotorod performance is a sensitive measure of early motor disease in GFAP-IL3 transgenic mice. The ability to detect the onset of mild motor deficits prior to the emergence of grossly observable symptomatology permits the use of this animal model for the study of therapeutic interventions.

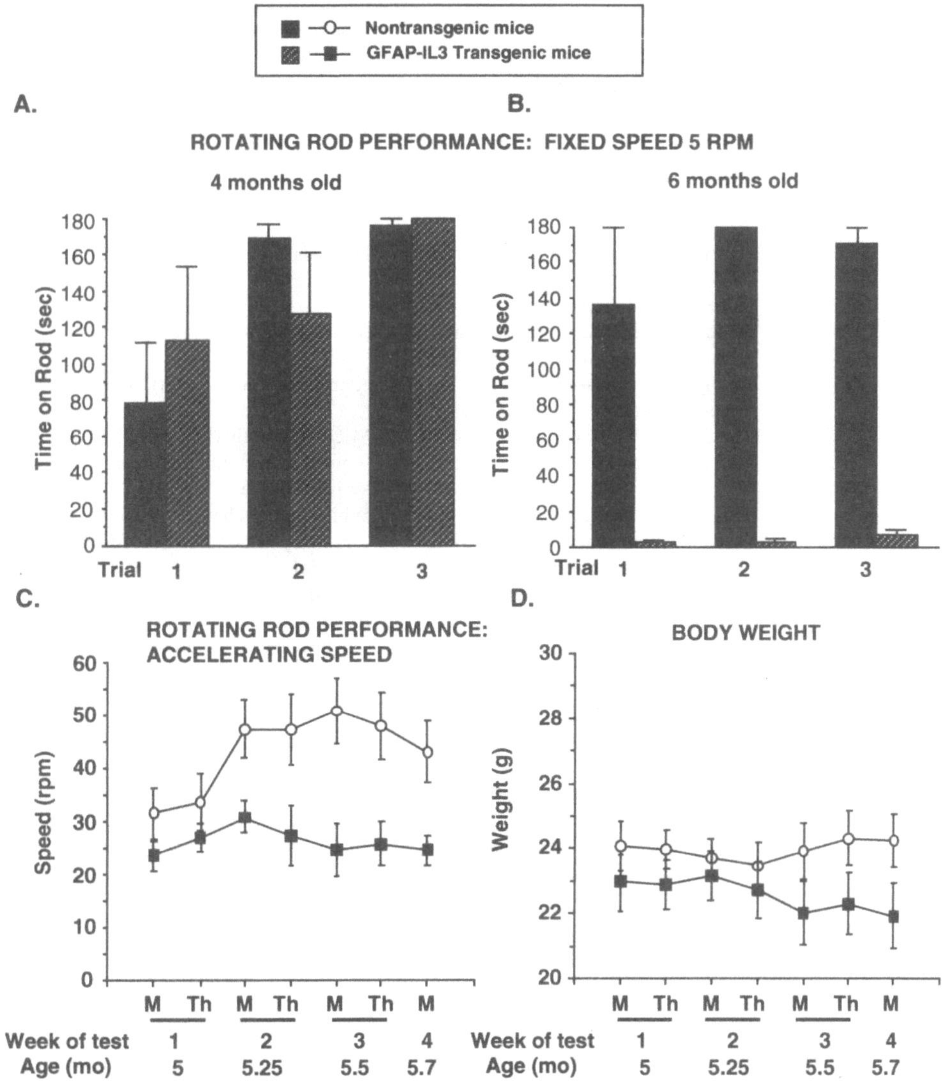

Figure 2. Rotorod deficit and body weight changes in GFAP-IL3 transgenic mice. A. Asymptomatic GFAP-IL3 mice at 4 months of age (N=5) perform equally well on a rotating rod (5 rpm) as normal controls of the same age (N=6). Values represent mean ± SEM time spent on rotating rod for 3 trials with a maximum possible duration of 180 sec/trial. B. GFAP-IL3 mice at 6 months of age exhibit a phenotype of neurologic disease (N=3) and demonstrate a significantly impaired ability to remain on the rotating rod compared with normal controls (N=4). C. Impaired performance on a rotating rod (20 rpm accelerating speed) appears between 5 and 5.25 months of age in GFAP-IL3 transgenic mice (N=6) compared with littermate controls (N=5). Test were conducted 2 times per week. Data were collapsed across 3 trials. Values represent the mean ± SEM speed at which the mice could no longer remain on the rod. D. Body weight differences (mean ± SEM) in the GFAP-IL3 transgenic mice compared with littermate controls are apparent by 5.5 months of age.

Table 1. Comparison of neuropathologic features in GFAP-IL6 and GFAP-IL3 transgenic mice

CNS alterations	GFAP-IL6 transgenic mice	GFAP-IL3 transgenic mice
Functional	Cognitive decline	(behavioral analysis in progress)
	Mild motor impairment	Major motor impairment
	Site-specific hippocampal pathophysiology	No hippocampal pathophysiology
Structural	Distribution of changes: diffuse-grey and white matter cerebellum>brain stem>basal ganglia >other brain regions	Distribution of changes: focal-white matter cerebellum=brain stem>other brain regions
	Neuronal loss and injury: early onset, diverse cerebellar neurons and hippocampal interneurons	Neuronal loss: late onset (analysis in progress)
	Vacuolar degeneration of neuronal dendrites and loss of dendritic spines	(analysis in progress)
	Astrogliosis (early-onset), non-proliferative	Astrogliosis (late-onset), proliferative
	Microglial activation including nodules, diffuse, non-proliferative	Microglial activation including nodules multi-nucleated giant cells, diffuse proliferative
	White-matter changes diffuse lesions secondary>primary demyelination axonal degeneration	White-matter changes focal lesions primary>secondary demyelination axonal preservation
	BBB disruption, early onset, diffuse	BBB disruption, late onset, localized
	Inflammatory infiltrates, mixed mononuclear cell, perivascular	Inflammatory infiltrates, predominantly, macrophage few mast cells, perivascular and focal white matter
	Angiogenesis	(analysis in progress)
Molecular	Upregulated cytokine gene expression (IL-1 and TNF-a)	Upregulated cytokine gene expression (IL-1 and TNF-a)
	Increased macrophage/microglial complement C3 expression	Increased macrophage/microglial MHC class II and complement C3 receptor
	Acute-phase protein synthesis	Acute-phase protein synthesis
	Complement C3 synthesis and deposition	(analysis in progress)

3. SUMMARY

These transgenic models (GFAP-IL6, GFAP-IL3): (1) indicate that expression of cytokines per se in the intact CNS can induce chronic progressive and cytokine-specific neural cell injury leading to unique functional deficits and, (2) recapitulate many of the structural and functional changes seen in human neurodegenerative diseases and inflammatory demyelinating diseases. Transgenic mice with cerebral expression of cytokines represent a valuable tool for advancing our understanding of the CNS pathobiology of cytokines and offer a unique resource for the development and testing of therapies aimed at abrogating the harmful actions of these important mediators.

4. ACKNOWLEDGMENTS

This work was supported by U.S. P.H.S. grants MH47680, MH50426, AG5131 and AG10689.

5. REFERENCES

1. Campbell, I.L., Abraham, C.R., Masliah, E., Kemper. P., Inglis, J.D., Oldstone, M.B.A. and Mucke, L. Neurologic disease induced in transgenic mice by cerebral overexpression of interleukin 6. *Proc. Natl. Acad. Sci. USA.* 90:10061-10065, 1993.
2. Chiang, C-S., Stalder, A.S., Samimi, A. and Campbell, I.L.. Reactive gliosis as a consequence of IL-6 expression in the brain. Studies in transgenic mice. *Dev. Neurosci.*, 16:212-221, 1994.
3. Campbell, I. L. Neuropathogenic actions of cytokines assessed in transgenic mice. *Int. J. Dev. Neurosci.*, 13:275-284, 1995.
4. Chiang, C-S., Powell, H.C., Gold, L., Samimi, A., and Campbell, I.L. Macrophage/microglial-mediated primary demyelination and motor disease induced by the CNS production of interleukin-3 in transgenic mice. *J. Clin. Invest.* in press, 1996.
5. Gold, L.H., Heyser, C.J. and Campbell, I.L. Progressive cognitive impairment in discriminated avoidance performance in GFAP-IL6 transgenic mice. *Neurosci. Abstr.* 21: 2110. 1995.
6. Gold, L.H., Brot, M.D., Polis, I., Schroeder, R.S., Tishon, A., de la Torre, J-C., Oldstone, M.B.A. and Koob, G.F. Behavioral effects of persistent lymphocytic choriomeningitis virus infection in mice. *Behav. Neural Biol.*, 62:100-109, 1994.
7. Steffensen, S.C., Campbell, I.L. and Henriksen, S.J. Site-specific hippocampal pathophysiology due to cerebral overexpression of interleukin-6 in transgenic mice. *Brain Res.*, 652:149-153, 1994.
8. Bellinger, F.P., Madamba, S.G., Campbell, I.L. and Siggins, G.R. Reduced long-term potentiation in the dentate gyrus of transgenic mice with cerebral overexpression of interleukin-6. *Neurosci. Lett.*, 198:95-98, 1995.
9. Jones, B.J. and Roberts, D.J. The quantitative measurement of motor inco-ordination in naive mice using an accelerating rota-rod. *J Pharm Pharmac* 20: 302-304, 1968.
10. Laffan, E.W., Lisciotto, C.A., Gapp, D.A. and Weldon, D.A. Development of rotorod performance in normal and congenitally hypothyroid mutant mice. *Beh Neural Biol* 52: 411-416, 1989.

IL1 BETA IMPAIRS RELATIONAL BUT NOT PROCEDURAL RODENT LEARNING IN A WATER MAZE TASK

Michael Gibertini*

Midwest Research Institute
425 Volker Blvd.
Kansas City, Missouri 64110

SICKNESS BEHAVIOR

The behavioral signs of infectious illness have been well-documented. They typically include anorexia, somnolence, decreased locomotor activity, decreased social and novel stimulus exploration, and decreased sexual behavior (Hart, 1988; Bluthe, Dantzer, and Kelley, 1991; 1992). It is thought that sickness behavior represents an organized set of responses that conserves metabolic energy, making it available for the febrile response (Hart, 1988; Dantzer, Bluthe, Kent, & Kelley, 1992). Proinflammatory cytokines secreted by activated macrophages and other immunocompetent cells appear to mediate sickness (Bluthe, Dantzer,& Kelley, 1991; Crestani, Seguy, & Dantzer, 1991; Cunningham & DeSouza, 1993; Spadaro & Dunn, 1990; Kent, Bluthe, Dantzer, Hardwick, Kelley, Rothwell, & Vannice, 1992; Masotto, Caspani, Grazia deSimone, Mengozzi, Scatturni, Sironi, Carenzi, & Ghezzi, 1992). Among these cytokines, interleukin-1-beta (IL1β) represents a major ascending communication link between the peripheral immune system and the central nervous system (e.g., Hall, O'Grady, & Menzies, 1992; Komaki, Arimura, and Koves, 1992).

In addition to the overt behavioral signs of sickness, an experiential component is likely including lassitude, malaise, fatigue, lethargy, depressed mood, and cognitive confusion or mental slowing. These experiential components are difficult to study systematically but evidence from clinical studies suggests cytokine involvement. For example, reports on the toxicities of exogenous cytokines used in cancer treatment highlight neurological complications including headache, lethargy, recent memory loss, expressive aphasia, diplopia, and transient amnesia (Gutierrez, Banks & Kastin, 1993; Morganti-Kossman, Kossman & Wahl, 1992; Oitzl, van Oers, Schobitz, & de Kloet, 1993; Fent & Zbinden, 1987). Less severe cognitive changes have also been reported to accompany infections such as rhinovirus (Dantzer, et al., 1992; Smith, Tyrrell, Coyle, & Higgins, 1988). Smith, et al. (1988)

*Phone: (816) 753-7600 ext 1516; Fax: (816) 753-7380.

AIDS, Drugs of Abuse, and the Neuroimmune Axis, Edited by Friedman *et al.*
Plenum Press, New York, 1996

suggest that interferon-alpha (IFNα) infusions may influence reaction time in humans. Cytokine-induced cognitive dysfunction, therefore, may be a febrile adjunct distinct from more overt behavioral changes.

Cytokines have complex effects in the CNS that are often difficult to separate experimentally. Changes in operant responding for food rewards after IL1 (Bluthe et al 1989) suggests that IL1 may influence learning. However, IL1 also affects eating, locomotion, and novel stimulus exploration, all of which may influence the cytokine/learning assessment. In the Morris water maze (MWM) paradigm (Morris, 1981; discussed in detail below), some parametric manipulations and measurements of behavioral tendencies can be used to dissociate the cognitive from other components of behavior (Brandeis, Brandys, and Yehud, 1989). However, the maze demands considerable effort, energy, and locomotor ability, all of which are diminished by cytokine administration. In addition, the stress of swimming in cold water with no obvious escape must certainly interact with the inherently stressful effects (Dunn, 1989) of cytokines themselves. Recently, Aubert et al. (1995), introduced a new paradigm for the study of cytokine influence on cognition; the so-called autoshaping paradigm (Messing et al., 1986; Sparber et al., 1991). This experimental procedure for rats requires little locomotion or exploration and the actual learning (autoshaping) is thought to be independent of the food reinforcement schedule. Aubert et al. (1995) used this method to demonstrate that pyrogens (including IL1) disrupt the acquisition of the autoshaped response. There is evidence that this learning paradigm is dependent on hippocampal activity and the authors interpret their findings as evidence that pyrogens affect hippocampal functioning.

There is much to learn about the effect of cytokines on information processing in laboratory animals. The first report of the MWM used in a study of cytokines and spatial learning (Oitzl, et al., 1993) was suggestive of an effect, despite the problems that sick animals may have with the water maze. Subsequently, a more comprehensive study (Gibertini, Friedman, Newton, and Klein, 1995) of learning in mice infected with *Legionella pneumophila* (Lp) indicated that sick animals have difficulty acquiring complex spatial memories and that this impairment may be mediated by peripheral IL1β. These data suggest CNS systems may be selectively responsive to immune system (IS) activation involving peripheral IL1β.

BRAIN SYSTEMS AND LEARNING

A great deal is known about the neurochemical and neuroanatomical substrates assessed by experimental paradigms of animal cognition. For purposes of this chapter, two major types of learning and memory will be described: relational and procedural. These types of memory are important because brain systems involved appear to be highly conserved across species (including humans) and because they are to a large extent both conceptually and neurobiologically nonoverlapping. Moreover, these distinct memory types are dissociable in the laboratory, allowing for the systematic examination of both environmental and physiological variables that may influence them. The effects of immune system activation on these experimental systems can be profitably studied for themselves, adding to our knowledge of the physiological regulation of behavior and behavior change. But they are also of interest for their ability to illuminate the conduits of IS-CNS communication, contributing to the eventual understanding of (1) in vivo IS regulation by CNS/ANS inputs and (2) the mechanisms underlying the behavioral, effective, and cognitive disturbances seen in patients suffering acute infectious and chronic inflammatory diseases.

Relational memory is a "brain-systems construct" (Squire and Zola-Morgan, 1991; Squire, et al., 1993) which is powerful in its ability to summarize the experimental data as well as the common experience of human memory. Relational memory is dependent on the integrity and adequate function of the hippocampus and related structures in the medial temporal lobe (Squire and Zola-Morgan, 1991; Zola-Morgan and Squire, 1993). Relational memory is acquired quickly, requiring few trials for mastery. It's somewhat unreliable and it is flexible (learning in one context can be expressed in another; Squire, et al., 1993). In human terms, relational memory is conscious and declarative (we *declare* a remembered item to ourselves or others). It is relational insofar as the hippocampus functions as an index that connects disparate inputs from brain areas mediating the varied and simultaneous perceptions of an event. It is where components of an experience, divided among the different sensory modalities and their projection areas, are conjoined and "bound together" to form the internal representation of a context or gestalt (Squire, 1992).

An example of relational learning in rats is the odor discrimination task (Eichenbaum et al., 1989). Rats are trained to respond to odor A and not B when the two are paired. Concurrently they are trained to respond to C and not D when these are paired. Rat's with hippocampal lesions can accomplish this, although not as efficiently as intact controls. However, when the odors are re-arranged (AD, CB), normal rats can flexibly respond to the correct odor in each case; lesioned animals treat the pairings as a new task and respond randomly. Presumably, the lesioned animals learn the task through simple habit formation (nonhippocampal, described below) which was confounded during the reversal phase of the experiment. Normal rats, on the other hand, are more efficient in both phases because they have access to a brain system which can construct a relationship and then enlarge that relationship once the context changes.

Human amnesiacs with hippocampal damage cannot (without great effort) learn new facts, cannot remember recent events, and cannot assemble and recall lists of words or objects, cannot place names with faces, etc. They can, however, remember information acquired premorbidly. New motor skills and habits can also be acquired. Interestingly, when an amnesiac is trained on a new set of facts, the ability to recall those facts is often "bound" in a hyperspecific way to the exact context in which those facts were learned. For example, an amnesiac trained on baseball facts in a question-and-answer format could learn the new facts but displayed the knowledge only when exact wordings from the original training sessions were employed (Schachter, 1985). This hyperspecificity is an example of the loss of flexibility in learning characteristic of animals (and humans) with hippocampal lesions.

Procedural memory (also called implicit memory) is a collection of memory types served by different (nonhippocampal) brain systems. It is slow, requiring many trials and much practice. It tends to be highly reliable and by extension, difficult to reverse. And it is highly inflexible. Habits and skills are acquired through procedural learning. In humans, the fact that procedural memory is independent of the hippocampal learning system is dramatically illustrated by hippocampal amnesics who are capable of learning an eye-hand coordination task if given over several trials. Amazingly, these patients can learn the task to normal levels but have no memory of any of the practice sessions or even that the task they can now perform normally was ever presented to them before. Other forms of procedural or implicit memory are priming (the ability to respond more quickly to a stimulus experienced recently than to a novel stimulus), and simple forms of classical and operant conditioning (Squire, 1992).

THE MORRIS WATER MAZE

The water maze test for rodent spatial and navigational memory was developed originally to study localization ability in the rat (Morris, 1981). Since that time, it has become a standard instrument for studying spatial memory in rodents (Brandeis, Brandys, and

Yehuds, 1989; McNamara and Skelton, 1993). The apparatus consists of a large (usually circular) pool with dimensions of 0.80-2.20 M diameter and 0.40-0.60 M high (Brandeis, et al., 1989). The water level is high enough to require continuous swimming (e.g., 0.25-0.40 M). The water is kept cool (18-26°C) and an escape platform (9-12 cm diameter) is placed 1 cm below the water. The water is generally rendered opaque with an opacifier such as milk powder. Under these conditions, the platform offers no local cues as to its location. Also, odor trails are eliminated and fixed response strategies are inefficient. The reinforcer in the system is escape from the cool water.

The water maze apparatus and procedures can be varied to emphasize different learning strategies and different neuroanatomical or neurochemical systems. The platform can be visible, invisible or removed for probes. The visible distal cues can be sparse or rich; the lights can be on or off. Platforms can be fixed or be moved to new locations between trials. In addition, the training and testing protocols can be spaced or massed; trial lengths can be varied. Motivation can be varied somewhat by changing water temperature or providing a warm drying chamber for the intertrial interval. By setting MWM parameters in various ways, investigators have demonstrated that hippocampal lesions produce a deficiency in place learning on the MWM; rats cannot find the hidden platform as readily as sham controls or rats with lesions in the neocortex. These deficits are independent of motor and motivational aspects of the procedure (see Brandeis, et al., 1989; McNamara and Skelton, 1993 for reviews). When spatial or relational memory demands are not so great (fixed start, fixed target, e.g.) then hippocampal function is not crucial to performance (Squire, 1992) presumably because water maze learning can also be mediated by several nonhippocampal-dependent learning processes (Squire, 1992; McDonald and White, 1993).

A commonly used MWM protocol is the standard reference memory paradigm. Here, the platform occupies a fixed (and hidden) location throughout acquisition training. The animal is started from any of several, randomly varied, entry points. Over several trials, the animal will learn the position of the platform and performance improves through an acquired ability to refer to an internal representation of the MWM (and its surrounds) in guiding swimming. This internal representation is richly loaded with visual projections (from repeated scannings of the walls and ceiling surrounding the maze) to the exclusion of other information because most other sensory input is not predictive of the location of the target. Thus accomplished performance in the MWM involves making a *reference* to a remembered *spatial relation* among objects in a distal *visual* field.

CYTOKINE EFFECTS ON WATER MAZE PERFORMANCE

The first attempt to demonstrate a direct effect of cytokines on learning in the MWM was undertaken by Oitzl, van Oers, Schobitz, and de Kloet, (1993). These investigators injected murine rIL1β or IL6 i.c.v. into male Wistar rats prior to training and testing in the MWM. They found that IL6 had no effect on water maze performance. IL1β, on the other hand, was associated with impaired performance on the day after the injection. These results may indicate that IL1β, but not IL6, interferes with the consolidation of spatial information which, in this protocol, is most evident during the first trial of the second day of training. It should also be noted that this study used i.c.v. injections and thus provides some information on a direct cytokine effect on hippocampal function.

In a recent study (Gibertini, et al., 1995), we used the MWM to study the effects of IL1β on spatial learning in mice infected with *Legionella pneumophila* (Lp). Lp is a gram-negative, facultative intracellular bacterium that is the cause of Legionnaires' disease and Pontiac Fever in humans (Yamamoto, Klein, & Friedman, 1993). This human pathogen also causes an immune reaction when injected into rodents (Yamamoto, Klein, Newton &

Friedman, 1992), although some mouse strains are more susceptible than others (Yamamoto, Klein, Newton, Widen & Friedman, 1988). To test the idea that cognition is affected during acute sickness, we used an experimentally-induced illness in the C57BL/6 mouse strain for two reasons: (1) the behavior of these mice in the MWM was well-characterized (Upchurch, et al., 1988); and (2) in this Lp-resistant strain, Lp organisms can be titrated to produce an acute, sub-lethal illness lasting two to three days that is reminiscent of severe but "self-limiting" bacterial infections in humans.

In these studies, we used a modified Morris Water Maze consisting of a round tank 1 M in diameter with vertical white polyvinylchloride sides 0.6 M high. The tank was filled to a depth of 15 cm with water (22°C to 25°C) that was rendered opaque with powdered milk. A round platform 10 cm in diameter constructed of galvanized steel and covered entirely with white surgical tape was positioned 0.5 cm below the surface of the water. This hidden platform was the target for all training trials and was permanently positioned in the center of the northwest quadrant of the pool. Training took place over 18 trials administered as six blocks of three 60 s trials. Three blocks of training were administered on each of two consecutive days. The compressed training schedule was dictated by the short illness period in this model. During training, each mouse was gently placed in the water in a randomly selected quadrant. If the mouse failed to find the platform in 60 s, it was placed on it for 10-15s. It was then placed into a drying chamber (37 °C). Performance was measured as the latency in seconds to locate, mount, and remain on the platform. After completion of the acquisition phase of the protocol, mice were allowed to recover for seven days. They were then tested for their recall of the platform position.

Figure 1 shows that, in these initial experiments, the control group improved over training blocks while the Lp group did not. Analysis of the slopes of the learning curves revealed a steep learning curve for the control animals and a flat curve (no performance change) for the Lp animals.

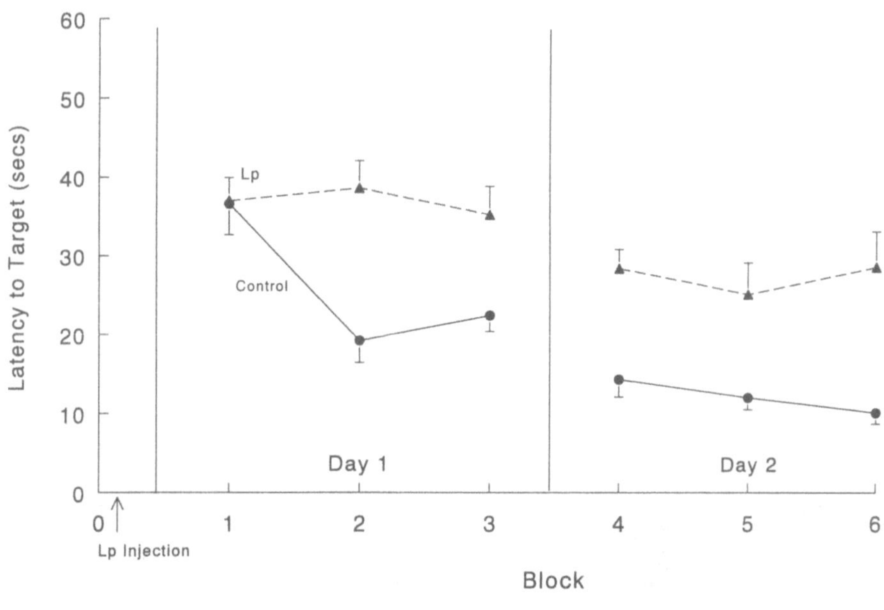

Figure 1. Water maze performance over three blocks of training on each of two consecutive days for mice infected on day 0 with Lp versus uninfected mice. Symbols denote mean latencies across three trials at each training block. Error bars are standard errors of the mean. From Gibertini, et al. (1995).

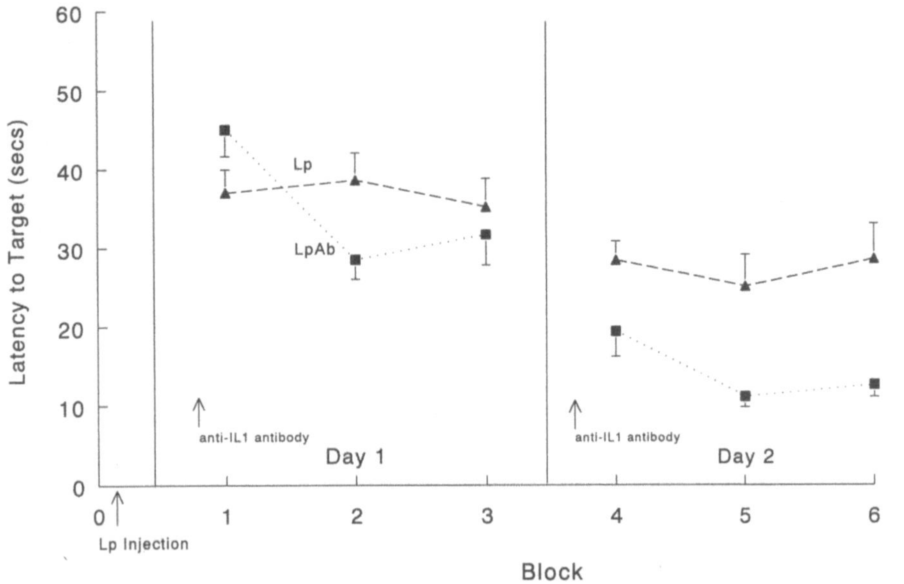

Figure 2. Water maze performance over three blocks of training on each of two consecutive days for mice infected on day 0 with Lp versus mice infected with Lp and then given anti-IL1 antibodies (LpAb) at the start of each of the training days. Symbols denote mean latencies across three trials at each training block. Error bars are standard errors of the mean. From Gibertini, et al., (1995).

In order to determine the role of IL1β in this effect, we treated some of the Lp-infected animals with anti-IL1 antibodies (100 μg/mouse, ip) 2-hours prior to the start of training. Figure 2 shows that this antibody treatment "normalized" the learning curve in the sick animals. We also tested IL1β directly by injecting well animals with rmIL1β (100 ng/mouse, ip) just prior to beginning training on this protocol. Figure 3 shows that, IL1β can have some effect on performance in the water maze. This is especially apparent during day 2 of training when the control mice show considerable improvement in the task and the IL1β mice do not.

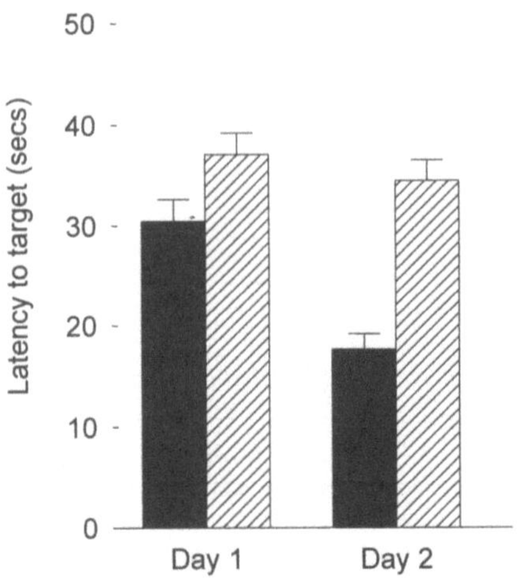

Figure 3. Random start protocol water maze performance over two days of training for the mice injected with IL1β (100 ng/mouse; ip; hatched bars) or saline (solid bars). Bars denote mean latencies across nine trials on each training day. Error bars are standard errors of the mean.

As noted above, the MWM is a highly flexible system, the parameters of which may be manipulated to highlight different aspects of behavior. In the standard reference memory version used in our studies, the demands on the spatial and relational memory systems can be varied by changing how the animal is introduced to a learning trial. If the animal is given a constant and unvarying place to enter the maze, the task of finding the platform over repeated trials becomes much easier than if the entry point is varied. The fixed-start protocol demands less of the hippocampus for successful solution to the puzzle. Animals may use a taxis (develop a habit involving certain movements that brings the animal to the goal) or a praxis (swim towards or away from a single visible object that results in bumping into the target) strategy to affect an escape from the water (Brandeis, et al., 1989). Diminishing latencies to target would represent refinements in one type of procedural learning or another but would involve the hippocampus little, if at all.

To test whether IL1β influenced this type of MWM protocol, we repeated the experiments discussed above with a single change made to the learning context: the animals were placed in the pool at the same point on each trial. For these experiments, animals were given rmIL1β (100ng/mouse, ip) 30 minutes prior to beginning training on each of the two acquisition training days. After a week's rest, they were given a retention test (30 s probe trial with no platform in the pool) followed immediately by another IL1β injection. Thirty minutes after this injection, mice were given an overtraining block (5 trials) followed by two reversal blocks. These reversal blocks were 3 trials each and presented a new problem to the mice insofar as the platform was in a new position in the pool. Figure 4 demonstrates that IL1β had little if any effect on learning the position of the platform under this protocol. As in other experiments, swimming speed and ability to find a visible platform were equivalent between the groups. The ease with which the sick mice found the hidden platform when the start position is fixed contrasts starkly with their performance when the start position varied (Figures 1 and 3). A likely explanation of this difference is that hippocampal functioning, presumably necessary for the more difficult random start protocol, is diminished in sick animals, disturbing their ability to learn complex relations in their environment but not simpler motor procedures.

A second parametric manipulation on the MWM instituted for these experiments was the inclusion of a reversal phase of training. This type of protocol allows the hippocampal dysfunction to be illuminated even when the original learning was acquired through nonhippocampal procedural mechanisms. During a reversal, the platform is moved to the opposite

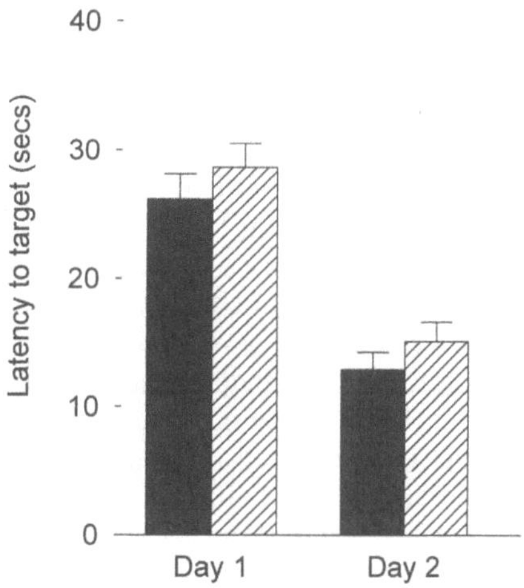

Figure 4. Fixed start protocol water maze performance over two days of training for the mice injected with IL1β (100 ng/mouse; ip; hatched bars) or saline (solid bars). Bars denote mean latencies across nine trials on each training day. Error bars are standard errors of the mean.

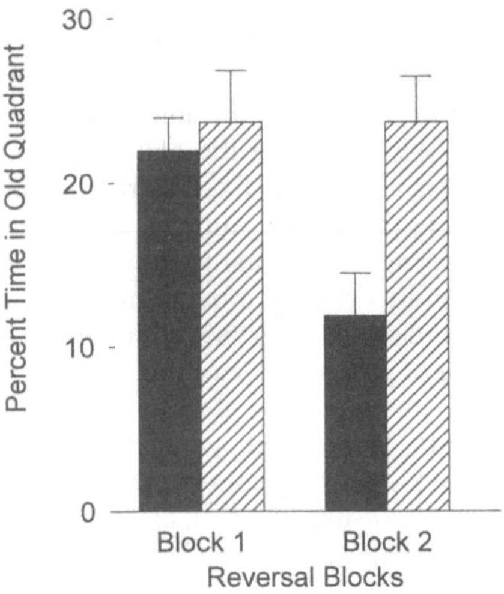

Figure 5. Probe trial after reversal training. Animals were injected with IL1β (100 ng/mouse, ip; hatched bars) or saline (solid bars), trained in a fixed start protocol and then subjected to a reversal of platform location. After 6 reversal trials, a 30s probe trial without a platform was conducted. Bars denote mean percent time searching in the old (platform no longer present) quadrant. Error bars are standard errors of the mean.

side of the pool and the animal must learn its position anew. Sick mice can learn the new task, albeit more slowly than well mice. Interestingly, the behavior of the mice with respect to the old target position is very characteristic of animals with hippocampal lesions (Squire, 1992). Specifically, the sick mice perseverated in the quadrant where the target had been, even while they were gradually learning the new position of the target. Control mice were much more flexibly involved with the task and more quickly abandoned the old quadrant in favor of searching in the new and correct quadrant (Figure 5). This behavioral inflexibility is characteristic of procedural (nonhippocampal) learning. The fixed-start reference memory with a reversal phase is thus a powerful tool for illuminating the brain systems affected and not affected by peripheral IL1β. The easy acquisition of the target position was not affected by IL1β presumably because the task could be done without calling upon the hippocampus. The reversal, on the other hand, demanded a relational learning (hippocampal) component (flexibility) and, in this phase of the protocol, clear differences between IL1-treated animals and controls arise.

IL1β AND THE HIPPOCAMPUS

IL1β can appear in the brain after infection or peripheral injection of LPS (Ban et al., 1992). Whether this occurs through intermediate steps involving cells of the circumventricular organs (Komaki et al. ,1992; Gotschall, et al., 1992), or through an ascending ANS sensory pathway (Bret-Dibat, et al., 1995), it is possible that hippocampus is ultimately affected by circulating IL1β . Interestingly, although it is thought that IL1β molecules do not traverse to the brain directly (Gotschall, et al., 1992), the IS-CNS signal mediated by peripheral IL1β may become transduced through release of central IL1β and expression on neurons of IL1β receptors. The intermediate steps involved in this transduction (and conservation of molecular function) represent an important area of study.

IL1β is associated with changes in hippocampal neurotransmitters. Intrahippocampal administration of IL1β increases extracellular 5-HT (Linthorst, et al.,1994) and decreases extracellular acetylcholine (Rada et al., 1991). Peripheral IL1β enhances NE and 5-HT turnover in the hippocampus (Zalcam, et al., 1994). In addition, IL1β depresses calcium currents in CA1 hippocampal neurons (Plata-Salaman and French-Mullen, 1992; 1994).

Katsuki, et al. (1990) found that IL1β inhibits long-term potentiation (LTP) in the mossy fiber-CA3 pathway of mouse hippocampus slice preparations. Bellinger, et al. (1993) suggested that IL1β enhances synaptic inhibitory mechanisms in the hippocampus and further demonstrated that IL1β modulates synaptic potentials and reduces LTP.

IL1β appears to have a role in normal hippocampal function. Peripheral IL1β or LPS can elicit IL1α and IL1β in the hippocampus (Ban et al., 1992). IL1 receptors are found in many brain regions. They are dense in the dentate gyrus (Takao, et al., 1990) and the pyramidal cell layer of the hilus and CA3 region of murine hippocampus (Cunningham et al., 1991). There is some evidence that these receptors are modulated by corticosteroids (Betancur et al., 1994). Also, the balance between glucocorticoid and mineralocorticoid receptors on hippocampal neurons may be influenced by peripheral IL1β (Schobitz et al., 1994; De Kloet, et al., 1994) in a way that leads to decreased hippocampal inhibition of the HPA axis, resulting in sustained glucocorticoid release during infection. The hippocampus may be a primary site of integration of cytokine and corticosteroid signals that affect both the physiological and the behavioral/cognitive response to infection.

SUMMARY AND IMPLICATIONS

The study of sickness behavior seeks to understand the mechanisms of IS-CNS communication. By developing animal models for one of the most important aspects of sickness behavior in people (cognitive dysfunction), we may eventually identify brain systems that may be involved in the *in vivo* regulation of immunity during infection. Such information will enhance our understanding of the components and mechanisms underlying the suffering of sick people across many dimensions (physical as well as mental and emotional). The work being undertaken on both a molecular and behavioral level should lead to new vistas for behavioral medicine and, ultimately, new therapeutics.

REFERENCES

Aubert, A., Vega, C., Dantzer, R., and Goodall, G. (1995). Pyrogens specifically disrupt the acquisition of a task involving cognitive processing in the rat. *Brain, Behavior, and Immunity, 9(2)*, 129-148.

Ban, E., Haour, F., & Lenstra, R. (1992). Brain interleukin 1 gene expression induced by peripheral lipopolysaccharide administration. *Cytokine, 4*, 48-54.

Bellinger, F.P., Madamba, S., & Siggins, G.R. (1993). Interleukin 1 beta inhibits synaptic strength and long-term potentiation in the rat CA1 hippocampus. *Brain Res, 628*, 227-234.

Betancur, C., Lledo, A., Borrell, J., & Guaza, C. (1994). Corticosteroid regulation of IL-1 receptors in the mouse hippocampus: effects of glucocorticoid treatment, stress, and adrenalectomy. *Neuroendocrinology, 59*, 120-128.

Bluthe, R.M., Dantzer, R., & Kelley, K.W. (1989). CRF is not involved in the behavioral effects of peripherally injected interleukin-1 in the rat. *Neuroscience Research Communications, 5*, 149-154.

Bluthe, R.M., Dantzer, R., & Kelley, K.W. (1992). Effects of interleukin-1 receptor antagonist on the behavioral effects of lipopolysaccharide in rat. *Brain Res, 573*, 318-320.

Bluthe, R.M., Dantzer, R., & Kelley, K.W. (1991). Interleukin-1 mediates behavioral but not metabolic effects of tumor necrosis factor α in mice. *European Journal of Pharmacology, 209*, 281-283.

Brandeis, R., Brandys, Y., & Yehuda, S. (1989). The use of the Morris water maze in the study of memory and learning. *International Journal of Neuroscience, 48*, 29-69.

Bret-Dibat, J., Bluthe, R., Kent, S., Kelley, K.W., and Dantzer, R. (1995). Lipopolysaccharide and interleukin-1 depress food-motivated behavior in mice by a vagal-mediated mechanism. *Brain, Behavior, and Immunity, 9(3)*; 242-246.

Crestani, F., Seguy, F., and Dantzer, R. (1991). Behavioral effects of peripherally injected interleukin-1: role of prostaglandins. *Brain Research, 542*, 330-335.

Cunningham, E.T. and De Souza, E.B. (1993). Interleukin 1 receptors in the brain and endocrine tissues. *Immunology Today, 14(4)*, 171-176.
Cunningham, E.T.J., Wada, E., Carter, D.B., Tracey, D.E., Battey, J.F., & De Souza, E.B. (1991). Localization of interleukin-1 receptor messenger RNA in murine hippocampus. *Endocrinology, 128*, 2666-2668.
de Kloet, E.R., Oitzl, M.S., & Schobitz, B. (1994). Cytokines and the brain corticosteroid receptor balance: relevance to pathophysiology of neuroendocrine-immune communication. *Psychoneuroendocrinology, 19*, 121-134.
Dantzer, R., Bluthe, R., Kent, S. and Kelley, K.W. (1992). Behavioral effects of cytokines. In N.J. Rothwell and R.D. Dantzer (Eds.) *Interleukin-1 in the brain.* Pergamon Press: Tarrytown, NY.
Dinarello, C.A. (1991). Interleukin-1 and interleukin-1 antagonism. *Blood,77(8)*: 1627-1652.
Dunn, A.J. (1989). Psychoneuroimmunology for the psychoneuroendocrinologist: A review of animal studies of nervous system-immune system interactions. *Psychoneuroendocrinology, 14(4)*; 251-274.
Eichenbaum, H., Matthews, P., Cohen, N.J. (1989). Further studies of hippocampal representation during odor discrimination learning. *Behavioral Neuroscience. 103*: 1207-1216.
Fent, K., Zbinden, G. (1987). Toxicity of interferon and interleukin. *TIPS, 8*, 100-104.
Fordyce, D.E. & Wehner, J.M. (1993). Physical activity enhances spatial learning performance with an associated alteration in hippocampal protein kinase C activity in C57BL/6 and DBA/2 mice. *Brain Res, 619*, 111-119.
Gibertini, M., Newton, C., Friedman, H., Klein, T.W. (1995). Spatial learning impairment in mice infected with Legionella pneumophila or administered exogenous interleukin-1-β. *Brain, Behavior, and Immunity, 9(2)*, 1113-128.
Gottschall, P.E., Komaki, G., and Arimura, A. (1992). Interleukin-1 activation of the central nervous system. In N.J. Rothwell and R.D. Dantzer (Eds.) *Interleukin-1 In the Brain.* Pergamon Press: Tarrytown, NY.
Gutierrez, E.G., Banks, W.A., & Kastin, A.J. (1993). Murine tumor necrosis factor alpha is transported from blood to brain in the mouse. *J Neuroimmunol, 47*, 169-176.
Hall, N.R.S., O'Grady, M.P. and Menzies, R.A. (1992). Cytokines and the central nervous system: links with mental disorders. in R. Kvetnansky, McCarty, R., and Axelrod, J. (Eds.) *Stress: Neuroendocrine and Molecular Approaches.* Gordon and Breach Science Publishers: New York.
Hart, B. L. (1988). Biological basis of the behavior of sick animals. *Neuroscience and Biobehavioral Reviews, 12*; 123-137.
Katsuki, H., Nakai, S., Hirai, Y., Akaji, K., Kiso, Y., & Satoh, M. (1990). Interleukin-1 beta inhibits long-term potentiation in the CA3 region of mouse hippocampal slices. *Eur J Pharmacol*, 181, 323-326.
Kent, S., Bluthe, R.M., Dantzer, R., Hardwick, A.J., Kelley, K.W., Rothwell, N.J., & Vannice, J.L. (1992). Different receptor mechanisms mediate the pyrogenic and behavioral effects of interleukin 1. *Proc Natl Acad Sci U S A, 89*, 9117-9120.
Komaki, G., Arimura, A., & Koves, K. (1992). Effect of intravenous injection of IL-1 beta on PGE2 levels in several brain areas as determined by microdialysis. *Am J Physiol, 262*, E246-E251.
Linthorst, A.C., Flachskamm, C., Holsboer, F., & Reul, J.M. (1994). Local administration of recombinant human interleukin-1 beta in the rat hippocampus increases serotonergic neurotransmission, hypothalamic-pituitary-adrenocortical axis activity, and body temperature. *Endocrinology, 135*, 520-532.
Masotto, C., Caspani, G., Grazia deSimone, M., Mengozzi, M., Scatturni, M., Sironi, M., Carenzi, A., and Ghezzi, P. (1992). Evidence for a different sensitivity to various central effects of interleukin-1 in mice. *Brain Research Bulletin, 28(2)*, 161-165.
Messing, R.B., Kleven, M.S., & Sparber, S.B. (1986). Delaying reinforcement in an autoshaping task generates adjunctive and superstitious behaviors. *Behavioral Processes, 13*; 327-338.
McDonald, R.J. and White, N.M. (1993). A triple dissociation of memory systems: Hippocampus, amygdala, and dorsal striatum. *Behavioral Neuroscience*, 107(1); 3-22.
McNamara, R.K. & Skelton, R.W. (1993). The neuropharmacological and neurochemical basis of place learning in the Morris water maze. *Brain Res Brain Res Rev, 18*, 33-49.
Morganti-Kossmann, M.C., Kossmann, T., & Wahl, S.M. (1992). Cytokines and neuropathology. *Trends Pharmacol Sci, 13*, 286-291.
Morris, R.G.M. (1981). Spatial localization does not require the presence of local cues. *Leaning and Motivation, 12*: 239-260.
Oitzl, M.S., van Oers, H., Schobitz, B., & de Kloet, E.R. (1993). Interleukin-1 beta, but not interleukin-6, impairs spatial navigation learning. *Brain Res, 613*, 160-163.
Plata-Salaman, C.R. & ffrench-Mullen, J.M. (1992). Interleukin-1 beta depresses calcium currents in CA1 hippocampal neurons at pathophysiological concentrations. *Brain Res Bull, 29*, 221-223.
Plata-Salaman, C.R. & ffrench-Mullen, J.M. (1994). Interleukin-1 beta inhibits Ca2+ channel currents in hippocampal neurons through protein kinase C. *Eur J Pharmacol, 266*, 1-10.

Rada, P., Mark, G.P., Vitek, M.P., Mangano, R.M., Blume, A.J., Beer, B., & Hoebel, B.G. (1991). Interleukin-1 beta decreases acetylcholine measured by microdialysis in the hippocampus of freely moving rats. *Brain Res, 550*, 287-290.

Schacter, D.L. (1985). Multiple forms of memory in humans and animals. In N.M. weinberger, J.L. McGaugh, and G. Lynch (Eds.) *Memory Systems of the Brain*. Guilford Press: New York.

Schobitz, B., Sutanto, W., Carey, M.P., Holsboer, F., & de Kloet, E.R. (1994). Endotoxin and interleukin 1 decrease the affinity of hippocampal mineralocorticoid (type I) receptor in parallel to activation of the hypothalamic-pituitary-adrenal axis. *Neuroendocrinology, 60*, 124-133.

Smith, A., Tyrrell, D., Coyle, K., and Higgins, P. (1988). Effects of interferon alpha in man: a preliminary report. *Psychopharmacology, 96*, 414-416.

Spadaro, F., and Dunn, A.J. (1990). Intracerebroventricular administration of interleukin-1 to mice alters investigation of stimuli in a novel environment. *Brain, Behavior, and Immunity, 4*, 308-322.

Sparber, S.B., Bollweg, G.L., & Messing, R.B. (1991). Food deprivation enhances both autoshaping and autoshaping impairment by a latent inhibition procedure. *Behavioral Processes, 23*; 59-74.

Squire, L.R. (1992). Memory and the hippocampus: A synthesis from findings with rats, monkeys, and humans. *Psychological Review, 99(2);* 195-231.

Squire, L.R., Knowlton, B., & Musen, G. (1993). The structure and organization of memory. *Annual Review of Psychology, 44*; 453-495.

Squire, L.R. & Zola-Morgan, S. (1991). The medial temporal lobe memory system. *Science, 253*; 1380-1385.

Takao, T., Tracey, D.E., Mitchell, W.M., & De Souza, E.B. (1990). Interleukin-1 receptors in mouse brain: characterization and neuronal localization. *Endocrinology, 127*, 3070-3078.

Upchurch, M. and Wehner, J. M. (1988). Differences between inbred strains of mice in Morris water maze performance. *Behavior Genetics, 18(1)*, 55-68.

Yamamoto, Y., Klein, T.W., & Friedman, H. (1993). Legionella and macrophages. In B.S. Zwilling and T.K. Eisenstein (Eds.) *Macrophage-Pathogen Interaction*. pp. 329-348, Marcel Dekker, Inc., New York, NY

Yamamoto, Y., Klein, T.W., Newton, C.A., & Friedman, H. (1992). Differing macrophage and lymphocyte roles in resistance to Legionella pneumophila infection. *J. Immunol, 148*, 584-589.

Yamamoto, Y., Klein, T.W., Newton, C.A., Widen, R., & Friedman, H. (1988). Growth of Legionella pneumophila in thioglycolate-elicited peritoneal macrophages from A/J mice. *Infect Immun, 56*, 370-375.

Zalcman, S., Green-Johnson, J.M., Murray, L., Nance, D.M., Dyçk, D., Anisman, H., & Greenberg, A.H. (1994). Cytokine-specific central monoamine alterations induced by interleukin-1, -2 and -6. *Brain Res, 643*, 40-49.

Zola-Morgan, S. & Squire, L.R. (1993). Neuroanatomy of memory. *Annual Review of Neuroscience, 16*: 547-463.

28

TNFα

A Neuromodulator in the Central Nervous System

Tracey A. Ignatowski, Bernice K. Noble, John R. Wright, Janet L. Gorfien, and Robert N. Spengler

Department of Pathology
State University of New York at Buffalo
School of Medicine and Biomedical Sciences
Buffalo, New York 14214

1. INTRODUCTION

Cytokines, key participants in immune/inflammatory processes, have recently been demonstrated to play a role in neural functions. Receptors for the cytokine tumor necrosis factor (TNFα) have been localized to many regions of the brain.[1] TNFα itself, along with another cytokine, interleukin-1, is contained in neuronal fibers/elements innervating various brain regions.[2,3] In addition, neurons grown *in vitro* are able to synthesize and secrete the cytokine interleukin-1β.[4] Therefore, it was of interest to determine whether fluctuations in cytokine content were associated with alterations in neuron function.

Recently, we have shown that both noradrenergic sensitivity to TNFα and TNFα production in the brain may be altered by the tricyclic antidepressant desipramine (DMI) or the α_2-adrenergic agonist clonidine.[5,6] DMI administration for one day produced an increase in TNFα mRNA in the locus coeruleus, a region of the brain containing noradrenergic nerve cell bodies, and an increase in TNFα levels distally in the hippocampus, a region containing noradrenergic nerve terminals. Those studies showed that TNFα may serve as a mediator of neurotransmitter release in the brain, and suggested that TNFα might be produced by the neuron itself.

Exogenous TNFα has been shown to inhibit [^{3}H]-norepinephrine (NE) secretion from potassium-depolarized, sympathetic neurons *in vitro*.[7] In addition, exogenous TNFα inhibited the release of [^{3}H]-NE from superfused brain slices after electrical stimulation.[5,8] Furthermore, in superfused brain slices from normal rats, blockade of α_2-adrenergic receptor activation intensified TNFα-induced inhibition of NE release.[5,6] After administration of DMI or clonidine, TNFα increased, rather than inhibited NE release from superfused brain slices, conditional on α_2-adrenergic receptor activation.[5,6] One aim of the present study was to identify the cellular source of the TNFα that is synthesized in distinct regions of the brain following DMI administration. The effect of TNFα on [^{3}H]-NE release was also investigated

AIDS, Drugs of Abuse, and the Neuroimmune Axis, Edited by Friedman *et al.*
Plenum Press, New York, 1996

in rats given DMI or clonidine for 1 or 14 days. The influence of α_2-adrenergic receptor activation on presynaptic sensitivity to TNFα was evaluated.

2. MATERIALS AND METHODS

2.1. Animals

Male Sprague-Dawley rats weighing 200-250 grams (Harlan Sprague Dawley, Inc., Indianapolis, IN) were maintained on a 12-hour light/dark cycle and were given food and water *ad libitum*. Rats were injected i.p., twice daily for either 1 day (acute) or 14 days (chronic) with the antidepressant drug DMI (10 mg/kg) or clonidine (0.6 mg/kg) dissolved in pyrogen-free saline, or with saline alone as controls. Rats in each treatment group, were randomly divided into two groups (see figure legends); brains were removed from rats decapitated 12 hours after the last injection. Brain slices were used for either field stimulation or immunoperoxidase staining.

2.2. Field Stimulation of Rat Hippocampal Slices

Superfusion studies were carried out according to established procedures.[5,6] Hippocampal slices, preloaded with [^{3}H]-NE (specific activity 59.7 Ci/mmol or 57.3 Ci/mmol at a final concentration of 330nM, NEN), were consecutively stimulated (4 Hz) at 16-min intervals for 2 min each in the absence and in the presence of cumulative concentrations of TNFα, with and without the α_2-adrenergic antagonist idazoxan (10^{-7}M). [^{3}H]-NE release, in excess of the spontaneous efflux of tritium, was determined. In order to establish frequency-response characteristics, consecutive field stimulations between 0.5 and 16 Hz for 2 min each were applied at 16-min intervals in the presence or absence of TNFα, clonidine or idazoxan.

2.3. Immunoperoxidase Staining

Immunolocalization of TNFα in brain tissue from control rats and rats administered DMI was performed by standard methods.[9] The polyclonal antiserum used for immunohistochemistry was prepared in our laboratory. It completely neutralized (1:500) the activity of human, rat, dog, and mouse TNFα, measured by means of the WEHI 164 subclone 13 cytotoxicity assay.[10] Titrations determined the proper dilutions of primary (1°) antibody (Polyclonal rabbit-anti-mouse TNFα, 1:25) and secondary (2°) antibody (Swine anti-rabbit immunoglobulin (IgG)-HRP conjugate antibody, 1:50, DAKO Corp.). Acetone-fixed, frozen sections were processed for immunoperoxidase staining using DAB as the chromogen (Sigma Chemical Co., St. Louis, MO). The DAB reaction product was intensified with imidazole.[11-13]

3. RESULTS

3.1. Field Stimulation of Rat Hippocampal Slices and the Effect of Exogenous TNFα

In brain slices obtained from controls the α_2-adrenergic antagonist idazoxan potentiated NE release. The α_2-adrenergic agonist clonidine inhibited NE release. Both responses

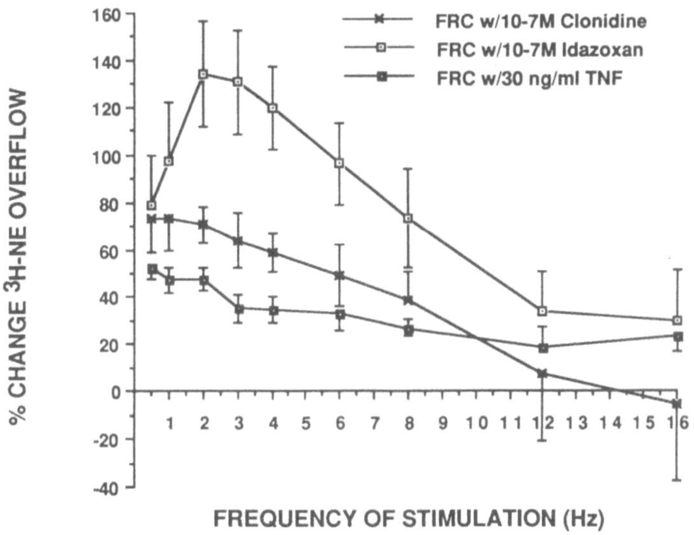

Figure 1. Frequency-response curves for the effects of clonidine, idazoxan, and TNFα on field-stimulated [^{3}H]-NE overflow, expressed as the percent change in [^{3}H]-NE release based on control values. Idazoxan (10^{-7}M), clonidine (10^{-7}M), or TNFα (30 ng/ml) was added *in vitro* to Krebs buffer perfusing experimental chambers 16 minutes before the onset of electrical field stimulation. Each point is the mean ± SEM. Three rats were used to generate each curve.

were frequency-dependent, diminishing at higher frequencies (Figure 1). Exogenous TNFα also inhibited NE release in controls, with greater potency at lower frequencies of stimulation when the α_2-adrenergic autoreceptor was less responsive to idazoxan, and therefore, appeared to be less activated. In a concentration-dependent manner, exogenous TNFα also decreased the fractional release (4 Hz) of [^{3}H]-NE during field stimulation of hippocampal slices obtained from controls.[5] TNFα inhibition of [^{3}H]-NE release was increased in the presence of idazoxan[5] (Figure 2).

In rats given DMI for 1 day the response of hippocampal slices to exogenous TNFα was not different from controls, as evidenced by similarities in the TNFα-concentration-effect curves (data not shown). However, after 14 days of DMI, TNFα enhanced rather than inhibited NE release (Figure 2). Also after 14 days DMI, blockade of α_2-adrenergic receptors by idazoxan reversed the response of the hippocampal slice to TNFα back to an inhibition of NE release, which was greater than that observed with control brain slices in the presence of idazoxan (Figure 2).

Following 1 day clonidine administration to rats, noradrenergic sensitivity to TNFα also reversed from an inhibition to a potentiation of NE release (Figure 2). After 14 days of clonidine, the TNFα-concentration-effect curve returned to control values (data not shown).[6] In the presence of idazoxan, however, the potentiation of NE release induced by TNFα seen after 1 day of clonidine, was reversed to an inhibition of NE release, which was a lesser inhibition than that observed for the control brain slices in the presence of idazoxan (Figure 2).

3.2. Endogenous TNFα Following DMI Administration to Rats

Constitutive levels of TNFα were found in specific brain regions of the rat, as previously described[5,6]. Those TNFα levels were depleted following 1 day of clonidine

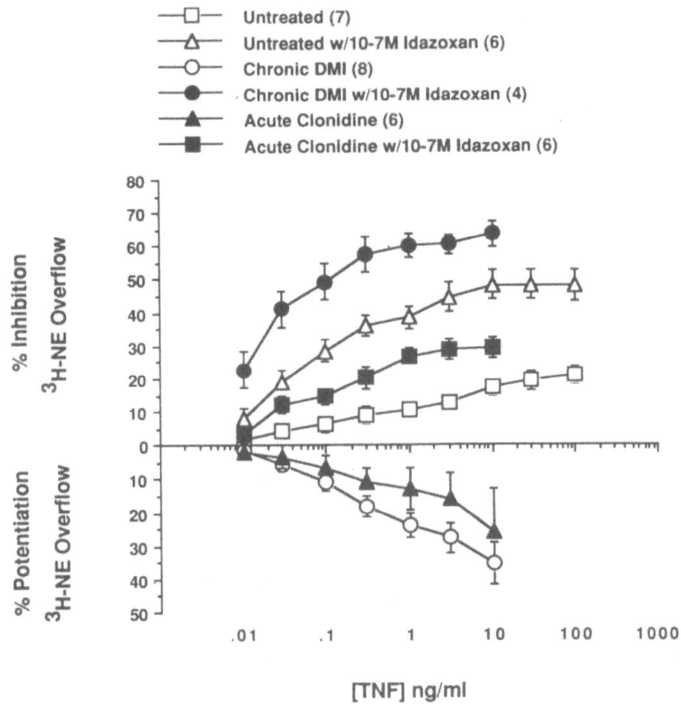

Figure 2. Regulation of the release of [^{3}H]-NE by TNFα during field stimulation of hippocampal slices. Electrical field stimulation (4 Hz, 100 mA, 26 V) was applied to isolated hippocampal slices from rats administered either 1 day (acute) of clonidine (0.6 mg/kg, i.p., twice daily) or 14 days (chronic) of DMI (10 mg/kg, i.p., twice daily), and the effects of idazoxan *in vitro*. Each point is the mean ± SEM with the number of rats in parentheses.

administration, with no change in TNFα mRNA levels[6]. In contrast, following 1 day of DMI administration, TNFα mRNA levels were increased in the locus coeruleus, and the levels of the bioactive TNFα were elevated in the hippocampus[5]. Neuronal TNFα immunoreactivity was observed in the hippocampus and in the area of the brainstem containing the locus coeruleus in control animals (7/7, Figures 3a and 4a). After 1-day DMI administration, cells were not positive for TNFα in either the hippocampus or the locus coeruleus (6/7, Figures

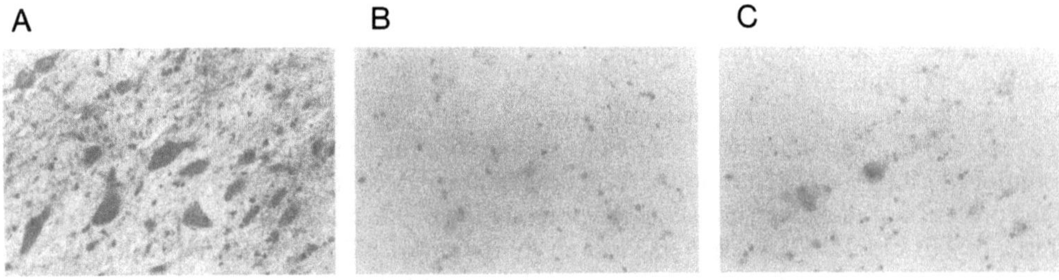

Figure 3. Series of immunoperoxidase stained brain slices obtained from the locus coeruleus. A. Control - TNFα-stained neuronal cell bodies (note perinuclear staining pattern) and positively stained neuronal fibers are evident throughout the section. B. Acute (1 day) DMI administration - lack of TNFα immunoreactive staining in a brain section taken from a similar region of the brain as in (A). C. Chronic (14 days) desipramine administration - intermediate TNFα staining evident in some of the neuronal cell bodies as compared to that stained under control conditions (A). Note: Same magnification (25X) and light intensity (70%) used for all pictures.

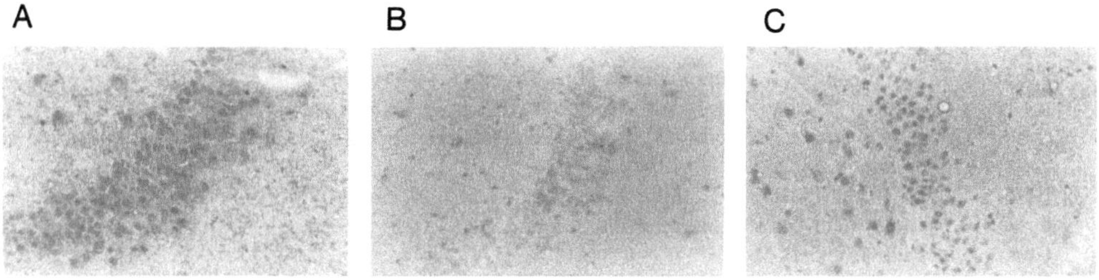

Figure 4. Immunoperoxidase stained rat hippocampal brain slices. A. Control - positive staining for TNFα in apical cell bodies and fibers throughout the section. B. Acute (1 day) desipramine administration - lack of TNFα staining in a brain section taken from a similar region of the brain as in (A). C. Chronic (14 days) desipramine administration - intermediate TNFα staining evident in some of the neuronal cell bodies as compared to that stained under control conditions (A). Note: Same magnification (25X) and light intensity (70%) used for all pictures.

3b and 4b). After 14 days of DMI, neuronal immunoreactive TNFα was present (although to a lesser extent) in those two brain regions (7/7, Figures 3c and 4c).

4. DISCUSSION

Analogous to α_2-adrenergic receptor activation, the cytokine TNFα inhibits NE release, not only in a concentration-dependent manner, but also in a frequency-dependent manner. Also, it was determined that α_2-adrenergic receptor activation and sensitivity plays a role in TNFα regulation of NE release. Of particular interest is that the switch from that of inhibition to potentiation of NE release by TNFα is common to both the antidepressant DMI and the α_2-adrenergic agonist clonidine; this switch was only observed after the period of administration when both may have antidepressant qualities.[5,6] Therefore, a switch in receptor coupling for the presynaptic α_2-adrenergic autoreceptor appears to be a mechanism of action for antidepressant drugs. Characterization of a neuromodulatory role for TNFα led to an investigation of whether the cytokine was present endogenously in the brain. Constitutive levels of TNFα (bioactive protein and mRNA) were found to exist in the rat brain,[5,6] and immunoperoxidase staining confirmed these findings. Interestingly, staining for TNFα was largely localized to neurons and processes, further substantiating the proposal that TNFα is either synthesized *de novo* or accumulated in and used by neurons. The staining pattern was similar in these sections; there was a marked perinuclear staining which is characteristic of cytokine accumulation in the Golgi organelle,[14] suggesting synthesis of TNFα by these neuronal cells. Taken together, there appears to be an augmentation in the production, as well as in the release of TNFα in response to 1-day DMI administration. The released TNFα would be diluted in the surrounding tissue and no longer detectable by this staining procedure, which preferentially stains concentrated or localized proteins. However, at the same time, increased levels of TNFα were ascertained from whole hippocampal homogenates by analysis in the WEHI 164 subclone 13 cytotoxicity assay. Therefore, these results demonstrate that not only is staining for TNFα immunoreactivity neuronally localized in the hippocampus and locus coeruleus of the rat brain, but that its expression is altered following the administration of an antidepressant. These observations, together with our previous findings, strongly support a functional role for the cytokine TNFα as a neuromodulator in the CNS.

REFERENCES

1. Kinouchi K., G. Brown, G. Pasternak, and D.B. Donner. 1991. Identification and characterization of receptors for tumor necrosis factor-alpha in the brain. Biochem. Biophys. Res. Comm. 181(3):1532-1538.
2. Breder, C.D., C.A. Dinarello, and C.B. Saper. 1988. Interleukin-1 Immunoreactive innervation of the human hypothalamus. Science. 240(4850):321-324.
3. Breder, C.D., M. Tsujimoto, Y. Terano, D.W. Scott, and C.B. Saper. 1993. Distribution and characterization of tumor necrosis factor-alpha-like immunoreactivity in the murine central nervous system. J. Comp. Neurol. 337(4):543-567.
4. Freidin, M., M.V.L. Bennett, and J.A. Kessler. 1992. Cultured sympathetic neurons synthesize and release the cytokine interleukin 1β. Proc. Natl. Acad. Sci. USA. 89:10440-10443.
5. Ignatowski, T.A. and R.N. Spengler. 1994. Tumor necrosis factor-α: presynaptic sensitivity is modified after antidepressant drug administration. Brain Res. 665:293-299.
6. Ignatowski, T.A., R.C. Chou, and R.N. Spengler. 1995. Changes in brain α_2-adrenergic autoreceptor sensitivity after clonidine administration are associated with changes in brain TNFα sensitivity. Brain Res. (Submitted).
7. Soliven, B. and J. Albert. 1992. Tumor necrosis factor modulates the inactivation of catecholamine secretion in cultured sympathetic neurons. J. Neurochem. 58:1073-1078.
8. Elenkov, I.J., K. Kovacs, E. Duda, E. Stark, and E.S. Vizi. 1992. Presynaptic inhibitory effect of TNF-α on the release of noradrenaline in isolated median eminence. J. Neuroimmunol. 41:117-120.
9. Noble, B., Ren, K., Taverne, J., Dipirro, J., Van Liew, J., Dijkstra, C., Janossy, G., and Poulter, L.W. 1990. Mononuclear cells in glomeruli and cytokines in urine reflect the severity of experimental proliferative immune complex glomerulonephritis. Clin. Exp. Immunol. 80:281-287.
10. Spengler, R.N., Chensue, S.W., Giacherio, D.A., Blenk, N., and Kunkel, S.L. 1994. Endogenous norepinephrine regulates macrophage-derived tumor necrosis factor alpha production from macrophages *in vitro*. J. Immunol. 152:3024-3031.
11. Scopsi, L. and L.I. Larsson. 1986. Increased sensitivity in peroxidase immunocytochemistry. A comparative study of a number of peroxidase visualization methods employing a model system. Histochemistry. 84:221-230.
12. Straus, W. 1982. Imidazole increases the sensitivity of the cytochemical reaction for peroxidase with diaminobenzidine at a neutral pH. J. Histochem. Cytochem. 30(5):491-493.
13. Trojanowski, J.Q., M.A. O'Brocka, and V.M.Y. Lee. 1983. A comparison of 8 different chromagen protocols for the demonstration of immunoreactive neurofilaments or glial filaments in rat cerebellum using the peroxidase-antiperoxidase method and monoclonal antibodies. J. Histochem. Cytochem. 31(10):1217-1223.
14. Sander, B., J. Andersson, and U. Andersson. 1991. Assessment of cytokines by immunofluorescence and the paraformaldehyde-saponin procedure. Immunological Reviews. 119:65-93.

29

DRUGS OF ABUSE AS POSSIBLE CO-FACTORS IN AIDS PROGRESSION

Summary of Panel Discussion

H. Friedman

University of South Florida College of Medicine
Tampa, Florida

A Panel Discussion on the question whether drugs of abuse act as possible co-factors in AIDS progression was presented at the Symposium on AIDS, Drugs of Abuse and Neuroimmune Axis. Panelists were well-known biomedical scientists in the area of drugs of abuse research. The first panelist was Dr. Harry Haverkos, Director of the AIDS Office at the National Institute on Drug Abuse. Dr. Clyde McCoy, Director of the Comprehensive Drug Research Center at the University of Miami School of Medicine and Dr. Paul Shapshak, Director of the Retrovirus Laboratory in the Department of Psychiatry at the University of Miami School of Medicine also were penalists. Dr. Shapshak is well known as a biomedical scientist studying the AIDS virus and the CNS. Dr. McCoy is a widely known epidemiologist. The third panelist was Dr. David Vlahov from the Johns Hopkins School of Public Health and a widely renown epidemiologist. Dr. Robert Donahoe, Director of the Psychoimmunology Laboratory at the Georgia Mental Health Institute and the Department of Psychiatry at Emory University was also a panelist. His expertise deals with virology and monkey models of AIDS. Dr. Phillip Peterson, Professor and Director of the Division of Infectious Diseases in the Department of Medicine at Hennepin County Medical Center in Minneapolis and the University of Minnesota Medical School, was also a panelist. His expertise deals with infectious diseases, including AIDS, and studies of how HIV affects the immune response as well as the CNS. Dr. Martin Adler, Professor of Pharmacology at Temple University School of Medicine was also a panelist and discussed the relationship between pharmacological principles and epidemiology in resolving the conflict between the dirth of epidemiological evidence that drugs of abuse are involved in AIDS progression and the disparity between numerous laboratory and experimental studies showing that drugs of abuse, in animal models, are major factors in suppressing the immune response and enhancing or augmenting HIV replication *in vitro*.

Dr. Haverkos pointed out that much has been learned in the last decade concerning the association of human immunodeficiency virus with AIDS, e.g., how the virus is transmitted and how the disease progresses from asymptomatic to symptomatic stages. It is widely accepted that interventions such as the use of AZT to arrest the replication of the virus and prophylaxis of opportunistic infections caused by organisms such as *P. carnii*, responsible for many pneumonias in AIDS patients, as well as other opportunistic infectious diseases in these patients have been developed in recent years and can alter the course of the illness. There is much evidence that other factors, including infections by opportunistic microorganisms such as those which cause sexually transmitted diseases, may be "co-factors" which have a role in promoting the various clinical responses in HIV-infected individuals. Although controversial, some investigators believe that there is a likelihood that various factors may serve in involving drugs of abuse as potential co-factors in AIDS progression. It is widely accepted that drugs of abuse, at least in experimental animals and *in vitro*, can cause immunosuppression and thus it is thought that such immunosuppression related to drugs of abuse may enhance AIDS progression. It is also believed by some substances used by individuals who are at high risk for AIDS, including inhalants such as nitrites, may be associated with HIV related Kaposi's sarcoma and this, in turn, may result in increased progression of the disease.

Drs. Clyde McCoy and Paul Shapshak have been studying epidemiological events associated with drugs of abuse use for many decades. Dr. McCoy has also been studying the effects of drugs of abuse on AIDS progression. He has examined data concerning the hypothesis that various drugs of abuse, including opiates and alcohol, which affect the immune system, may accelerate the progression of AIDS and susceptibility to infectious diseases associated with AIDS. Extensive review of the literature suggests that a majority of studies to date have failed to suggest a relationship between drugs of abuse consumption and progression of AIDS. It should be pointed out, however, that the results in the literature could be confounded by several factors, including differences in terminology between epidemiologists and basic scientists as well as study design features of epidemiologic investigations (including small sample sizes, measures of drug use, non-randomized designs, lack of longitudinal panels and lack of cause-effect relationships, i.e., unknown date of infection). It was stressed that interpretation of results is especially difficult due to the confounding effects of poly drug use by high risk drug abusers. It is necessary to address such shortcomings, especially clearer definition of terms and greater caution in drawing conclusions from epidemiologic findings, as well as considering the advantages of multiple disciplinary results.

Dr. David Vlahov has published a number of journal papers, widely accepted by other epidemiologists, indicating that there is no evidence linking drugs of abuse with progression of AIDS. He summarized his own work in Baltimore, using a cohort of AIDS patients (the ALIVE study), the Bronx cohort (Montefiore), and the Italian seroconverter study to examine the possible effect of injected drugs on the rate of immunosuppression and clinical progression to AIDS in patients infected with HIV. The results of these studies were consistent in suggesting that the frequency of drug use or comparisons between injection drug users vs. non-injection drug users did not show an increased rate of CD4 cell decline or the rate of decline of immune activation markers, the rate of progression to AIDS, or different estimations of the AIDS incubation period. He pointed out that while the lack of differences due to injection drug use could be related to a series of methodological considerations, the consistency of results across studies in human populations is noteworthy. Nevertheless, most of the panelists agreed that further epidemiologic studies taking into consideration the facts pointed out by other speakers are important in relating the epidemiological studies to animal studies, as well as other published studies, suggesting that drugs of abuse, especially opiates, may be involved in AIDS progression.

Dr. Robert Donahoe reviewed work in his laboratory, as well as in other laboratories, with a monkey model of AIDS, i.e., SIV infection. He reviewed studies concerning a monkey model of opiate dependency and infection with the Simian AIDS virus and indicated that the immunological effects of opiates include enhanced as well as decreased susceptibility to virus infection. Data from his monkey model suggest the importance of proper maintenance of opiate dependency to faciliate anti-SIV responses and that opiate withdrawal may be a critical factor in exacerbating the retrovirus infection in the monkeys. He reported a possible dichotomous effect of opiate administration in the monkeys, i.e., in some cases withdrawal of opiates from the monkeys made them more susceptible to more rapid replication of the AIDS virus . His study, as well as the results of other studies, suggest that opiate addiction may have a variable impact on HIV infection dependent upon the degree of the opiate dependency, along with other variables inherent in the addiction millieu. Results of studies with monkeys have important implications for epidemiological assessments of the association of AIDS with opiate addiction as well as for clinicians using opiates therapeutically in various medical situations and for clinicians treating heroin addicts and AIDS patients. His results with monkeys show that long term treatment with opiates may have significant effects not only on the immune response but also the susceptibility to infection with an AIDS inducing virus associated not only with active opiate use but also the opiate withdrawal.

Dr. Phillip Peterson, a clinician and basic scientist, reviewed work from his laboratory as well as other laboratories showing that opiates can promote the expression of HIV *in vitro*. His laboratory has studied the effects of morphine on HIV expression in cell cultures in order to examine whether opiates can accelerate the progression of HIV infection. For this purpose, his laboratory infected peripheral blood mononuclear cells with HIV-1 and determined whether these cells would induce mitogen activated normal human peripheral blood cells to express more virus. His laboratory also studied whether a chronically infected human cell line co-cultured with human fetal brain cells would cause replication of the virus *in vitro*. Expression of the virus was assessed by quantitating the p24 antigen level of the virus in co-culture supernatants. His laboratory found that although morphine had no direct effect on HIV expression in these culture systems, the expression of the virus was markedly potentiated by morphine. The effect of the morphine was blocked by a μ receptor antagonist, indicating an opiate receptor mechanism was involved. His results also support the view that morphine may enhance HIV replication by induction of tumor necrosis factorα production which, in turn, mediates the biochemical mechanism for enhancing viral expression. The *in vitro* findings from his laboratory support the belief that opiates accelerate the progression of HIV infection.

Dr. Martin Adler then discussed the possible reasons for the apparent disparity between epidemiologic and basic science results. He suggested a number of possibilities for the disagreement. He pointed out that immunological studies in both animals and *in vitro* models have proven to be predictive of effects in humans. Animal experiments are quite conclusive that opiates and other drugs of abuse affect the immune response and that there is an acceleration of HIV replication *in vitro*. Thus it seems logical to believe there is an effect in humans as well and it is actually illogical to believe otherwise. Basic scientists, especially in pharmacological studies, have always been concerned with the role of drug interactions, dose response studies, pharmacokinetics, frequency and duration of doses and genetic factors. Epidemiological results also must take into consideration such factors and, moreover, studies with humans, especially drug abusers, must consider the poly-drug use by the subjects, the duration of injection, doses of the drug, the type of drugs used, etc. It is apparent that the design of various experiments by biomedical scientists and the questions asked must take into account these variables and be answered by accepted research designs and statistical procedures. It is also apparent that epidemiological studies must take into account variations among populations and the design of the questions being asked, as well as many other variables. Although it appears that there is a great deal of disagreement between basic scientists studying the immune dysfunctions associated with use of drugs of abuse and the effects of drugs of abuse on AIDS progression and the results of epidemiological studies with various cohorts of patients having HIV infection or active AIDS, the disagreements are resolvable to determine whether or not drugs of abuse use may be associated with more rapid progression of the disease or with opportunistic infectins associated with AIDS.

With the onset of AIDS in the early 1980's in the United States and throughout the world many attempts have been made to assess the possible "co-factor" relationship of use of illicit drugs with susceptibility of individuals to the AIDS virus. Approximately a fifth of all AIDS patients in this country are known to be intravenous drug abusers. It has been shown that the AIDS virus can be spread by contaminated needles or equipment used by drug abusers. In addition, it is widely accepted that heroin or morphine per se are immunosuppressive, at least in animal models or *in vitro*. It is also known that many AIDS patients are not intravenous drug abusers but may abuse other drugs like marijuana, cocaine or even alcohol. Thus it is widely believed by basic biomedical scientists that use of such drugs may serve as co-factors in AIDS progression. There is a concerted effort by a number of investigators to examine in detail the mechanisms by which such drugs compromise the immune response in general, and particularly, in concert with immunosuppressive viruses such as the retrovirus which causes AIDS. Nevertheless, it is still not known definitively that drugs of abuse have a role in accelerating the course of disease. Much more work must be done in patient populations, as well as in laboratory settings, to answer the important question of whether drugs of abuse are involved in more rapid AIDS progression.

INDEX

MIX
Papier aus verantwortungsvollen Quellen
Paper from responsible sources
FSC® C105338

If you have any concerns about our products,
you can contact us on
ProductSafety@springernature.com

In case Publisher is established outside the EU,
the EU authorized representative is:
Springer Nature Customer Service Center GmbH
Europaplatz 3, 69115 Heidelberg, Germany

Printed by Libri Plureos GmbH
in Hamburg, Germany